BASIC PHARMACOKINETICS

CRC PRESS
PHARMACY EDUCATION
SERIES

Basic Pharmacokinetics
Mohsen A. Hedaya

Essentials of Law and Ethics for Pharmacy Technicians, Second Edition
Kenneth M. Strandberg

Pharmacy: What It Is and How It Works, Second Edition
William N. Kelly

Basic Pharmacology: Understanding Drug Actions and Reactions
Maria A. Hernandez and Appu Rathinavelu

Managing Pharmacy Practice: Principles, Strategies, and Systems
Andrew M. Peterson

Essentials of Human Physiology for Pharmacy
Laurie Kelly

Essential Math and Calculations for Pharmacy Technicians
Indra K. Reddy and Mansoor A. Khan

Pharmacoethics: A Problem-Based Approach
David A. Gettman and Dean Arneson

Pharmaceutical Care: Insights from Community Pharmacists
William N. Tindall and Marsha K. Millonig

Essentials of Pathophysiology for Pharmacy
Martin M. Zdanowicz

Quick Reference to Cardiovascular Pharmacotherapy
Judy W. M. Cheng

Essentials of Pharmacy Law
Douglas J. Pisano

Pharmacokinetic Principles of Dosing Adjustments: Understanding the Basics
Ronald D. Schoenwald

Pharmaceutical and Clinical Calculations, Second Edition
Mansoor A. Khan and Indra K. Reddy

Strauss's Federal Drug Laws and Examination Review, Fifth Edition Revised
Steven Strauss

Inside Pharmacy: Anatomy of a Profession
Raymond A. Gosselin and Jack Robbins

Understanding Medical Terms: A Guide for Pharmacy Practice, Second Edition
Walter F. Stanaszek, Mary J. Stanaszek, Robert J. Holt, and Steven Strauss

Pharmacokinetic Analysis: A Practical Approach
Peter I. D. Lee and Gordon L. Amidon

BASIC PHARMACOKINETICS

MOHSEN A. HEDAYA

CRC Press
Taylor & Francis Group
Boca Raton London New York

CRC Press is an imprint of the
Taylor & Francis Group, an informa business

CRC Press
Taylor & Francis Group
6000 Broken Sound Parkway NW, Suite 300
Boca Raton, FL 33487-2742

Printed in the United States of America on acid-free paper
10 9 8 7 6 5 4 3 2

International Standard Book Number-10: 1-4200-4671-3 (Hardcover)
International Standard Book Number-13: 978-1-4200-4671-7 (Hardcover)

Visit the Taylor & Francis Web site at
http://www.taylorandfrancis.com

and the CRC Press Web site at
http://www.crcpress.com

Dedication

To my wife and three sons for allowing me the time to complete this textbook

Table of Contents

Chapter 11

Chapter 14

Chapter 15

Chapter 16

Chapter 17

Foreword

Basic Pharmacokinetics is an introductory text designed to take the reader on a journey into this discipline using interactive learning. As such, it is not only a textbook—it also is a self-instructional computer-assisted medium for active learning. Indeed, the tutorial materials included in the accompanying compact disk have received an award from the American Association of Colleges of Pharmacy for innovation in teaching.

This volume and its companion CD are intended for students and practitioners in the health professions who need to comprehend the concepts and principles related to how the body absorbs, distributes, metabolizes, and excretes drugs. A quantitative understanding of these processes is a prerequisite for dosage regimen design and, in particular, to recognize how a variety of patient characteristics (age, disease, pharmacogenomics, etc.) and other factors may dictate specific dosage requirements.

The materials addressed in the text and the accompanying disk introduce the learner to the concepts that underlie the field of pharmacokinetics. Following a brief introduction to the field, the author addresses drug disposition on intravenous dosing, oral drug administration, and the principle of steady state. Subsequent topics include drug elimination, the effect of disease and other sources of variability in pharmacokinetics, and the consequences expected when nonlinear disposition complicates pharmacokinetic behavior. The author provides a detailed discussion of clearance, focusing on physiological considerations and linking this parameter to potential drug interaction scenarios through a discussion of the role of high or low intrinsic clearance and changes in free fraction in plasma.

The learning modules in the CD closely support and complement the text, providing the learner with an opportunity to assess his or her understanding of the principles presented. After identifying a set of learning objectives, each of the modules presents the student with three options: an introduction that is linked to the corresponding material in the text; a simulation tool that permits the learner to visually inspect pharmacokinetic behavior of a drug; and a self-assessment section that tests the learner's knowledge through a series of questions related to the topic, providing feedback as necessary. Of note, the simulation component allows the user to select parameter sets through adjustable sliders, provides the option of either a linear or logarithmic y-axis display, and accommodates multiple curves plotted on the same graph, demonstrating how a change in a particular parameter alters the plasma concentration–time profile of the drug in question.

Because pharmacokinetics is a quantitative discipline, it is sometimes tempting for an instructor to resort to a presentation of equations and relationships without fully exploring the underlying concepts. Although the key mathematical relations are certainly included in this author's textual materials, the additional interactive environment that the student encounters creates a positive educational experience.

The author's reliance on active learning, his use of examples illustrating important pharmacokinetic principles, and particularly the thoughtful simulation tools he has developed make this text and its companion CD an extremely effective and enjoyable introduction to the field of pharmacokinetics.

Ronald J. Sawchuk
Minneapolis, Minnesota

Preface

Pharmacokinetics is a discipline that has been expanding to become an essential component of all the processes involved in drug development, from drug discovery and preclinical evaluation to the clinical use of drugs. Pharmacokinetic studies are performed to make sure that the drug reaches its site of action in an adequate amount and by a suitable route. Also, pharmacokinetic studies are important in evaluating the different drug dosage forms after different routes of administration. Furthermore, individualization of the drug therapy based on the patient's specific conditions can increase the chance of treatment success. Individualization of drug therapy is mainly based on applying the basic pharmacokinetic principles to calculate the proper dosing regimen for each individual patient. This expansion in the field of pharmacokinetics has been accompanied by the use of complex experimental techniques and the utilization of sophisticated approaches in data analysis and interpretation. Despite this progress, the basic pharmacokinetic concepts remain the backbone of all these new developments in the field of pharmacokinetics. Thorough understanding of the basic pharmacokinetic concepts is essential before getting into more involved and applied areas of pharmacokinetics. All health-care professionals are usually exposed to basic pharmacokinetic principles during their education, with pharmacists and pharmaceutical scientists recognized as the most knowledgeable in the field. The primary intent of developing this textbook is to present the basic pharmacokinetic principles in a simple, clear, and easy format for beginning pharmacokinetic learners.

The pharmacokinetic parameters that determine the drug blood concentration–time profile are related by mathematical expressions. This makes understanding the pharmacokinetic concepts a bit difficult for those who do not have a good mathematical background and increases the need for more effective approaches in presenting the pharmacokinetic principles. Graphical presentations and computer simulations allow visualization of the interplay between the different pharmacokinetic parameters by observing how the change in one or more of the pharmacokinetic parameters of the drug is reflected on the drug concentration–time profile in the body. This visual appreciation has proven important in understanding the basic pharmacokinetic principles. This book consists of two parts: textual printed materials and highly interactive computer-based presentations. The printed materials and the computer-based presentations provide a useful combination for learners to grasp and understand basic pharmacokinetic principles. The computer-based information is presented in a self-instructional format, which introduces the concepts utilizing highly interactive graphical presentations and simulations. This presentation style is an attractive learning medium for students and provides a teaching–learning environment that can complement the printed materials. The students' perception of the computer-based presentations can be summarized by a comment made by one of my students: "The computer-based modules provided learning experiences that cannot be duplicated by textbooks." The information in this textbook covers the basic pharmacokinetic principles that have been covered in numerous textbooks. However, every effort was made to make presentation of the basic principles clear and simple. Practice problems and solved examples are included in each chapter and each module to reinforce the learning process. I hope that this book is beneficial for beginning pharmacokinetic learners.

Mohsen A. Hedaya, Pharm.D., Ph.D.

The Author

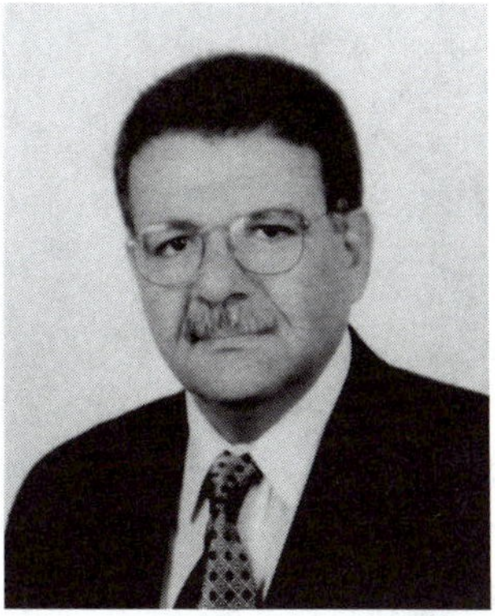

Mohsen A. Hedaya, Pharm.D., Ph.D., is currently professor and chair of the Department of Clinical Pharmacy, Faculty of Pharmacy, Tanta University, Egypt.

Dr. Hedaya received his bachelor of science degree in pharmacy (1980) from Tanta University, Egypt, and his doctor of pharmacy (1984) and doctor of philosophy (1989) degrees from the University of Minnesota in the United States. He worked as a postdoctoral research fellow at the University of Minnesota, and in 1990 he was appointed as a lecturer of clinical pharmacy, Faculty of Pharmacy, at Tanta University. In 1993, he joined the College of Pharmacy at Washington State University in the United States as an assistant professor of pharmaceutical sciences. After returning to Egypt in 1999, Dr. Hedaya worked as an associate professor and then professor of clinical pharmacy, Faculty of Pharmacy, at Tanta University.

Dr. Hedaya is a member of numerous national and international scientific associations, and he has received several prestigious awards, such as the Innovation in Teaching Award from the American Association of Colleges of Pharmacy and the National Encouragement Award in Biomedical Sciences from the National Academy for Scientific Research in Egypt. He has published about 30 scientific articles in national and international journals and has given over 30 presentations at national and international scientific meetings. Dr. Hedaya's areas of special interest include pharmacokinetics and pharmacodynamics modeling and simulations, bioanalytical method development and validation, bioequivalence study design and data analysis, and the development and assessment of computer-based instructional materials for pharmaceutical education. The computer-based educational materials developed by Dr. Hedaya in the area of pharmacokinetics are currently used by more than 250 educational, research, and industrial institutions around the world.

1 Introduction to Biopharmaceutics and Pharmacokinetics

OBJECTIVES

After completing this chapter you should be able to:

- Understand the difference between biopharmaceutics, pharmacokinetics, and pharmacodynamics
- Describe the major differences between linear and nonlinear pharmacokinetics
- Describe the general approaches utilized in pharmacokinetic modeling
- Describe how pharmacokinetic simulations can be used to illustrate the basic pharmacokinetic principles

1.1 INTRODUCTION

Biopharmaceutics is the science that deals with the relationship among the drug physicochemical properties, the dosage form characteristics, the route of drug administration, and the availability of the drug to the site of drug action.

The physicochemical properties determine the drug stability, solubility, membrane permeability, and drug affinity to different tissue components. Knowledge of drug stability is important in determining the storage and manufacturing conditions and the route of drug administration. For example, heat-sensitive drugs should be stored at low temperature, moisture-sensitive drugs are manufactured using dry procedures, and acid-labile drugs are not administered orally in the form of conventional tablets. The drug solubility is important in selecting the solvent used in liquid formulation and in determining the drug absorption because the drug has to be in solution before crossing the biological membrane. Hydrophilic compounds are highly soluble in biological fluids, but they have poor membrane permeability; lipophilic compounds have low solubility in biological fluids but have good membrane permeability. So, a balance has to exist between the lipophilicity and the hydrophilicity of the compound for adequate transport across biological membranes.

The drug properties are also important in determining the dosage form and the route of drug administration. The design of dosage form affects the rate of drug release from the dosage form and influences the rate of availability of the drug at the site of absorption, which is the major factor affecting the rate of drug absorption.

The rates of drug absorption and elimination determine the time course of the drug in the body and the site of action, which is important in determining the resulting therapeutic effects.

Pharmacokinetics is the study of the kinetics of drug absorption, distribution, and elimination. Studying the rate of absorption of the drug is important because faster drug absorption leads to faster onset of drug effect, which is necessary in the treatment of acute conditions and in emergency situations. Faster drug absorption may not be required during multiple drug administrations for the treatment of chronic diseases. Studying the extent of drug absorption is important because the amount of the drug responsible for producing the drug effect is not the total dose administered but the amount of the drug which is absorbed and becomes available for the drug site of action.

Studying the drug distribution is important because the drug has to be distributed to the site of action to produce its effect. For example, an antibiotic can be useful in the treatment of meningitis only if the antibiotic is distributed to the central nervous system. Also, studying the rate of drug elimination is necessary to determine the frequency of drug administration. Drugs that are eliminated faster require frequent drug administration to maintain effective drug concentrations all the time during multiple drug administrations. Studying the organs responsible for drug elimination is also necessary to determine the required dosage adjustment in patients with organ dysfunction. Each process (absorption, distribution, metabolism, and excretion) is associated with one or more parameters that are dependent on the drug, drug product, and the patient. These are the pharmacokinetic parameters, and they determine the rate or the extent of the different processes.

Clinical pharmacokinetics is the field of applying the basic pharmacokinetic principles in the individualization of drug therapy. This usually involves the use of drug blood concentration as a guide for the design of the appropriate dosage regimen for each individual patient.

Pharmacodynamics is the time course for the drug effect and the relationship between the drug concentration and the observed therapeutic effects. Studying the pharmacodynamics of the drug is important in determining the change in the drug effect caused by the change of the time course of the drug in the body.

1.2 APPLICATION OF BIOPHARMACEUTIC AND PHARMACOKINETIC PRINCIPLES IN BIOMEDICAL FIELDS

1.2.1 Drug Formulation Design

Biopharmaceutical principles are used to determine the factors that can affect the rate and the extent of drug absorption after administration by different routes. This can help in designing the drug formulation to ensure optimal absorption characteristics.

1.2.2 Drug Dosage Form Design

Biopharmaceutical principles are used to determine the mechanism of absorption and transfer of drug molecules to the site of action. This can help in the development of new dosage form and in determining the best route of administration to achieve the optimal therapeutic effect.

1.2.3 Pharmacological Testing

Pharmacokinetic principles are used to assess the relationship between the drug concentration and pharmacological activities. This is important to determine how much and how often the drug should be administered.

1.2.4 Toxicological Testing

Pharmacokinetic principles are used to assess tissue accumulation of drugs and how it is related to drug toxicity.

1.2.5 Evaluation of Organ Function

Pharmacokinetic principles are used to evaluate the function of eliminating organs. For example, inulin is eliminated entirely by the kidney, and the rate of inulin elimination can be used to assess kidney function.

1.2.6 Dosing Regimen Design

Pharmacokinetic principles are used to design the dosing regimen (dose and dosing interval of a specific drug product) to achieve the maximum therapeutic effect with minimal toxicity.

1.3 DRUG CONCENTRATION–TIME PROFILE

Studying the rates of drug absorption, distribution, and elimination allows characterization of the time course of the drug concentration in the body. The time course of the drug in the body is related to the time course of the drug therapeutic effect. The therapeutic outcome after drug administration is determined by the kinetics of drug absorption, distribution, and elimination.

Administration of the same dose of different drugs to the same individual will produce different drug concentration–time profiles. This is because different drugs have different rates of absorption, distribution, and elimination. Also, administration of the same dose of a drug to different individuals will produce different drug concentration–time profiles. This is because the same drug can be absorbed, distributed, and eliminated at different rates in different individuals. So, it is important to determine the factors that can affect the absorption, distribution, and elimination of each drug.

1.4 LINEAR AND NONLINEAR PHARMACOKINETICS

1.4.1 Linear Pharmacokinetics

Linear pharmacokinetics is also known as dose-independent or concentration-independent pharmacokinetics because the pharmacokinetic parameters such as half-life, total body clearance, and volume of distribution are constant and do not depend on the drug concentration or the drug amount in the body. The absorption, distribution, and elimination processes of the drug that affect the drug concentration–time profile inside the body follow first-order kinetics. The change in drug dose results in proportional change in the drug concentration–time profile in the body.

1.4.2 Nonlinear Pharmacokinetics

Nonlinear pharmacokinetics is also known as dose-dependent or concentration-dependent pharmacokinetics because the pharmacokinetic parameters such as half-life, total body clearance, and possibly volume of distribution are dependent on the drug concentration and the drug amount in the body. At least one of the pharmacokinetic processes (absorption, distribution, and elimination) that affect the drug concentration- time profile inside the body is saturable and does not follow first-order kinetics. The change in drug dose results in disproportional (more than proportional or less than proportional) change in the drug concentration–time profile in the body.

1.5 PHARMACOKINETIC MODELING

The goal of pharmacokinetic data analysis is to estimate the pharmacokinetic parameters that determine the rates of drug absorption, distribution, and elimination. Estimation of these parameters requires the assumption of a specific pharmacokinetic model. Pharmacokinetic models allow quantitative (mathematical) description of the rates of drug absorption, distribution, and elimination after administration. Modeling allows prediction of the drug pharmacokinetic behavior after administration of different dosing regimens and prediction of the changes in drug pharmacokinetic behavior caused by physiological and pathological changes.

1.5.1 Compartmental Modeling

In compartmental modeling, the body is divided into one or more compartments. The model describes the distribution of the drug between the compartments and drug elimination from one or more of the compartments. These models differ in the number of compartments and the arrangement of the compartments relative to each other. Compartmental modeling is data-based modeling. This is because the measured plasma concentration after drug administration is used to choose the best pharmacokinetic model that can describe the pharmacokinetic behavior of the drug.

1.5.2 Physiological Modeling

In physiological modeling, the body is divided into a series of organs or tissue spaces, and the model describes the uptake and disposition of the drug in each of these organs. Building the model depends on knowledge of the organ size, the organ blood flow, the drug uptake to each organ, and drug elimination from different organs. This modeling technique is useful because it can predict the difference in the drug pharmacokinetics in different species by changing the size, the blood flow, and the elimination parameters for the different species. Also, these models can be used to predict the change in drug pharmacokinetics caused by physiological and pathological changes.

1.5.3 Noncompartmental Approach

The noncompartmental approach does not assume any specific model, but it uses the total body clearance, mean residence time, and volume of distribution to describe the rate of drug disposition.

1.6 PHARMACOKINETIC SIMULATION

Pharmacokinetic simulations involve graphical presentation of the drug blood concentration–time profile in the body given specific values for the pharmacokinetic parameters. For example, the plasma concentration–time profile after a single intravenous dose administration can be described by the following equation:

$$Cp = \frac{Dose}{Vd}\, e^{-kt} \tag{1.1}$$

where Cp is the drug plasma concentration at any time t, Vd is the volume of distribution, and k is the elimination rate constant. The volume of distribution and the elimination rate constants are two pharmacokinetic parameters. The plasma concentration–time profile can be simulated by substituting for the values for each of the parameters and then calculating the plasma concentration at different time points. The calculated plasma concentrations at the different time points are plotted to show the plasma concentration–time profile. By choosing different values of the pharmacokinetic parameters, pharmacokinetic simulations can be used to visualize the effect of changing one or more pharmacokinetic parameters on the drug concentration–time profile.

QUESTIONS

1.1. What is the difference between pharmacokinetics and pharmacodynamics?
1.2. What is meant by the pharmacokinetic parameter?
1.3. Please describe the major differences between linear and nonlinear pharmacokinetics.
1.4. What are the advantages of using physiological pharmacokinetic models?
1.5. Simulations can be used to describe the effect of changing one or more pharmacokinetic parameters on the plasma concentration–time profile. Please discuss.

2 Drug Pharmacokinetics Following Single Intravenous Administration

OBJECTIVES

After completing this chapter you should be able to:

- Describe the plasma concentration–time profile after a single intravenous (IV) administration
- Identify the factors that affect the plasma concentration–time profile after a single IV drug administration
- Determine the pharmacokinetic parameters after a single IV drug administration
- Analyze the effect of changing one or more of the pharmacokinetic parameters on the plasma concentration–time profile after a single IV drug administration
- Utilize the mathematical expressions to calculate the plasma concentration at any time after a single IV drug administration
- Calculate the appropriate IV dose required to achieve a specific drug concentration

2.1 INTRODUCTION

During IV administration, the drug is directly introduced into the systemic circulation. The drug is distributed to all parts of the body and then eliminated through one or more of the elimination pathways. Drug distribution and elimination occur simultaneously at different rates/extents depending on the pharmacokinetic parameters of the drug. The volume of distribution of the drug describes the extent of drug distribution to different tissues, which is dependent on the affinity of the drug to these tissues. The drug total body clearance describes the efficiency of the different eliminating organs, such as the liver and the kidney, in eliminating the drug. Other parameters such as the drug half-life and the elimination rate constant determine the rate of decline of the drug profile in the body. In the following discussion, the different pharmacokinetic parameters that affect the drug profile in the body are discussed individually.

2.2 ELIMINATION RATE CONSTANT

2.2.1 Rate of Drug Elimination

The rate of a process is the velocity at which it occurs. If the amount of a drug (A) in the body is decreasing with time because of elimination, then the rate of elimination is expressed as –dA/dt. The negative sign is used because the drug amount is decreasing. The rate of elimination is determined experimentally by measuring the decrease in the amount of the drug A at given time intervals. The units of the rate of elimination are units of mass per time (e.g., mg/hr, g/day, or mg/min).

2.2.1.1 Rate Constant for Drug Elimination

The rate constant for the elimination process is a constant that influences the rate of the elimination process. The way the rate constant influences the rate of elimination is dependent on the order of the elimination process.

2.2.2 Order of Drug Elimination

Drug elimination can follow zero-order kinetics or first-order kinetics. Most drugs are eliminated by first-order kinetics in the range of doses used clinically.

2.2.2.1 Zero-Order Elimination

In zero-order elimination, the rate of elimination is constant and is equal to the zero-order elimination rate constant K_0. The zero-order elimination rate constant has units of mass/time. If the amount of drug A is decreasing at a constant rate, then the rate of change of the amount of drug in the body dA/dt is expressed as

$$\frac{dA}{dt} = -K_0 \tag{2.1}$$

where K_0 is the zero-order elimination rate constant. Integration of Equation 2.1 yields the following expression:

$$A = A_0 - K_0\, t \tag{2.2}$$

where A is the amount of the drug at any time t, and A_0 is the amount of drug at time zero. Equation 2.2 describes a linear relationship between the amount of the drug A and time t. A plot of the amount of the drug versus time on a Cartesian graph paper yields a straight line as in Figure 2.1. The y-intercept is equal to A_0, and the slope is equal to $-K_0$.

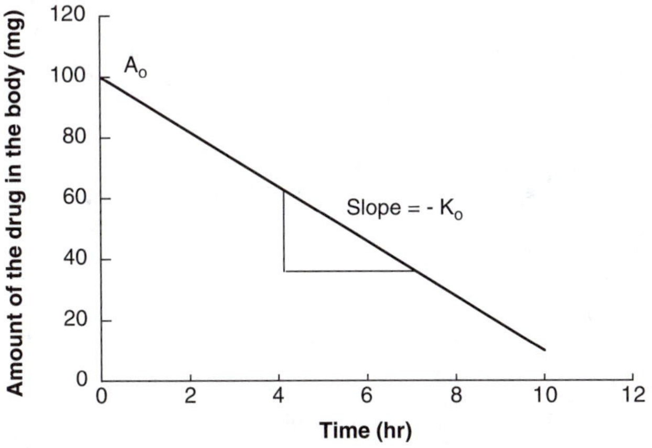

FIGURE 2.1 A plot of the amount of the drug versus time on the Cartesian scale when the elimination of the drug follows zero-order kinetics.

EXAMPLE

A drug is known to decompose in acidic medium by a zero-order process. After addition of 500 mg of the drug in a beaker that has 0.01*N* HCl, the following data were obtained:

Time (hr)	Amount of Drug Remaining (mg)
2	432
4	356
8	221

1. Calculate the zero-order decomposition rate constant of this drug.
2. What will be the amount of the drug remaining after 12 hr?

Answer

1. For calculation of the zero-order decomposition rate constant:
   Plot the amount of the drug versus time on Cartesian graph paper.
   Draw the best line that goes through the three data points.
   Calculate the slope of the line by taking two points on the line you drew (do not calculate the slope from two of the given data points): Slope = $\frac{y_2 - y_1}{x_2 - x_1}$
   From Figure 2.2, the calculated slope = $-K_0$ = −36.6 mg/hr. So, the zero-order decomposition rate constant = 36.6 mg/h.
2. To calculate the amount of the drug remaining after 12 hr, substitute in Equation 2.2 for the value of K_0 and time:

$$A = A_0 - K_0 t$$

Amount remaining after 12 hr = 500 mg − 36.6 mg/hr × 12 hr = 60.8 mg

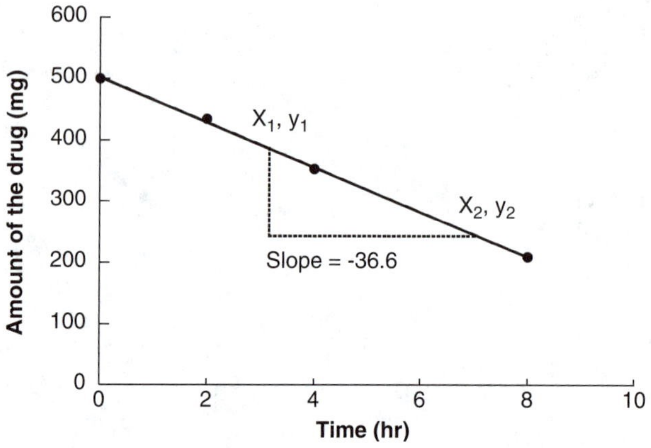

FIGURE 2.2 A plot of the amount of the drug remaining (undecomposed) versus time on the Cartesian scale.

2.2.2.2 First-Order Elimination

In first-order elimination, the rate of elimination is dependent on the elimination rate constant k and the amount of the drug in the body A. The first-order elimination rate constant has units of time^{-1}. When the drug elimination process follows first-order kinetics, the rate of change of the amount of drug in the body dA/dt is expressed as

$$\frac{dA}{dt} = -\text{k A} \tag{2.3}$$

where k is the first-order elimination rate constant. The amount of the drug in the body decreases with time because of drug elimination. Also, the rate of drug elimination decreases with time because of the decrease in drug amount in the body. This is because the rate of drug elimination at any time is dependent on the elimination rate constant (constant) and the amount of drug in the body (decreases with time). A plot of the amount of drug in the body versus time on the Cartesian scale is a curve with decreasing slope as shown in Figure 2.3.

Equation 2.3 describes the rate of change of the amount of the drug in the body with time. Integration of Equation 2.3 yields the following expression:

$$\ln \text{A} = \ln \text{A}_0 - \text{kt} \tag{2.4}$$

Equation 2.4 describes a linear relationship between ln A and time. A plot of ln A versus time on Cartesian graph paper yields a straight line. The y-intercept is equal to ln A_0, and the slope is –k, as shown in Figure 2.4.

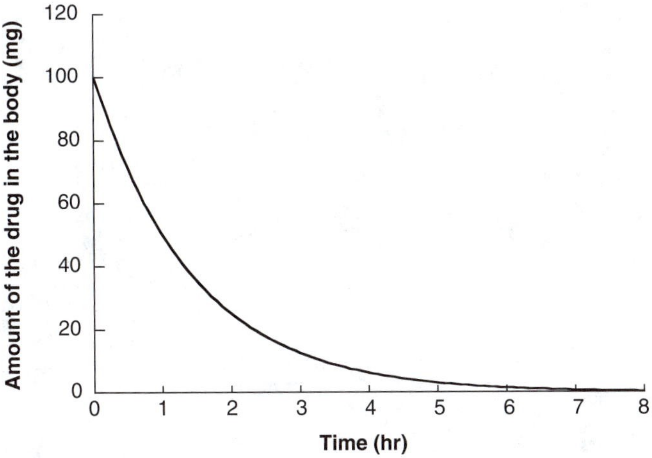

FIGURE 2.3 A plot of the amount of the drug versus time on the Cartesian scale when the elimination of the drug follows first-order kinetics.

Because ln A = 2.303 log A, Equation 2.4, which describes the natural logarithm of the amount of the drug in the body at any time, can be expressed as

$$\log A = \log A_0 - \frac{k\ t}{2.303} \tag{2.5}$$

Equation 2.5 describes a linear relationship between log A and time. A plot of log A versus time on Cartesian graph paper yields a straight line. The y-intercept is equal to log A_0, and the slope is –k/2.303 as in Figure 2.5.

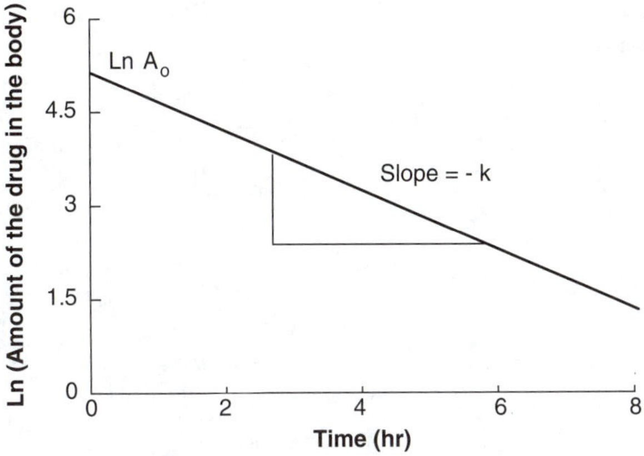

FIGURE 2.4 A plot of the natural logarithm of the amount of the drug versus time on the Cartesian scale when the elimination of the drug follows first-order kinetics.

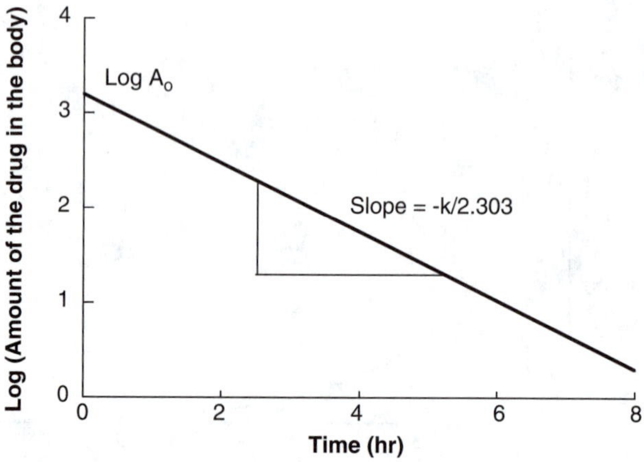

FIGURE 2.5 A plot of the logarithm of the amount of the drug versus time on the Cartesian scale when the elimination of the drug follows first-order kinetics.

Taking the anti-ln of Equation 2.4 yields the following equation:

$$A = A_0 \, e^{-kt} \tag{2.6}$$

This is an exponential (nonlinear) expression that describes the change in the amount of the drug in the body with time. Plotting the amount of drug in the body versus time on semilog graph paper will give a straight line. The y-intercept is equal to A_0, and the slope is $-k/2.303$ as in Figure 2.6.

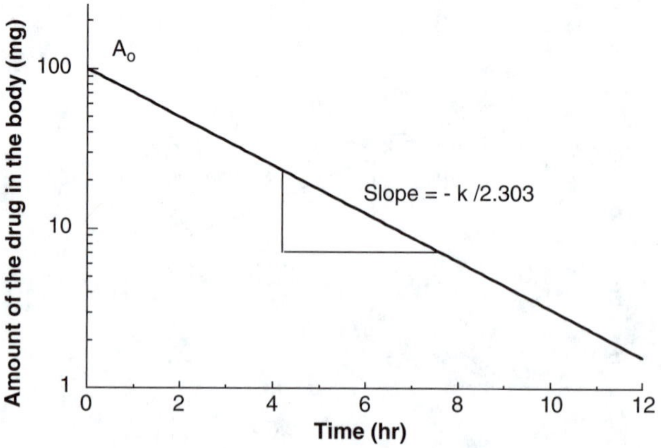

FIGURE 2.6 A plot of the amount of the drug versus time on the semilog scale when the elimination of the drug follows first-order kinetics.

2.2.3 Determination of the First-Order Elimination Rate Constant *k*

The first-order elimination rate constant k can be determined by measuring the amount of the drug in the body at different time points after a single IV administration.

- Plotting ln A versus time on Cartesian graph paper, the slope of the resulting line = −k.
- Plotting log A versus time on Cartesian graph paper, the slope of the resulting line = −k/2.303.
- Plotting A versus time on semilog graph paper, the slope of the resulting line = −k/2.303.

The slope of a straight line is determined by choosing two points on the line and the slope will be

$$\text{Slope} = \frac{y_2 - y_1}{x_2 - x_1} \tag{2.7}$$

However, the slope of the line plotted on a semilog graph paper will be

$$\text{Slope} = \frac{\log y_2 - \log y_1}{x_2 - x_1} \tag{2.8}$$

2.2.4 Mathematical Expressions That Describe the Amount of the Drug in the Body When Elimination Process Follows First-Order Elimination

Equations 2.4 to 2.6 describe the time course for the amount of the drug in the body after a single IV administration when the elimination process follows first-order kinetics. These equations can be written in a more general form:

$$\ln A_2 = \ln A_1 - k\,t \tag{2.9}$$

$$\log A_2 = \log A_1 - \frac{k\,t}{2.303} \tag{2.10}$$

$$A_2 = A_1\, e^{-k\,t} \tag{2.11}$$

where A_1 and A_2 are the amount of drug in the body at two different time points, the difference between the two time points is t, and k is the first-order elimination rate constant. These three equations can be used in calculating useful pharmacokinetic information.

Example

Ampicillin is an antibiotic that is eliminated from the body by a first-order process. Equations 2.9 to 2.11 can be used to solve the following four different questions:

1. Calculate the amount of ampicillin remaining in the body 6 hr after IV administration of a single 500-mg dose if the first-order elimination rate constant is $0.53\ hr^{-1}$.

Answer

$$A_2 = A_1\ e^{-kt}$$

$$\text{Amount remaining} = 500\ \text{mg}\ e^{-0.53\ hr^{-1}\ 6\ hr}$$

$$\text{Amount remaining} = 20.8\ \text{mg}$$

2. Calculate ampicillin first-order elimination rate constant if the amount of ampicillin remaining in the body 6 hr after administration of a single IV dose of 500 mg was 20.8 mg.

Answer

$$A_2 = A_1 e^{-kt}$$

$$20.8\ \text{mg} = 500\ \text{mg}\ e^{-k\,6\ hr}$$

$$\frac{20.8\ \text{mg}}{500\ \text{mg}} = e^{-k\,6\ hr}$$

$$\ln\ \frac{20.8}{500} = \ln\ e^{-k\,6\ hr}$$

$$-\ 3.179 = -\ k\ 6\ hr$$

$$k = 0.53\ hr^{-1}$$

3. Calculate the time required for the amount of ampicillin in the body to decrease to 20.8 mg after IV administration of a single 500-mg dose if the first-order elimination rate constant is $0.53\ hr^{-1}$.

Answer

$$A_2 = A_1\ e^{-kt}$$

$$20.8\ \text{mg} = 500\ \text{mg}\ e^{-0.53\ hr^{-1} t}$$

You can solve for t, which will be 6 hr.

4. Calculate the IV bolus dose of ampicillin administered if the amount of ampicillin remaining in the body after 6 hr was 20.8 mg, and the first-order elimination rate constant of ampicillin is $0.53\ hr^{-1}$.

Answer

$$A_2 = A_1\ e^{-kt}$$

$$20.8\ \text{mg} = A_1\ e^{-0.53\ \text{hr}^{-1}\ 6\ \text{hr}}$$

You can solve for A_1 which will be 500 mg.

Please note that Equation 2.11 was used to solve the questions; however, Equations 2.9 and 2.10 can also be used to solve the questions.

2.2.5 Clinical Importance of the Elimination Rate Constant

When comparing a group of drugs, a larger elimination rate constant means a faster rate of drug elimination from the body. Drugs that are eliminated rapidly from the body have a shorter duration of effect after single-dose administration. This is because the amount of the drug in the body will fall below the effective level quickly. During multiple administrations, drugs that are eliminated rapidly from the body will need to be given more frequently to maintain an effective drug level in the body; slowly eliminated drugs should be given less frequently. For example, penicillin G is eliminated from the body quickly, so it is usually administered every 4–6 hr, and a drug like digoxin, which is eliminated slowly from the body, is usually administered once every day.

Patients who have dysfunction in the organ responsible for the elimination of a drug usually eliminate the drug at a slower rate compared to patients with a normally functioning eliminating organ (Figure 2.7). So, patients with dysfunction in the eliminating organs require smaller doses of the drug (or doses should be administered

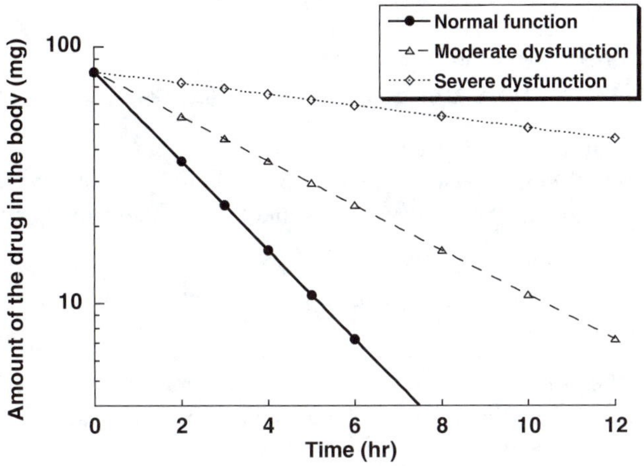

FIGURE 2.7 The amount of the drug-time profile in patients with different degrees of eliminating organ dysfunction. Patients with eliminating organ dysfunction eliminate the drug at a slower rate compared to patients with normal organ function.

less frequently) compared to patients with a normally functioning eliminating organ. For example, patients with kidney failure require smaller doses of aminoglycoside antibiotics compared with patients with normal kidney function. This is because the aminoglycoside antibiotics are eliminated by the kidney, and kidney dysfunction slows the rate of their elimination.

2.2.6 Summary

- The first-order elimination rate constant is the rate constant for the elimination of the drug from the body. It determines how fast the drug is eliminated from the body.
- The first-order elimination rate constant is a dependent pharmacokinetic parameter that depends on the total body clearance and the volume of distribution of the drug (two pharmacokinetic parameters discussed in Sections 2.3 and 2.5).
- This rate constant represents the rate constant for drug elimination through all routes of drug elimination, such as metabolism, renal excretion, and other routes.
- The first-order elimination rate constant has units of time^{-1}.

2.3 VOLUME OF DISTRIBUTION

After IV administration, the drug is distributed via the systemic circulation to all parts of the body, leaving only a fraction of the administered dose in the sampling compartment (the blood). Drugs are not distributed equally to all tissues because different drugs have different affinities to different tissues. This means that the amount of the drug, and hence the concentration of the drug, in the sampling compartment will be different for different drugs depending on the administered dose and the drug distribution characteristics.

2.3.1 Relationship between Drug Amount in the Body and Drug Blood Concentration

If a known amount of the drug is added to a beaker that contains a solvent, then the resulting concentration is dependent on the volume of the solvent. The relationship among the drug amount, drug concentration, and the volume can be expressed as

$$\text{Drug concentration} = \frac{\text{Amount}}{\text{Volume}} \tag{2.12}$$

Similarly, when a certain amount of the drug is administered as a single IV dose, the drug is distributed to all parts of the body, and the resulting drug concentration can be expressed as

$$\text{Drug concentration} = \frac{\text{Drug amount in the body}}{\text{Vd}} \tag{2.13}$$

The volume of distribution Vd is the parameter that relates the amount of the drug in the body to the drug concentration in the blood. Because the drug is not distributed equally to all parts of the body as the drug usually has different affinities to different tissues, the volume of distribution does not represent a real volume. In other words, we can say that the body behaves as if it has a volume equal to the volume of distribution. The volume of distribution is often known as the apparent volume of distribution. The physicochemical properties of the drug and the affinity of the drug to the blood and tissue components will influence the volume of distribution of the drug. Drugs that are extensively distributed to the tissues usually have a larger volume of distribution. The volume of distribution is an independent pharmacokinetic parameter that does not depend on other parameters.

The drug blood concentration is determined by dividing the amount of the drug in the body by the volume of distribution. So, dividing the equations that describe the amount of the drug-time profile (Eqs. 2.4 to 2.6) by the volume of distribution yields the equations that describe the drug blood concentration–time profile. When the drug elimination follows first-order kinetics, the drug blood concentration–time profile after a single IV bolus dose can be described by the following equations:

$$\ln Cp = \ln Cp_0 - kt \tag{2.14}$$

$$\log Cp = \log Cp_0 - \frac{k\,t}{2.303} \tag{2.15}$$

$$Cp = Cp_0\ e^{-k\,t} \tag{2.16}$$

2.3.2 Drug Protein Binding and Volume of Distribution

The affinity of the drug to any tissue is determined from factors such as the lipid solubility of the drug, the binding of the drug to the plasma proteins, and the binding of the drug to different tissue components. When the drug reaches the systemic circulation, it can bind to plasma proteins such as albumin, α-1-acid glycoprotein, and lipoprotein. The extent of protein binding in blood can range from 0% when the drug is not bound to plasma protein to more than 99% when the majority of the drug is bound to plasma protein. This is dependent on the affinity of the drug to the plasma protein. The binding of the drug molecule to plasma protein is reversible, and ratio of the free (unbound) drug concentration to the total (bound and unbound) drug concentration is relatively constant for a given drug in a given individual.

The free (unbound) drug molecules are the pharmacologically active moiety because the free molecules can cross biological membranes and can bind to drug receptors. So, the intensity of the pharmacological effect is dependent on the free drug concentration rather than the total drug concentration. However, because the free fractions (ratio of the free drug concentration to the total drug concentration) for most drugs is relatively constant for each drug, the total drug concentration in plasma is also related to the intensity of the pharmacological effect. Measuring the free drug

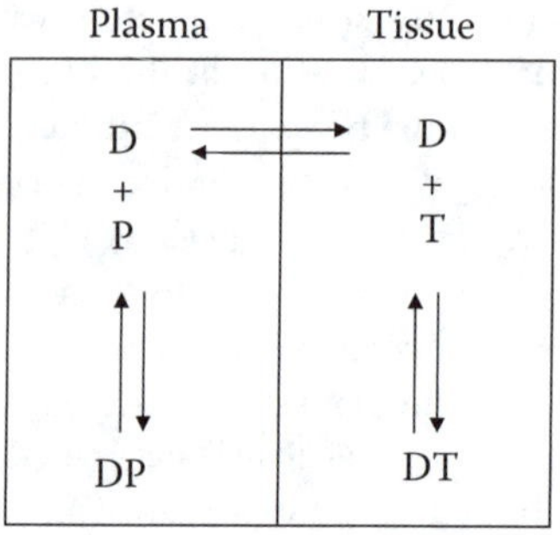

FIGURE 2.8 A diagram representing the distribution of the drug between the plasma and the tissues. D is the free (unbound) drug molecule in plasma and tissue, P is the plasma protein, DP is the drug bound to plasma protein, T is the tissue components to which the drug can bind, and DT is a drug molecule bound to tissue components.

concentration will be necessary to monitor the therapeutic effect of the drug in certain pathological conditions, which can affect the amount of circulating plasma protein or alter the affinity of the drug to plasma protein, such as in liver diseases and renal failure.

A simple model that describes the distribution of drugs in plasma and tissues is presented in Figure 2.8. Free drug molecules in plasma can distribute to different tissues depending on their lipid solubility, which determines their ability to cross biological membranes. Once free drug molecules are distributed to tissues, a new equilibrium is established in plasma to maintain the constant binding of the drug to plasma proteins. Also, the drug molecules distributed to the tissues can bind to different tissue components to an extent that is dependent on the affinity of the drug molecules to different tissue components. The binding of the drug to tissue components is also reversible, and the ratio of the free to total drug concentration is relatively constant for a given drug in a given tissue.

When the drug is distributed to tissues and equilibrium is established between the drug in plasma and the drug in the tissues, the free drug concentration in plasma should be equal to the free drug concentration in the tissues. However, the total (free and bound) drug concentrations in plasma and tissues are usually different and depend on the relative affinities of the drug to plasma proteins and to tissue components. Drugs that are highly bound to tissue components (i.e., have high affinity to the tissues and have small free [unbound] fraction in tissues) usually have a large volume of distribution. Based on this discussion, the volume of distribution of the drugs is dependent on the volume of the vascular volume, the volume of the tissues where the drug is distributed, and the affinity of the drug to the plasma and tissue components. Because the affinity of the drug to the plasma and tissue components can be related to the free fraction of the drug in plasma and tissues, the volume of distribution can be expressed as follows:

$$Vd = V_p + V_t \left(\frac{F_p}{F_t} \right) \tag{2.17}$$

where Vd is the volume of distribution, V_p is the volume of the plasma, V_t is the volume of the tissues, F_p is the free fraction of the drug in plasma, and F_t is the free fraction of the drug in tissues. This relationship indicates that changes in the plasma protein binding or the tissue binding can lead to changes in the drug volume of distribution.

Patients with liver diseases usually have lower plasma protein concentrations, which can significantly reduce drug binding to plasma protein and increase the free fraction of the drug. Also, drug–drug interactions that can result in displacement of one drug from its protein binding sites can lead to increase in the free fraction of the drug. According to Equation 2.17, these conditions can lead to an increase in the volume of distribution of the drug if the drug tissue binding is not affected. On the other hand, conditions that can decrease the drug tissue binding (increase free fraction in tissues) without affecting the plasma protein binding can decrease the drug volume of distribution.

2.3.3 Determination of Volume of Distribution

The volume of distribution can be calculated from the relationship between the drug amount in the body and the resulting drug concentration. However, it is usually impossible to measure the amount of the drug in the body. The only time we know the amount of drug in the body is right after drug administration (at time zero), when the amount of drug is equal to the dose. Immediately after IV administration, Equation 2.13 can be written as

$$Cp_0 = \frac{Dose}{Vd} \tag{2.18}$$

where Cp_0 is the drug blood concentration at time zero. Because it is practically impossible to measure the blood concentration at time zero, the initial drug concentration can be estimated graphically as in Figure 2.9. The drug concentrations measured after administration of a single IV dose of the drug are plotted on semilog graph paper. The best-fitted line is drawn and is back-extrapolated to the y-axis. The y-intercept is the initial drug concentration (Cp_0). The volume of distribution is calculated from a rearrangement of Equation 2.18:

$$Vd = \frac{Dose}{Cp_0} \tag{2.19}$$

The volume of distribution has units of volume (e.g., liters). Because the volume of distribution depends on the weight of the patient, the volume of distribution can be related to the body weight, for example, volume/weight (e.g., L/kg).

2.3.4 Clinical Importance of Volume of Distribution

Most drugs have a specific therapeutic range in which the drug is most likely to be effective with minimum adverse effects. So, the goal is to achieve a specific drug

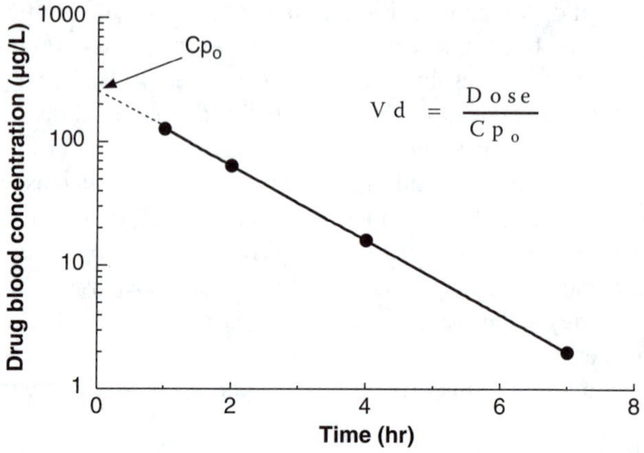

FIGURE 2.9 The best line that fits the plasma concentration obtained after IV bolus administration is back-extrapolated to the y-axis to calculate the plasma concentration at time zero Cp_0.

blood concentration. The volume of distribution allows calculation of the dose required to achieve a certain blood concentration of the drug, as in Equation 2.20:

$$\text{Dose} = Cp_{\text{desired}} \times Vd \tag{2.20}$$

The volume of distribution also allows calculation of the expected drug blood concentration achieved after administration of a certain dose. Increasing the dose in a given patient results in a proportional increase in the initial drug blood concentration (because Vd is constant), and the drug blood concentration–time profiles decline with the same slope because the elimination rate constant is similar (Figure 2.10).

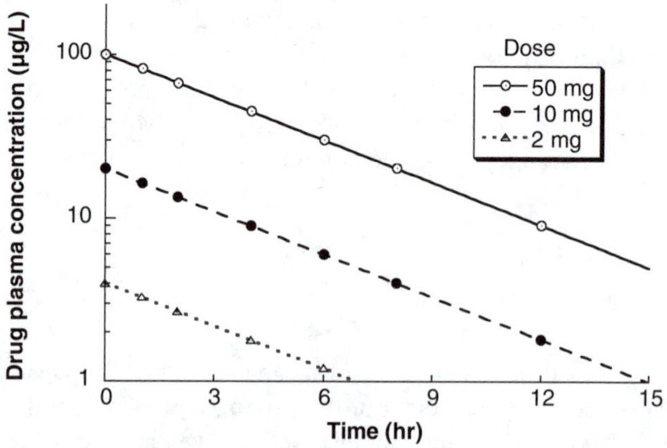

FIGURE 2.10 The plasma drug concentration–time profile after administration of increasing doses of the same drug in the same individual. The initial plasma concentration is proportional to the administered dose, and the slopes of the profiles are similar, indicating that the elimination rate constant is dose independent.

Drugs that are extensively distributed to the tissues will have a large volume of distribution and will require larger doses to achieve a certain drug blood concentration.

2.3.5 Summary

- The volume of distribution is the apparent volume in which the drug can be distributed.
- The volume of distribution is the factor that relates the amount of drug in the body to the concentration of the drug in the sampling site. It is not an actual volume; however, it is a hypothetical volume determined by the drug distribution behavior.
- The volume of distribution ranges from 3–5 L to more than 25 L/kg. Drugs with higher affinity for tissues have higher volume of distribution. The volume of distribution has units of volume or volume/weight.

2.4 HALF-LIFE

The half-life $t_{1/2}$ is defined as the time required for the drug amount in the body or the drug blood concentration to decrease by one half (50%).

2.4.1 Half-Life during Zero-Order and First-Order Elimination

2.4.1.1 Zero-Order Elimination

When drug elimination follows zero-order kinetics, the half-life depends on the amount (and the concentration) of the drug and the zero-order elimination rate constant. In other words, the time required for the concentration of drug in plasma to decrease from 100 to 50 μg/L is longer than the time required for the drug plasma concentration to decrease from 50 to 25 μg/L, as in Figure 2.11.

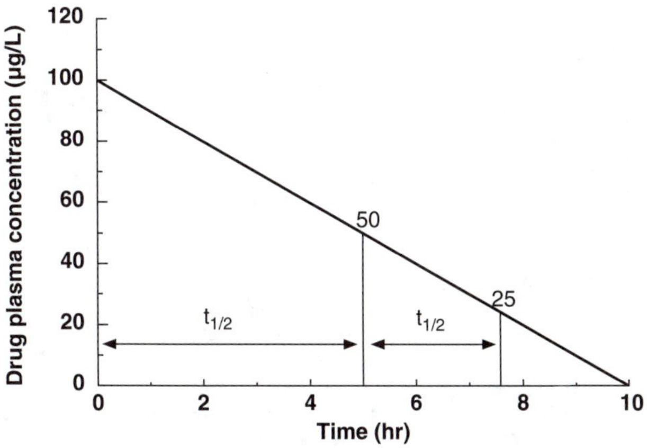

FIGURE 2.11 The half-life of the drug is dependent on the drug concentration when the drug elimination process follows zero-order kinetics.

The half-life when the elimination process follows zero-order kinetics is proportional to the initial drug amount (A_0) or drug concentration and is inversely proportional to the zero-order elimination rate constant K_0.

$$t_{1/2} = \frac{0.5\, A_0}{K_0} \tag{2.21}$$

2.4.1.2 First-Order Elimination

When the elimination process follows first-order kinetics, the half-life of the drug is constant and is related to the elimination rate constant. In other words, the time required for the drug plasma concentration to decrease from 100 to 50 μg/L is the same as the time required for the drug plasma concentration to decrease from 15 to 7.5 μg/L, as illustrated in Figure 2.12. The half-life when the elimination process follows first-order kinetics is constant and can be determined from the first-order elimination rate constant from the following equation:

$$t_{1/2} = \frac{0.693}{k} \tag{2.22}$$

2.4.2 Graphical Determination of Half-Life

The blood concentrations are measured at different time points after a single IV bolus dose of the drug. Draw the blood concentrations versus time on semilog graph paper and draw the best line that goes through the samples. Starting at any point on the line, find out the time required for the y-coordinate of this point to decrease by 50% as in Figure 2.13. This is the half-life.

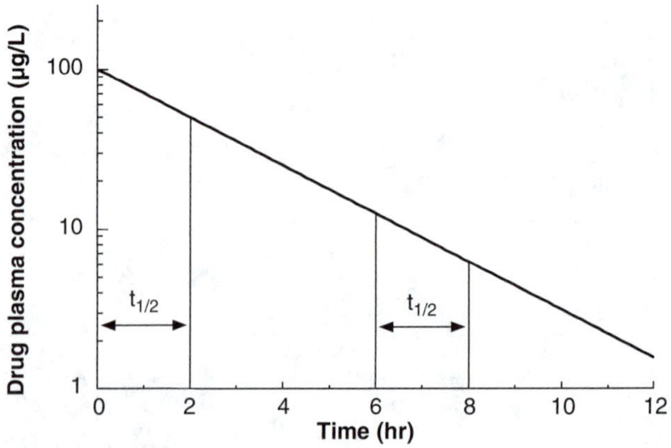

FIGURE 2.12 The half-life of the drug is independent of the drug concentration when the drug elimination process follows first-order kinetics.

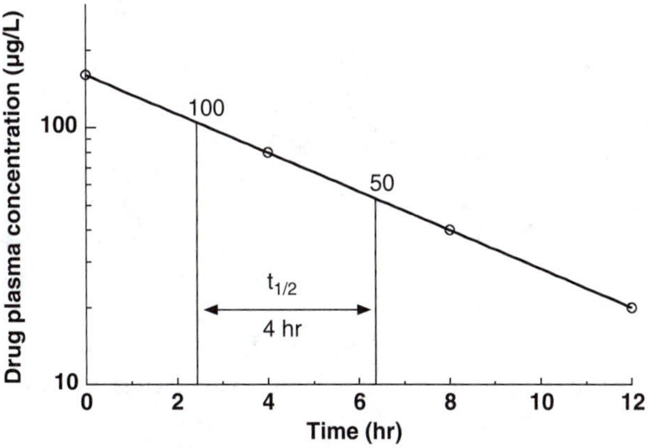

FIGURE 2.13 Graphical determination of the half-life.

2.4.3 Clinical Importance of Half-Life

The half-life is the parameter that reflects the rate of drug elimination, similar to the elimination rate constant. Drugs that have a short half-life (large elimination rate constant) are eliminated from the body faster than drugs with a long half-life (Figure 2.14). Drugs that have a short half-life need to be given more frequently during multiple administrations; drugs with a long half-life should be given less frequently. Also, drugs given to patients who have a dysfunction of the organ responsible for the elimination of a drug have a longer half-life compared to those given to patients with normal function of the eliminating organ. For example, the half-life of aminoglycoside is much longer in patients with kidney failure compared to the half-life in patients with normal kidney function. This is because the aminoglycoside antibiotics are eliminated primarily by the kidney.

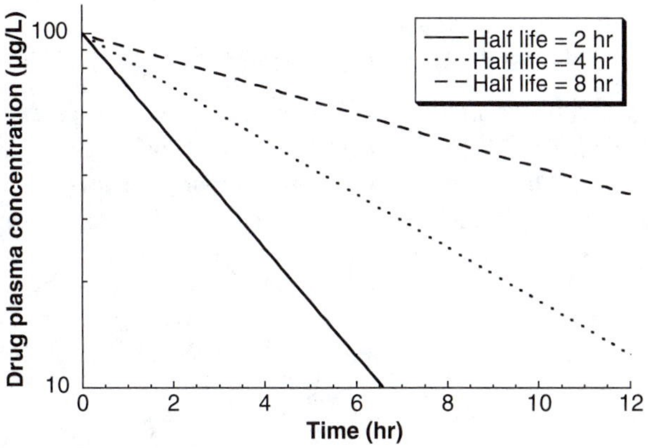

FIGURE 2.14 Drugs with shorter half-lives are eliminated faster than drugs with longer half-lives.

2.4.4 Summary

- The half-life is the time required for the amount of the drug in the body or the plasma concentration of the drug to decrease by 50%.
- The half-life and the first-order elimination rate constant are dependent on the total body clearance and the volume of distribution.
- The half-life of a drug is constant within a patient (dose and concentration independent) when the drug elimination process follows first-order kinetics. However, different patients may have different half-lives for the same drug.
- The half-life is an important parameter because it indicates how fast the drug is eliminated from the body. Drugs with shorter half-lives are eliminated faster than those with longer half-lives.
- The half-life has units of time.

2.5 TOTAL BODY CLEARANCE

The *total body clearance* CL_T is defined as the volume of plasma or blood that is completely cleared from the drug per unit time. The CL_T is a measure of the efficiency of all eliminating organs in metabolizing/excreting the drug. The CL_T has units of volume/time (e.g., L/hr or ml/min). It can also be expressed in units of volume/time/weight (e.g., L/hr/kg or ml/min/kg). The total body clearance of a drug in a particular patient is constant and is independent of drug concentration as long as the drug elimination process follows first-order kinetics.

The CL_T represents the overall clearance of the drug from the body by all eliminating organs. *Organ clearance* represents the clearance of the drug by a specific organ. For example, the *renal clearance* can be defined as the volume of plasma or blood completely cleared from the drug per unit time by the kidney. So, the CL_T is the sum of the clearances of all eliminating organs as expressed in Equation 2.23:

$$CL_T = \text{Renal clearance} + \text{Hepatic clearance} + \text{Lung clearance} + \ldots \quad (2.23)$$

2.5.1 Relationship between Total Body Clearance, Volume of Distribution, and the Elimination Rate Constant

The total body clearance and the volume of distribution of the drug (the two independent pharmacokinetic parameters) are the two parameters that determine the drug elimination rate constant and half-life (the dependent pharmacokinetic parameters) as in Equations 2.24 and 2.25:

$$\frac{CL_T}{Vd} = k \quad (2.24)$$

and

$$\frac{CL_T}{Vd} = \frac{0.693}{t_{1/2}} \tag{2.25}$$

So, the total body clearance can be calculated from the volume of distribution and the elimination rate constant by rearrangement of Equation 2.24:

$$CL_T = k \,.\, Vd \tag{2.26}$$

The total body clearance can also be calculated from the drug excretion rate and the drug blood concentration as in Equation 2.27:

$$\frac{\text{Drug excretion rate}}{\text{Blood drug concentration}} = \frac{dA/dt}{Cp} = CL_T \tag{2.27}$$

2.5.2 Determination of Total Body Clearance

A single IV bolus dose is administered to an individual, and serial blood samples are obtained after drug administration. The drug concentrations in the blood samples are measured and plotted on semilog graph paper. The elimination rate constant and the volume of distribution of the drug are determined as described before. The total body clearance is calculated from the volume of distribution and the elimination rate constant according to Equation 2.26.

The total body clearance can be calculated according to Equation 2.27 from the drug elimination rate and the drug blood concentration. However, it is practically difficult to measure the overall rate of drug elimination from the body. It is only possible to calculate the rate of drug elimination by a specific organ such as the rate of drug elimination by the kidney in urine. So, this method can be suitable in such cases to measure the renal clearance of drugs as follows:

$$CL_{Renal} = \frac{\text{Renal excretion rate}}{\text{Drug blood concentration}} \tag{2.28}$$

2.5.3 Total Body Clearance and Volume of Distribution Are Independent Pharmacokinetic Parameters

The total body clearance of a drug is determined by the intrinsic ability of the eliminating organs to excrete or metabolize the drug. For example, if the drug is metabolized by the liver, then the metabolic clearance is determined from the activity of the metabolizing enzymes and the factors that can help the drug to come in contact with the enzymes. Also, the renal clearance of a drug is determined from the ability of the kidney to excrete the drug in the urine. On the other hand, the volume of distribution of the drug is dependent on the physicochemical properties of the drug, which influence the affinity of the drug for the different tissues. For example, drugs with high affinity for distribution to different tissues have a larger volume of distribution; drugs that are poorly distributed to tissues have a small volume of distribution.

Based on this discussion, changes in the ability of an organ to eliminate the drug can affect the clearance of the drug without affecting its volume of distribution. Also, changes that affect the distribution of the drug to different tissues can affect the volume of distribution of the drug without affecting its clearance. For this reason, the total body clearance and the volume of distribution are considered the independent pharmacokinetic parameters. The total body clearance and the volume of distribution together will determine the elimination rate constant and the half-life of the drug according to Equations 2.24 and 2.25. So, the elimination rate constant and the half-life are considered the dependent pharmacokinetic parameters. Two different drugs may have similar CL_T; however, because of the difference in the Vd, the drug with the larger Vd will have a longer $t_{1/2}$ (and smaller k). Similarly, two drugs may have similar Vd, and the drug with the lower CL_T will have a longer $t_{1/2}$ (and smaller k).

It is important to note that the CL_T is not a measure of the rate of drug elimination. Higher CL_T does not always mean a faster rate of drug disappearance from the body (larger k and shorter half-life). This is because the Vd will need to be considered in determining the rate of drug elimination.

Example

Gentamicin:	$CL_T = 0.07$ L/hr/kg	Vd = 0.2 L/kg	$t_{1/2} = 2.0$ hr
Rifampin:	$CL_T = 0.2$ L/hr/kg	Vd = 1 L/kg	$t_{1/2} = 3.46$ hr

The total body clearance of rifampin is higher than that of gentamicin. However, because the rifampin Vd is larger, the rate of decrease of the plasma rifampin concentration is slower than that of gentamicin (smaller k, longer half-life).

2.5.4 Clinical Importance of Total Body Clearance

For the same drug (the same Vd), a decrease in drug CL_T means a slower rate of drug elimination. So, patients with different degrees of eliminating organ dysfunction who are taking the same drug eliminate the drug at different rates and may require dosage adjustment according to the degree of dysfunction. The CL_T of the drug can be used as a monitoring parameter for the function of the eliminating organ of the drug.

The clearance of some specific markers can be used to determine the function of the eliminating organ of this marker. For example, creatinine is an endogenous byproduct of muscle metabolism that is excreted only by the kidney. The clearance of creatinine is used as a measure of kidney function. A decrease in kidney function results in lower creatinine clearance.

2.5.5 Summary

- The total body clearance is the volume of the plasma or blood that is completely cleared from the drug per unit time. It has units of volume/time or volume/time/weight.

- The total body clearance for a drug is constant within a patient (dose and concentration independent) when the elimination processes follow first-order kinetics.
- The total body clearance is a measure of the efficiency of all eliminating organs in eliminating the drug, and it is the sum of all organ clearances (i.e., CL_T is the sum of the renal clearance, hepatic clearance, and all other organ clearances).
- The elimination rate constant and the half-life (the dependent pharmacokinetic parameters) are dependent on (are determined from) the total body clearance and the volume of distribution (the independent pharmacokinetic parameters).

2.6 AREA UNDER THE CURVE

The *area under the curve* (AUC) is the integral of the blood concentration with respect to time from time zero to time infinity. It has units of mass-time/volume.

$$\int_{t=0}^{t=\infty} Cp\, dt = AUC \tag{2.29}$$

2.6.1 Factors Affecting Area Under the Curve after a Single IV Bolus Dose

Integrating Equation 2.16, which describes the blood concentration–time profile after administration of a single IV bolus dose, yields the value of the AUC:

$$AUC\ |_{t=0}^{t=\infty} = \frac{Cp_0}{k} \tag{2.30}$$

Because Cp_0 is equal to the dose/Vd, the AUC after administration of a single oral dose can be expressed as

$$AUC\ |_{t=0}^{t=\infty} = \frac{Dose}{k\ Vd} = \frac{Dose}{CL_T} \tag{2.31}$$

Based on Equation 2.31, the AUC after administration of a single IV bolus dose is directly proportional to the administered dose as in Figure 2.15 and is inversely proportional to the CL_T as in Figure 2.16. Patients with different degrees of eliminating organ dysfunction have different clearance values for the same drug. Patients with severe dysfunction usually have lower clearance; those with normal function have higher clearance. So, after administration of the same IV dose, a higher AUC is observed in patients with lower clearance, and a lower AUC is seen in a patient with higher clearance (Figure 2.16).

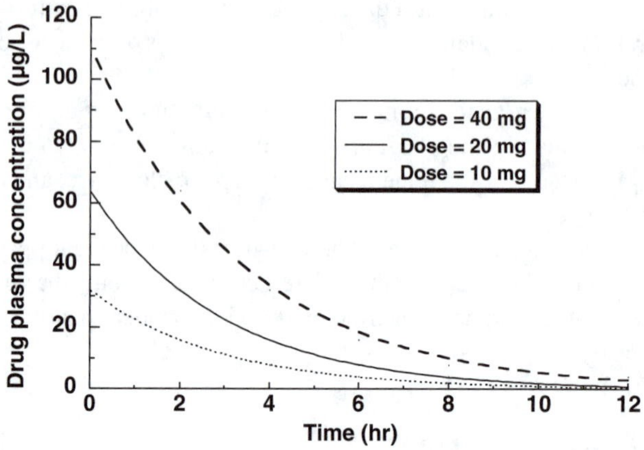

FIGURE 2.15 The area under the plasma concentration–time curve is proportional to the administered dose.

Please note that administration of different drugs to the same group of individuals will result in different AUCs because the different drugs have different CL_T. Drugs with smaller clearance produce a higher AUC; those with higher clearance produce a smaller AUC.

2.6.2 Calculation of Area Under the Curve after a Single IV Bolus Dose

The drug concentrations measured after administration of a single IV dose of the drug are plotted on a semilog graph paper. The best fitted line is drawn and is back-extrapolated to the y-axis. The y-intercept is the initial drug concentration (Cp_0).

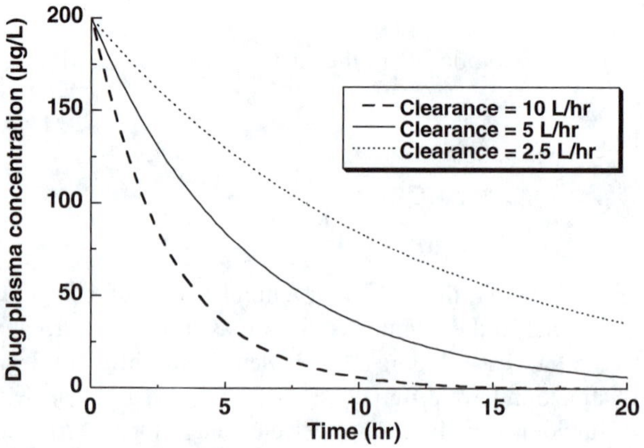

FIGURE 2.16 The area under the plasma concentration–time curve is inversely proportional to the total body clearance.

The elimination rate constant (k) is calculated from the slope of the best fitted line, or from the half life of the drug. The AUC is calculated from Equation 2.30. This method can be used only for calculation of the AUC after administration of a single IV bolus dose. A more general method for calculation of the AUC after all routes of administration is called the trapezoidal rule and will be discussed in chapter five of this book.

2.6.3 Clinical Importance of Area Under the Curve

Since the AUC is directly proportional to the administered IV bolus dose, the AUC is usually used to compare the amount of the drug that reaches the systemic circulation after different routes of administration. The AUC can also be used to compare the clearance of a drug in different individuals after administration of the same dose.

Example

After IV bolus administration of 1000 mg amoxicillin, the following plasma concentrations were obtained:

Time (hr)	Concentration (mg/L)
0	72
1	45
3	18
5	7.1
7	2.8

1. Using a graphical method, calculate the Vd, $t_{1/2}$, k, CL_T, and AUC of amoxicillin.

Answer

Plot the plasma concentrations of amoxicillin versus time on semilog graph paper.

Draw the best line that goes through the plasma concentrations and back-extrapolate the line to the y-axis.

From Figure 2.17, the $Cp_0 = 72$ mg/L:

$$Vd = \frac{Dose}{Cp_0} = \frac{1000\ mg}{72\ mg/L} = 13.89\ L$$

The half-life is determined by taking any drug concentration (e.g., 38 mg/L) and calculating the time required for this concentration to decrease by 50%. From Figure 2.17, the half-life is 1.5 hr.

$$k = \frac{0.693}{t_{1/2}} = \frac{0.693}{1.5\ hr} = 0.462\ hr^{-1}$$

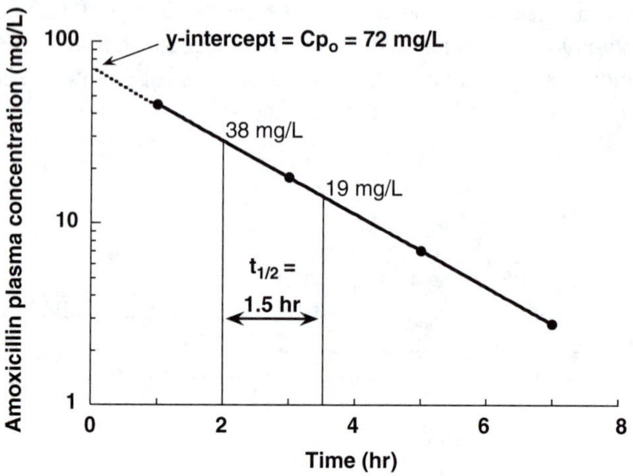

FIGURE 2.17 A plot of the plasma concentration–time curve.

Note that it is possible to calculate the elimination rate constant k from the slope of the line (Slope = –k/2.303). Then, the half-life is calculated from k.

$$CL_T = k\ Vd = 0.462\ hr^{-1} \times 13.89\ L = 6.417\ L/hr$$

$$AUC = \frac{Cp_0}{k} = \frac{72\ mg/L}{0.462\ hr^{-1}} = 155.8\ mg\text{-}hr/L$$

or

$$AUC = \frac{Dose}{CL_T} = \frac{1000\ mg}{6.417\ L/hr} = 155.8\ mg\text{-}hr/L$$

2.7 FACTORS AFFECTING THE DRUG BLOOD CONCENTRATION–TIME PROFILE AFTER A SINGLE IV BOLUS DOSE

After an IV bolus drug administration, the initial drug concentration depends on the dose and Vd of the drug. When the drug elimination process follows first-order kinetics, the amount of the drug in the body and the drug plasma concentration decline at a rate dependent on the elimination rate constant k.

2.7.1 Dose

Administration of increasing doses in the same individual produces higher Cp_0 and AUC; however, the dose does not affect k, Vd, or CL_T.

2.7.2 Volume of Distribution

Administration of the same dose of the same drug to a group of individuals who have different Vd results in lower initial drug concentrations Cp_0 in the individuals with larger Vd. The difference in the rate of elimination of the drug (k and half-life) in these individuals will depend on whether CL_T is similar in these individuals. This is because k and $t_{1/2}$ depend on both CL_T and Vd.

2.7.3 Total Body Clearance

Administration of the same dose of a drug to a group of individuals who have different CL_T results in different rates of decline of the blood drug concentration if Vd is similar in these individuals. Individuals with higher CL_T eliminate the drug at a faster rate (larger k and shorter $t_{1/2}$) and will have lower AUC.

PRACTICE PROBLEMS

2.1. Two different drugs were administered to the same individual in different doses on different occasions, and the half-lives were calculated after each drug administration.

Dose (mg)	Drug A Half-life (hr)	Drug B Half-life (hr)
40	6	4
60	6	6
80	6	8

a. Which of the two drugs is eliminated by first-order process? Why?
b. Calculate the elimination rate constant for the drug that is eliminated by a first-order process.
c. Describe how the rate of elimination, the elimination rate constant, and the half-life change with the change in dose for both drugs.

2.2. A single 400-mg IV bolus dose of an antibiotic was administered to a patient. The amounts of the drug determined at different times after drug administration were as follows:

Time (hr)	Amount (mg)
0	400
2	378
4	356
8	312
12	268
18	202
24	136

a. Does the elimination process follow zero-order or first-order kinetics?
b. What is the rate constant for the elimination process?
c. What is the half-life of the drug immediately after drug administration?
d. What is the rate constant for the elimination process if the dose was 600 mg?
e. What is the amount of the drug in the body 20 hr after drug administration?
f. What is the amount of the drug in the body 40 hr after drug administration?

2.3. A single IV bolus dose of a drug was administered to a patient, and the amount of the drug in the body was determined at different time points after drug administration.

Time (hr)	Amount (mg)
0.5	396
1	315
2	198
4	79
8	12.4
12	1.96

a. What is the order of the elimination process of this drug?
b. What is the rate constant for the elimination process?
c. What is the dose of the drug administered to this patient?
d. What is the equation that describes the amount of the drug-time profile in the body?
e. Calculate the amount of drug in the body 10 hr after administration.
f. What is the half-life of the drug immediately after drug administration?

2.4. A single 1000-mg IV bolus dose of an antibiotic that is eliminated by a first-order process was administered to a patient, and the following blood concentrations were obtained:

Time (hr)	Blood Concentration (mg/L)
0	33.3
1	26.5
2	21.0
4	13.2
6	8.33
8	5.25
12	2.08

a. Graphically estimate $t_{1/2}$, k, Vd, and CL_T.
b. Calculate the AUC after administration of the 1000 mg.

c. What is the initial drug concentration Cp_0, $t_{1/2}$, k, Vd, CL_T, and AUC if the administered dose was only 500 mg?
d. What is the dose required to achieve a Cp_0 of 50 mg/L?

2.5. The following blood concentrations were measured after administration of a single 200-mg IV bolus dose of a drug that is eliminated by a first-order process:

Time (hr)	Blood Concentration (mg/L)
1	1.85
2	0.858
3	0.397
4	0.184
6	0.039

a. Graphically estimate $t_{1/2}$, k, Vd, CL_T, and AUC.
b. Calculate mathematically and graphically the time when the blood drug concentration is exactly 0.5 mg/L.
c. What is the initial drug concentration Cp_0, $t_{1/2}$, k, Vd, CL_T, and AUC if the administered dose was only 400 mg?
d. Calculate mathematically the drug blood concentration after 10 hr of drug administration.

2.6. Draw the line that represents the following plasma concentration-time relationship on semilog graph paper.

$$Cp = 25\ e^{-0.099t}$$

2.7. After administration of a single 400-mg IV bolus dose of a drug, a plot of the blood concentration–time profile on semilog graph paper is linear with a slope of $-0.1\ hr^{-1}$ and a y-intercept of 1 mg/L.
a. Calculate $t_{1/2}$, k, Vd, CL_T, and AUC for this drug.
b. What are the slope and y-intercept if the dose was 1000 mg?
c. What is the length of time required for the initial drug concentration to decrease to 0.25 mg/L after administration of the 400-mg dose?
d. What is the smallest dose required to achieve a blood drug concentration above 1 mg/L for 6 hr after drug administration?

2.8. A single IV bolus dose of 5 mg/kg was administered to a patient. A semilog plot of the plasma concentration–time profile was linear with a y-intercept of 10 mg/L and a slope of $-0.06\ hr^{-1}$.

a. Calculate $t_{1/2}$, k, Vd, CL_T, and AUC for this drug.
b. What are the slope and y-intercept if the dose was 20 mg/kg?
c. What is the length of time required for the initial drug concentration to decrease to 1 mg/L after administration of 5 mg/kg?
d. What is the dose required to achieve a blood drug concentration above 1 mg/L for 12 hr after drug administration?

2.9. The following are the pharmacokinetic parameters for a group of drugs:

Drug	Vd	Elimination Rate Constant
Theophylline	0.45 L/kg	$0.11\ hr^{-1}$
Ampicillin	0.3 L/kg	$0.6\ hr^{-1}$
Quinidine	3 L/kg	$0.08\ hr^{-1}$
Propranolol	5 L/kg	$0.15\ hr^{-1}$
Procainamide	2 L/kg	$0.23\ hr^{-1}$
Lidocaine	1.3 L/kg	$0.4\ hr^{-1}$

a. Which drug is eliminated the fastest after IV administration? Why?
b. Which drug will produce the highest initial drug concentration if the same doses of the drugs are administered by IV bolus dose? Why?
c. Which drug has the highest CL_T? Why?
d. Which drug will require the highest dose to achieve a Cp_0 of 15 μg/L? Why?
e. Which drug will require frequent administration (more doses every day) to maintain the drug concentration in the therapeutic range all the time? Why?

2.10. A patient received a single 600-mg IV bolus dose of a drug that is eliminated mainly by the kidney by a first-order process. Two weeks later, the patient developed acute kidney disease and received another 600-mg IV bolus dose of the same drug. The following drug concentrations were obtained after administration of the drug before and after developing the renal disease:

Time (hr)	Drug Concentration (mg/L) Before Renal Disease	Drug Concentration (mg/L) After Renal Disease
1	21.2	25.5
2	15.0	21.2
4	7.5	15.0
6	3.75	10.6
8	1.88	7.5
12	0.469	3.75

a. Calculate the $t_{1/2}$, k, Vd, CL_T, and AUC for this drug before and after developing renal disease.
b. Explain the differences in the pharmacokinetic parameters for the two occasions.

2.11. A single 800-mg dose of a drug was given by IV bolus administration, and the plasma concentrations were determined. A plot of the plasma concentration–time profile was linear on semilog graph paper. The y-intercept of the plot was 20 mg/L, and the slope of the line was $-0.043\ hr^{-1}$.

a. Calculate the $t_{1/2}$, k, Vd, CL_T, and AUC for this drug.
b. Calculate the blood drug concentration 14 hr after drug administration.
c. What is the slope of the plasma concentration–time profile on a semilog scale if a dose of 400 mg was given by IV bolus?
d. Calculate the initial plasma concentration if the dose of this drug was 400 mg by IV bolus.

2.12. A general anesthetic drug has a volume of distribution of 15 L and a minimum effective concentration of 2 μg/ml (the drug is effective as long as the drug concentration is above 2 μg/ml). After administration of 120 mg of the drug as an IV bolus dose to a patient, the drug produced an anesthetic effect (drug was effective) for 6 hr.
a. Calculate the half-life of this drug
b. Calculate the minimum effective concentration for the drug if the dose was 400 mg.
c. Calculate the expected duration of effect if an IV bolus dose of 240 mg was administered.
d. Calculate the lowest dose that will produce an effect for 3 hr.
e. Calculate the expected duration of effect if 20 mg was given as an IV bolus dose.

3 Drug Absorption Following Oral Administration: Biopharmaceutical Considerations

OBJECTIVES

After completing this chapter you should be able to:

- Describe the different mechanisms for drug absorption after oral administration
- Describe how the gastrointestinal tract (GIT) physiology and physicochemical drug properties affect the absorption of drugs after oral administration
- Describe the factors that affect drug dissolution after oral drug administration and recommend approaches to improve drug dissolution and hence drug absorption
- Analyze the different factors that can affect the drug absorption and recommend the strategies that can improve drug absorption

3.1 INTRODUCTION

Drug absorption is the process of drug movement from its site of administration to the extracellular compartment of the body. There are three major routes of drug administration: enteral, parenteral, and topical. The intravenous (IV) and intra-arterial routes are the only routes of administration that guarantee complete entrance of drug to the systemic circulation because the drug is administered directly into the systemic circulation. All other routes of administration can have bioavailability ranging from 0% if no drug reaches the systemic circulation to 100% if the entire dose reaches the systemic circulation.

Because the majority of drugs are administered orally, the following discussion focuses on drug absorption from the GIT. After administration in the form of a solid dosage form, the dosage form has to disintegrate, and the drug has to dissolve in the GIT fluids. Once the drug is in solution in the GIT, it will be ready to be absorbed.

Drugs have to cross the GIT membrane to reach the systemic circulation, where they can be distributed to all parts of the body, including their site of action. In this chapter, we discuss the different factors that can affect the passage of the drug from the site of drug administration until it reaches the systemic circulation. These factors include the physiological properties of the site of drug administration, the physicochemical properties of the drug, and the properties of the drug dosage form.

3.2 PHYSIOLOGICAL FACTORS AFFECTING ORAL DRUG ABSORPTION

3.2.1 Nature of the GIT Membrane

Dissolved drug molecules within the GIT lumen will have to cross the GIT membrane to reach the systemic circulation. Generally, the structure of the biological membrane consists of a phospholipid bilayer with interdispersed carbohydrates and integral protein groups. The membrane also contains small aqueous pores or channels. A drug can cross the GIT membrane by different mechanisms.

3.2.1.1 Passive Diffusion

Passive diffusion is a process by which the molecules are transported from higher concentration to lower concentration according to the concentration gradient. The diffusion process is called passive because it does not require energy, and the driving force for the diffusion process is the concentration gradient. The rate of drug transport across the biological membranes is governed by Fick's law of diffusion.

$$\text{Rate of diffusion} = \frac{dA}{dt} = \frac{D\,S\,K}{h}(C_{GIT} - C_p) \tag{3.1}$$

where dA/dt is the rate of drug diffusion across the membrane, D is the diffusion coefficient, S is the membrane surface area, K is the partition coefficient, h is the thickness of the membrane, and $(C_{GIT} - C_p)$ is the difference in drug concentration in the GIT and the plasma.

Examining Fick's law can help illustrate the factors affecting the rate of diffusion of a compound across the biological membrane by passive diffusion (e.g., drug absorption by passive diffusion). The rate of drug absorption by passive diffusion increases with the increase in the drug lipid solubility, the increase in the surface area available for drug absorption, the increase in concentration gradient between the GIT and the plasma, and decreases with the increase in the thickness of the GIT membrane.

When the drug is absorbed from the GIT, it reaches the systemic circulation, where it is distributed to all parts of the body. Distribution of the absorbed drug to all parts of the body dilutes the drug concentration in the systemic circulation and makes the drug concentration in plasma low relative to the drug concentration in the GIT side. This will always make the drug concentration in the GIT side much higher than the drug concentration in the plasma side, which is known as the *sink condition*. In this case, Fick's law can be simplified to

$$\text{Rate of diffusion} = \frac{dA}{dt} \cong \frac{D\,S\,K}{h}\ C_{GIT} \tag{3.2}$$

Because the parameters D, S, K, and h are the same for a specific system, this equation represents a first-order diffusion with the rate of diffusion proportional to the drug concentration in the GIT. This can also explain why the oral absorption of most drugs from solution follows first-order kinetics.

3.2.1.2 Carrier-Mediated Transport

Carrier molecules can be involved in the transport of the drug across the GIT membrane. These carrier molecules are specific for the transport of a particular drug or a group of drugs from the mucosal to the serosal side of the membrane. Because there is an infinite number of carrier molecules, the process of carrier-mediated transport is saturable. This means that the rate of drug transport increases as the drug concentration increases until it reaches a plateau at high drug concentration. The GIT has specialized carriers for the transport of specific compounds, such as amino acids, glucose, peptides, and neocleocides. Structurally related compounds can be transported by the same carrier system, and these compounds can compete for the same carrier molecules. So, some drugs can competitively inhibit the absorption of other drugs or compounds if they are absorbed by the same carrier system.

Carrier-mediated transport can be active transport, by which the drug is transported against the concentration gradient, that is, from lower to higher concentration. The active transport process requires energy. The other kind of carrier-mediated transport is facilitated diffusion, by which the drug transport is according to the concentration gradient, that is, from higher to lower concentration. The facilitated diffusion process does not require energy.

3.2.1.3 Paracellular

Small molecules can cross the membrane paracellularly via the aqueous pores in the membrane.

3.2.1.4 Other Mechanisms

Other mechanisms include pinocytosis, phagocytosis, presorption, potocytosis, and ion pair transport.

3.2.2 Gastrointestinal Physiology

The major components of the GIT are the buccal cavity, esophagus, stomach, small intestine, large intestine (colon), and rectum. These GIT segments differ from each other with respect to the anatomical structure, transit time, secretions, and pH.

3.2.2.1 Buccal Cavity

Drugs can be absorbed from the buccal cavity. However, the buccal cavity is not a major site for absorption of orally administered drugs because of its short transit time and the relatively small surface area. Dosage forms designed to deliver drugs through the buccal cavity are retained by sublingual administration or by adhesion of the dosage form to the surface of the cavity. Drug absorption from the buccal cavity has the advantage of direct absorption to the systemic circulation (it does not pass through the liver).

3.2.2.2 Esophagus

Orally administered drugs are not absorbed from the esophagus because of its short transit time, thick membrane, and small surface area.

3.2.2.3 Stomach

The stomach pH is between 1.0 and 3.0, which makes it suitable for the absorption of weak acids such as aspirin and highly permeable compounds such as ethanol. This pH can cause the decomposition of many acid-labile drugs, such as peptide drugs (e.g., insulin) and some antibiotics (e.g., penicillin G). The stomach has a relatively small surface area compared to the small intestine (the main site of absorption of most drugs) and relatively short transit time when the drug is administered on an empty stomach. These two factors explain the limited role of the stomach in the absorption of drugs.

The gastric emptying rate is an important factor in determining the rate at which the drug reaches the intestine, where most of the drugs are absorbed. This makes the gastric emptying rate the main factor in determining the rate of absorption for most drugs. The gastric emptying rate can be delayed by food, especially fatty meals and food with high viscosity. Diseases such as pyloric stenosis, gastroenteritis, and gastroesophageal reflux can also slow the gastric emptying rate. Narcotic analgesics and drugs with an anticholinergic effect such as atropine, propantheline, tricyclic antidepressants, and chloropromazine can delay the gastric emptying rate. Any factor that can delay the gastric emptying rate will result in delaying the rate of drug absorption. This delay in the rate of drug absorption may represent a problem when rapid onset of drug effect is required.

3.2.2.4 Small Intestine

The small intestine consists of three segments: duodenum, jejunum, and ileum. The pH of the small intestine ranges from 6.0 to 6.5 in the duodenum and from 7.0 to 8.0 in the rest of the small intestine, which makes it suitable for the absorption of drugs that are not ionized in this pH (weak bases). However, because of the large surface area of the small intestine as a consequence of the presence of the villi and the microvilli, the small intestine is the main site of absorption for most drugs.

The proximal segment of the small intestine has more surface area per unit length, has more carrier-mediated transport system, and has larger aqueous pore size compared to the distal segment of the small intestine. The intestinal transit time ranges from 3 to 4 hr, which is important when designing a delayed-release dosage form. Dosage forms designed to release the drugs over a period of 6 hr or more will have low bioavailability unless the dosage form is retained in the stomach or the drug has good absorption from the large intestine. Some diseases (e.g., diarrhea) and drugs (e.g., metoclopramide) can shorten the intestinal transit time, which can significantly affect the absorption of drugs that have a small window of absorption (have a specific site for absorption).

3.2.2.5 Large Intestine

Drug absorption in the large intestine is limited because it does not have a large surface area similar to that of the small intestine. However, because the residence time in the large intestine is long, residual drug absorption can occur for some drugs. This can lead to prolonged drug absorption.

3.2.2.6 Rectum

The rectum is the last segment of the GIT; it can be used for rectal drug administration in the form of suppositories. Many drugs can be absorbed from the rectum directly to the systemic circulation (without passing through the liver).

3.2.3 Effect of Food on Drug Absorption

The effect of food on drug absorption is different depending on the characteristics of the drug, the site of drug absorption, and the type of food consumed. Generally, food can affect the rate or the extent (amount) of drug absorption. The extent of absorption of some drugs, such as griseofulvin, is increased when administered with fat-rich meals, while the absorption of tetracyclines is significantly reduced when administered with or right after eating dairy products. Food can increase the gastric pH, which may increase or decrease the dissolution of the drug depending on the drug properties, and stimulates the secretion of bile salts, which can enhance the solubility of lipid-soluble drugs.

Generally, the rate of drug absorption is slower when the drug is administered with or immediately after food. This is mainly because of the delay in the gastric emptying rate, which prolongs the time required to reach the intestine, where most drugs are absorbed. The food contents and food consistency determine the effect of food on the gastric emptying rate. Fat-rich meals delay the gastric emptying rate more than balanced meals; bulk and viscous meals delay gastric emptying more than liquid meals.

3.2.4 Pathological Conditions Affecting Drug Absorption

Many diseases and pathological conditions have been associated with modification of the drug absorption process. Gastroenteritis and diarrhea can significantly affect gastrointestinal motility and gastrointestinal transit time. This can lead to significant alteration of the absorption of drug administered in the form of prolonged-release products. Conditions that can alter the gastric pH such as achlorhydria in elderly patients can significantly delay the rate of dissolution of basic drugs in the stomach, leading to slow or incomplete drug absorption. Diseases that can affect the nature of the gut wall such as Crohn's disease and celiac disease can significantly affect the absorption of some drugs. Also, drugs used in the treatment of chronic diseases can affect the absorption of other drugs. For example, drugs with an anticholinergic effect or side effect such as tricyclic antidepressants and phenothiazines can significantly delay the rate of drug absorption of many drugs. Also, the antiemetic drug metoclopramide can enhance the rate of absorption of some drugs, such as atenolol.

3.3 PHYSICAL FACTORS AFFECTING ORAL DRUG ABSORPTION

Drugs can be absorbed only if they are available in solution at the site of absorption. The absorption of drugs administered in solution form is influenced mainly by the physicochemical properties of the drug, which determine the ability of the drug to cross the membrane. When the drug is administered in a solid dosage form, the dosage form will have to disintegrate first to release the particles containing the drug, and then the drug will have to dissolve before it can be absorbed as illustrated in Figure 3.1. So, drug absorption is dependent on the physicochemical properties of the drug, the solubility of the drug, and the dosage form characteristics.

The overall absorption process consists of series of processes starting from disintegration, then dissolution, and then permeation across the membrane. So, the rate of the overall absorption process is determined from the rate of the slowest process. The slowest step in a series of processes is called the *rate-limiting step*. For a drug with poor aqueous solubility, the dissolution rate of the drug is usually slow, and the absorption rate of such a drug is dependent on the dissolution rate of the drug. On the other hand, the rate-limiting step for the absorption of drugs with high aqueous solubility is the rate of permeation across the membrane because it is usually the slowest step. Controlled-release dosage forms are dosage forms designed to release the drug at a certain rate. The rate of drug absorption is controlled by controlling the rate of release of the drug from the dosage form.

3.3.1 Drug Physicochemical Properties

3.3.1.1 Drug Lipid Solubility

The lipid solubility or the lipophilicity of drugs is measured by the partition coefficient of the drug between an organic solvent like octanol and water. Drugs have

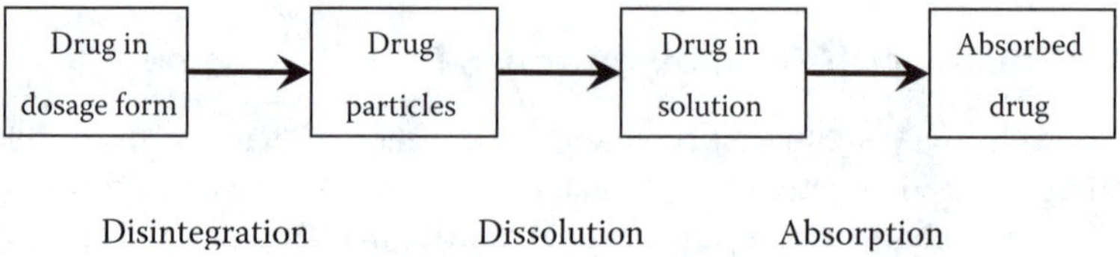

FIGURE 3.1 The processes involved in the absorption of drugs administered as solid dosage forms.

to possess reasonable lipid solubility to be absorbed across the GIT membrane by passive diffusion because of the lipoid nature of the biological membranes. Studies have demonstrated good correlation between the partition coefficient and the fraction of dose absorbed in a series of compounds from the same chemical class.

Many drugs are not absorbed after oral administration despite availability at the site of action in solution because they are highly hydrophilic and are not able to cross the GIT membrane. Examples of these drugs are the aminoglycoside antibiotics, which are not absorbed in the GIT to any extent, and the antiviral drugs gancyclovir and acyclovir, which have limited absorption after oral administration. On the other hand, highly lipophilic drugs have limited absorption after oral administration because of their poor dissolution in the aqueous contents of the GIT lumen. So, the drugs have to possess a balance between hydrophilicity to dissolve in the GIT lumen and lipophilicity to cross the GIT membrane.

3.3.1.2 pH Partition Theory

Another factor that can influence drug absorption is the pH partition theory. This theory describes the relationship among the drug pK_a, the pH at the absorption site, and the lipid solubility of the drug. The pH of the GIT ranges from 1.0 to 3.0 in the stomach and from 6.0 to 7.0 in the small intestine. Because most drugs are either weak acids or weak bases, the percentage of the drug ionized and un-ionized will be different in different parts of the GIT. Because the un-ionized form of the drug is more lipophilic compared to the ionized form, the absorption of drugs is usually different in the different parts of the GIT. For example, weak acids will be un-ionized in the acidic pH of the stomach and are absorbed in the stomach better than weak bases, which are mostly ionized in the acidic pH of the stomach. Also, weak bases are mostly un-ionized in the intestinal pH and are absorbed in the intestine better than weak acids, which are usually ionized in the intestine. The relationship between the pK_a of the drug and the percentage of drug ionized and un-ionized at different pH is described by the Henderson-Hasselbalch equation. For weak acids,

$$pK_a - pH = \log \frac{(\text{un-ionized})}{(\text{ionized})} = \log \frac{(HA)}{(A^-)} \tag{3.3}$$

For weak bases,

$$pK_a - pH = \log \frac{(\text{ionized})}{(\text{un-ionized})} = \log \frac{(HB^+)}{(B)} \tag{3.4}$$

If you examine these equations, then you find that when the pH of the medium is equal to the pK_a of the drug, 50% of the drug will be present in the ionized form and 50% in the un-ionized form. If a weak acid is dissolved in a medium with pH that is 1 unit lower than the pK_a of the drug, then 90% of the drug will be in the un-ionized form and 10% in the ionized form.

This discussion suggests that weak acids are absorbed better in the stomach, and weak bases are absorbed better in the small intestine. However, there are many other factors that need to be considered, including the large surface area of the small intestine, which makes the small intestine the major site of drug absorption for most drugs, including weak acids. There are an abundance of other factors that make application of the pH partition theory in describing or predicting the absorption of drug not an easy task. These factors include the possible absorption of ionized molecules, the difference between the pH at the surface of the membrane (at the absorption site) and the pH in the GIT lumen, and the presence of the stagnant layer at the surface of the membrane. So, it is important to note that this discussion is a simple description of a complex process.

3.3.2 Dissolution of the Drug

Drugs in the solid dosage form have to be dissolved before they can be absorbed. When the dissolution of a drug is the slowest process involved in drug absorption, the absorption of the drug will be dissolution rate limited. In other words, the rate of drug dissolution will control the rate of the overall absorption process. In 1897, Arthur Amos Noyes and Willis Rodney Whitney described the dissolution rate dc/dt of any solid compound.

In this dissolution model, it was assumed that the drug is present in the form of solid particles with total surface area equal to S, and the solid particles are surrounded by an unstirred (stagnant) layer of the solvent. The thickness of the unstirred layer is h, and the diffusion coefficient of the drug in this unstirred layer is equal to D. The drug concentration on the surface of the solid particles is equal to the saturation solubility of the drug C_s, and the drug concentration in the bulk solvent is C. The drug is dissolved in the solvent right on the surface of the particles. The dissolved drug molecules then diffuse through the unstirred layer to reach the bulk solution. The driving force of this diffusion process is the concentration gradient (C_s – C). As the process continues, more drug will be dissolved from the surface of the particles, and the drug concentration increases in the bulk solution. This process is presented in Figure 3.2 and can be described by the Noyes–Whitney equation:

$$\frac{dc}{dt} = \frac{D\,S}{h}(C_s - C) \tag{3.5}$$

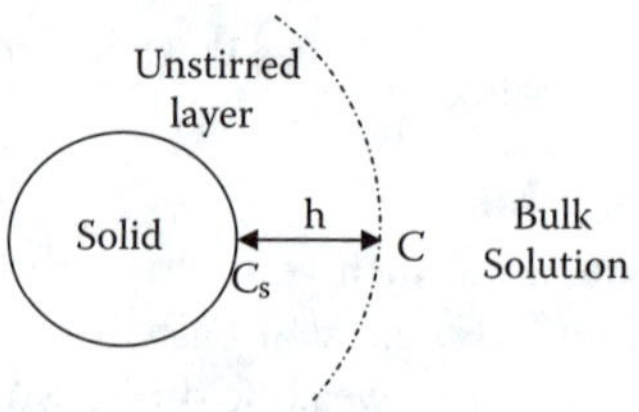

FIGURE 3.2 A model that describes the dissolution of drug from a spherical particle.

This equation describes the parameters that determine the rate of drug dissolution. It is important to discuss these parameters to understand how the rate of drug dissolution can be modified.

3.3.2.1 Surface Area

The rate of drug dissolution increases with increasing surface area of the solid particles. The surface area can be increased by particle size reduction. The solubility of poorly soluble drugs can be increased by using a micronized form of the drug. It is well documented that the dissolution rate, the absorption rate, and the amount of the drug absorbed can be increased when the drug used in the formulation has a small particle size.

3.3.2.2 Diffusion Coefficient

The diffusion coefficient of the drug through the dissolution medium is inversely related to the viscosity of the dissolution medium. So, the dissolution rate of the drug is inversely related to the viscosity of the dissolution medium. Food, food consistency, and food composition are some of the factors that can affect the viscosity of GIT contents and hence the drug dissolution rate after oral administration.

3.3.2.3 Thickness of the Unstirred Layer

The thickness of the unstirred layer inversely affects the dissolution rate of the drug. Agitation can disturb the unstirred layer, resulting in reduction of its thickness and increasing the dissolution rate.

3.3.2.4 Drug Solubility

The intrinsic solubility of a specific compound in a certain solvent or dissolution medium is usually constant. However, there are several factors that can modify the solubility and hence the absorption of some drugs. These factors include the following:

Gastrointestinal pH: The weak acids and weak bases usually have different solubility in different parts of the GIT, depending on the pH. Weak bases are usually more soluble in the acidic environment of the stomach; weak acids are more soluble in the alkaline pH of the intestine. Modification of the gastric pH by administration of antacids or food can significantly affect the dissolution rate of weak bases in the stomach. Antacids have been shown to decrease the dissolution rate of ketoconazole. Also, protein-rich food has been shown to increase the gastric pH, which can decrease the rate and extent of absorption of basic drugs such as atenolol and indinavir.

Salts: The drugs used in pharmaceutical formulations can be in the form of the free acid/free base or in the form of the salt of these acids or bases. For example, the nonsteriodal anti-inflammatory drug diclofenac is the free acid, and diclofenac sodium and diclofenac potassium are the salts. Also, quinidine is the free base, and quinidine sulfate and quinidine phosphate are the salts. Whether the drug is administered in the form of the salt or the free acid/base, the same active moiety of the drug will be present in the blood after its absorption. However, salts are usually more soluble than free acid/base, and even different salts of the same drug can have different solubility. So, for poorly soluble drugs, the use of salts can increase the drug dissolution and absorption rates. This means that the plasma concentration–time profile of the drug and the drug pharmacological response may be different depending on the salt used in the formulation. So, the choice of the salt form of the drug is an important step in drug formulation.

Crystal form: Many drugs exhibit a property known as *polymorphism*, which means that the drug can exist in more than one crystalline form. Although the chemical nature of the drug is similar in different crystalline forms, these forms can have substantially different physical properties, including different solubility. The drug solubility is usually higher when the drug exists in the amorphous form compared to the crystalline form. So, the dissolution rate of the drug and the absorption rate can be different depending on the crystalline form used in the drug formulation. This means that the plasma concentration–time profile of the drug and the drug pharmacological response may be different depending on the crystalline form used in the formulation.

Complexation: The solubility of a drug can be enhanced by addition of complexing agents to the formulation. Cyclodextrins have been used to increase the solubility of poorly soluble drugs by the formation of inclusion complexes. This approach has been used to increase the absorption rate of some drugs. It is important to note that complexation does not always increase the dissolution rate of the drug. For example, tetracyclines form an insoluble complex with calcium, resulting in significant reduction in its extent of absorption.

The factors described can affect the drug dissolution rate. Some of these factors can be controlled, and some cannot be controlled. So, it is important to modify the controllable factors to achieve the most favorable drug dissolution rate and ensure the optimal rate and extent of drug absorption.

3.4 DOSAGE FORM CHARACTERISTICS

Drugs administered in the form of solution are ready to be absorbed once they reach the site of their absorption, and drugs administered in the form of suspension will have to dissolve first before they can be absorbed. Also, drugs administered in solid dosage forms such as tablets and capsules will have to disintegrate to granules or small particles first before they can be dissolved and then absorbed. So, it is generally acceptable that the rate of drug absorption usually decreases from solution to suspension to capsules to tablets. Although this is the general rule, there are situations for which this rule does not apply. So, the characteristics of the dosage forms are important in determining the rate and the extent of drug absorption.

3.4.1 Types of Oral Dosage Forms

3.4.1.1 Solutions

Drug absorption after administration of solutions is usually rapid because the drug in solution is ready to be absorbed once it reaches the site of absorption. The rate-determining step in drug absorption after administration of solutions is the rate at which the drug reaches the site of absorption or the rate of permeation across the membrane. Sometimes, the dissolved drug may precipitate in the GIT because of unfavorable conditions that may affect the drug solubility. For example, weak acids administered in solution may precipitate once they reach the stomach because of the acidic pH, which decreases the solubility of most weak acids. In most cases, the precipitated drug will usually redissolve without any absorption problems.

3.4.1.2 Suspensions

Suspensions contain the drug in the form of fine particles dispersed in the formulation vehicle with the aid of a suspending agent. The dispersed particles have to dissolve before the drug can be absorbed. The dissolution rate of the drug when administered in the form of suspension is usually dependent on the particle size, with fine particles dissolving faster than larger particles.

3.4.1.3 Capsules

Hard gelatin capsules contain the uncompressed drug and additives inside the capsule shell. Once the capsule shell is disrupted by the aqueous environment of the GIT, the capsule content is released, and drug starts to dissolve. The capsule contents disperse rapidly and expose a large surface area to the GIT contents, resulting in a rapid dissolution rate. This makes the rate of drug absorption faster when administered in the form of a capsule compared to tablets.

3.4.1.4 Tablets

Tablets usually contain the active drug ingredients in addition to many other additives compressed together into a single dosage unit. These additives include diluents, filling agent, disintegrating agent, granulating agents, lubricants, coloring agents, and others. After administration of a drug in the form of a tablet, the drug dissolution is slow because of the small effective surface area of the tablet. The tablet usually disintegrates to small fragments, resulting in an increase of the effective surface area and the rate of dissolution. The drug surface area and the drug dissolution rate increase further with the disintegration of the granules. So, the rate of tablet disintegration is an important factor in determining the drug dissolution and drug absorption rates. The disintegration rate of tablets is dependent on the tablet additives and the manufacturing procedures. So, tablets are usually subjected to disintegration and dissolution tests as part of quality control after manufacturing.

3.4.1.5 Coated Tablets

Coated tablets are tablets covered by a special covering such as a sugar coating, film coating, or enteric coating. The reason for coating the tablet is to improve some of the tablet characteristics, such as unpleasant taste or odor, or to improve the appearance. The coat of enteric-coated tablets is stable in the acidic medium of the stomach and can dissolve rapidly in the alkaline environment of the small intestine. The idea is to protect the tablet ingredients from the acidic medium in the stomach and release the tablet contents in the intestine. The coating of these tablets has to dissolve first before the drug can disintegrate and dissolve.

3.4.1.6 Sustained-Release Tablets

These are tablets formulated to release the active ingredient at a slow rate. So, the rate-determining step in the drug absorption after administration of sustained-release tablets is the rate of release of the drug from the dosage form. The use of sustained-release tablets can be beneficial because they can decrease the fluctuations in the drug concentration during multiple drug administrations. These formulations can also decrease the frequency of drug administration for drugs with short half-lives.

3.4.2 In Vitro Disintegration Test

Solid dosage forms should disintegrate to small particles or granules before the drug is dissolved and then absorbed. *Complete disintegration* is defined as that state in which any residue of the unit, except fragments of insoluble coating or capsule shell, remaining in the screen of the test apparatus is a soft mass having no palpably firm core (*USP XXIII*, 1995).

The apparatus used in the disintegration test consists of a set of open-ended tubes. The lower end of each tube is covered with a woven stainless steel wire with a specific mesh size. The tubes can move vertically up and down at a certain rate and are placed in a vessel containing enough disintegration medium to completely cover both sides of the tubes. The temperature of the disintegration medium is adjusted at 37°C.

One unit of the solid dosage form is placed in each tube, and the vessel is filled with the disintegration fluid adjusted at 37°C (usually simulated gastric fluid). The tubes move up and down at a specific rate. After a specific time, the apparatus is stopped, and the tubes are checked for any remaining solid fragments of the dosage form. When the dosage form is completely disintegrated, all the particles will move across the tube's lower wire cover, and the tubes will not contain any solid fragments. However, when the disintegration process is not complete, the tubes will contain some residue of solid fragments that is too large to pass across the tube's lower wire cover. Different test specifications are given for the different solid dosage forms (immediate-release tablets, coated tablets, enteric-coated tablets, and sublingual tablets).

3.4.3 In Vitro Dissolution Test

The idea of in vitro dissolution testing is to determine the rate and extent of dissolution of the drug from its dosage form under certain controlled conditions.

Some of the controlled factors include the size and shape of the dissolution vessel, the dissolution medium (different pH), the rate of agitation, and the temperature. Some of the official methods used for in vitro dissolution testing of solid dosage forms include the rotating basket, paddle, and other methods.

3.4.3.1 Rotating Basket

The rotating basket method involves placing the solid dosage form in a basket completely immersed under the dissolution medium. The temperature of the dissolution medium is controlled at 37°C, and the basket is rotated at different speeds with a metal shaft. Samples can be drawn at different time points to determine the concentration of the drug in the dissolution medium, which reflects the amount of drug dissolved at different time points. The dissolution rate can then be calculated.

3.4.3.2 Paddle Method

The dissolution vessel is a round-bottom vessel that has a rotating paddle. The temperature of the dissolution medium and the speed of paddle rotation can be controlled. The dosage form can be placed in the vessel, and then serial samples from the dissolution medium are drawn to calculate the drug dissolution rate.

3.4.3.3 Other Methods

There are other official and unofficial methods that are used to determine the dissolution rate.

3.4.3.4 Dissolution Requirements

The dissolution requirements for solid dosage forms are expressed by the percentage of the drug that should dissolve during certain periods of time. For example, 75% of the drug in the dosage form should dissolve in 45 min. This required limit can be different for different drugs.

3.4.3.5 Correlation of In Vitro Drug Dissolution with In Vivo Drug Absorption

The in vitro dissolution testing is a valuable test for the quality control of the solid dosage forms. However, the correlation between the in vitro dissolution rate and the in vivo absorption rate does not always exist. Good correlation between the dissolution rate and the in vivo absorption rate has been reported for controlled-release drug products. For immediate-release solid dosage forms, good correlation usually exists between in vitro dissolution and in vivo absorption when the dissolution rate of the drug is the rate-determining step for drug absorption (low-solubility, high-permeability drugs).

QUESTIONS

3.1. Describe the different mechanisms involved in drug absorption.

3.2. The different parts of the GIT have different physiological and anatomical characters that can influence the absorption of drugs. Please discuss.

3.3. Discuss briefly the effect of food on drug absorption.

3.4. Enumerate the different factors that can affect the rate of drug dissolution. Please indicate which of these factors can be modified to enhance the drug dissolution and hence absorption.

3.5. It is generally acceptable that the rate of drug absorption from different dosage forms is usually in the order of solution > suspension > capsule > tablet. Please explain.

3.6. Please describe the value of performing the in vitro disintegration and dissolution tests for solid dosage forms.

4 Drug Pharmacokinetics Following Single Oral Drug Administration: Rate of Drug Absorption

OBJECTIVES

After completing this chapter you should be able to:

- Describe how the rate and the extent of drug absorption after oral administration affect the onset and the duration of drug effect
- Calculate the drug half-life after oral administration
- Analyze how the change in the absorption rate constant affects the plasma concentration–time profile after a single oral administration
- Estimate the absorption rate constant utilizing the method of residuals and the Wagner–Nelson method

4.1 INTRODUCTION

Administration of the drug by any route that does not involve direct introduction of the drug into the systemic circulation is called *extravascular drug administration.* This includes oral, rectal, buccal, sublingual, transdermal, intramuscular, subcutaneous, inhalation, and other routes. We discuss drug absorption after oral administration; however, the same principles can be applied for the other extravascular routes of administration. The drug has to be absorbed from the site of administration to the systemic circulation and then distributed to all parts of the body to produce its pharmacological effect. The rate and extent of this absorption process is important. The rate of absorption influences the rate at which the drug appears in the systemic circulation after drug administration and is determined from the absorption rate constant k_a. The extent of drug absorption represents the fraction of the administered dose that reaches the systemic circulation and is a measure of the drug bioavailability F. In this chapter, we discuss the rate of drug absorption; the extent of drug absorption is discussed in the next chapter.

The rate and extent of drug absorption to the systemic circulation after oral drug administration determine the onset and the intensity of drug effect as illustrated in Figure 4.1. The assumption is that the plasma drug concentration has to exceed the minimum effective concentration (MEC) to produce the effect, and the intensity of

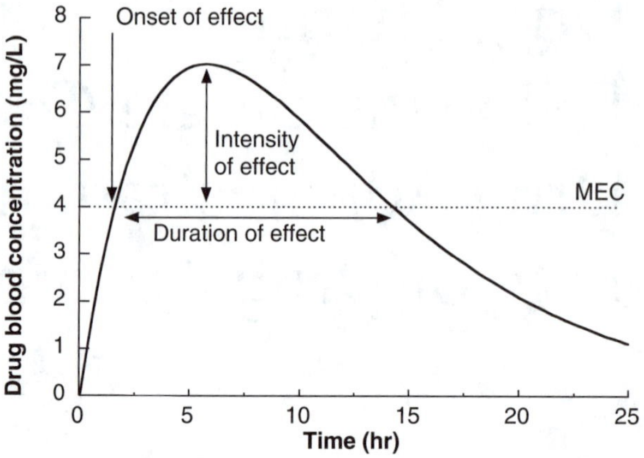

FIGURE 4.1 The relationship between the plasma concentration–time profile and the onset, intensity, and duration of the therapeutic effect of the drug.

the effect is correlated with the plasma drug concentration. Rapid drug absorption results in faster onset of drug effect. Larger extent of drug absorption (higher bioavailability) results in higher plasma drug concentration, which produces more intense effect. Also, the drug plasma concentration will stay above the MEC for a longer time, which will result in prolonged duration of effect.

After administration of a solid dosage form, the drug has to be in solution before it can be absorbed to the systemic circulation. So, tablets and capsules have to disintegrate to granules, and the drug in the granules has to dissolve before it can cross the membrane to reach the systemic circulation. Once the drug is in the systemic circulation, it is distributed to all parts of the body, including the site of action and the eliminating organs. The rate constant that describes the overall absorption process is the absorption rate constant, (k_a). The absorption rate constant after administration of different dosage forms of the same drug can be different because of the differences in the formulation characteristics.

4.2 DRUG ABSORPTION AFTER ORAL ADMINISTRATION

The absorption of most drugs follows first-order kinetics; however, the absorption of some drugs is described better by zero-order kinetics. So, the following discussion assumes first-order absorption. After oral administration, the drug is introduced to the gastrointestinal tract (GIT). The amount of drug in the GIT A_i after oral administration declines exponentially at a rate dependent on the k_a if the absorption process follows first-order kinetics as expressed in Equation 4.1 and presented in Figure 4.2.

$$A_i = \text{Dose } e^{-k_a t} \tag{4.1}$$

Because the rate of any process that follows first-order kinetics is determined from the product of the rate constant for the process and the amount available for the

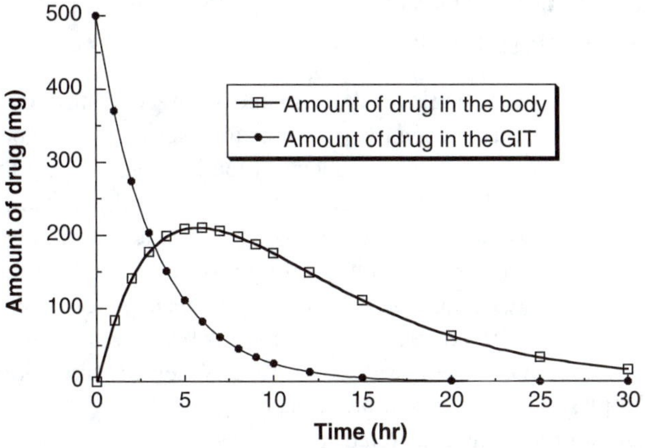

FIGURE 4.2 The drug amount-time profile in the GIT and inside the body after a single oral administration of the drug.

process, the rate of change of the amount of the drug in the body (A) depends on the rate of drug absorption (k_aA_i) and the rate of drug elimination (k A).

$$\frac{dA}{dt} = k_aA_i - k\,A \tag{4.2}$$

Initially, the rate of drug absorption is larger than the rate of drug elimination, so the amount of the drug in the body increases. After some time, the rate of drug elimination becomes larger than the rate of drug absorption, and the amount of drug in the body decreases as in Figure 4.2.

By integrating Equation 4.2,

$$A = \frac{A_i\, k_a}{k_a - k}\,(e^{-kt} - e^{-k_a t}) \tag{4.3}$$

and

$$A = \frac{F\,D\,k_a}{k_a - k}\,(e^{-kt} - e^{-k_a t}) \tag{4.4}$$

where A is the amount of the drug at any time t, D is the orally administered dose, F is the fraction of the dose that reaches the systemic circulation (i.e. the absolute bioavailability), k_a is the first-order absorption rate constant, k is the first-order elimination rate constant. Dividing Equation 4.4 by the volume of distribution Vd gives the equation that describes the drug blood concentration–time profile:

$$Cp = \frac{F\,D\,k_a}{Vd\,(k_a - k)}\,(e^{-kt} - e^{-k_a t}) \tag{4.5}$$

4.3 PLASMA CONCENTRATION–TIME PROFILE AFTER A SINGLE ORAL DOSE

After administration of a single oral drug, the drug concentration–time profile includes an absorption phase when the rate of drug absorption is larger than the rate of drug elimination. The plasma drug concentration increases during the absorption phase. A maximum value C_{max} is reached when the rate of drug absorption is equal to the rate of drug elimination. The time when C_{max} is achieved is called the t_{max}. The t_{max} can be used to compare the rate of drug absorption of different drugs, with shorter t_{max} indicating faster drug absorption. After the C_{max}, drug absorption continues, but the plasma drug concentration decreases because the rate of drug elimination is larger than the rate of drug absorption. When the absorption process is completed, the plasma drug concentration decreases at a rate dependent on the rate of the elimination process as illustrated in Figure 4.3.

When the plasma concentration is at its maximum value (the peak), the rate of change of the plasma concentration is equal to zero. The rate of change in plasma concentration can be obtained by differentiating Equation 4.5 and making the results equal to zero:

$$\frac{dCp}{dt} = \frac{d}{dt}\left(\frac{F\,D\,k_a}{Vd\,(k_a - k)}\,(e^{-kt} - e^{-k_a t})\right) = 0 \tag{4.6}$$

This can be simplified to

$$-ke^{-kt} + k_a e^{-k_a t} = 0 \tag{4.7}$$

$$ke^{-kt} = k_a e^{-k_a t} \tag{4.8}$$

$$\ln k - kt = \ln k_a - k_a t \tag{4.9}$$

The time at C_{max} is equal to t_{max}

$$t_{max} = \frac{\ln k_a - \ln k}{k_a - k} = \frac{\ln (k_a / k)}{k_a - k} = \frac{2.303 \log\ (k_a / k)}{k_a - k} \tag{4.10}$$

So, the time to achieve the maximum plasma drug concentration is dependent on both the absorption rate constant k_a and the elimination rate constant k. The C_{max} can be calculated by substituting for the time in Equation 4.5 by t_{max}:

$$C_{max} = \frac{F\,D\,k_a}{Vd\,(k_a - k)}\,(e^{-kt_{max}} - e^{-k_a t_{max}}) \tag{4.11}$$

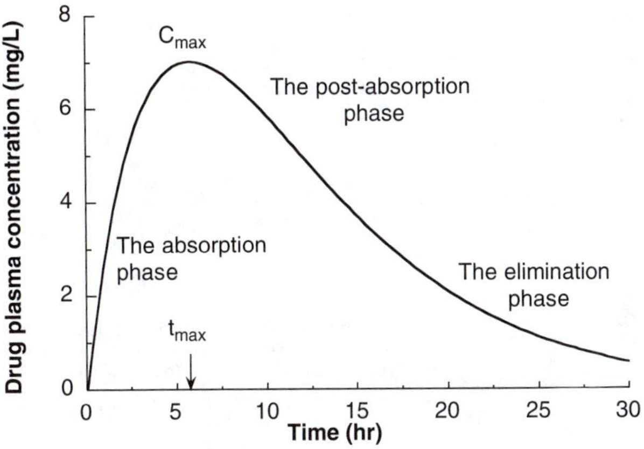

FIGURE 4.3 The plasma drug concentration–time profile after administration of a single oral dose of the drug.

When the plasma drug concentration-time curve is plotted on semilog graph paper, the elimination phase will be linear because the plasma drug concentration decreases at a rate dependent on the elimination rate constant. The elimination rate constant and the half-life can be determined only when the absorption process is completed and the drug concentration declines because of the elimination process. When the drug concentration declines linearly on semilog plot, this indicates that the absorption process is completed.

The elimination rate constant can be determined from the slope of the linear part of the curve. The slope is equal to –k/2.303. The half-life can also be determined by measuring the time required for any drug concentration in the linear part of the curve to decrease by 50%. When the linear part of the curve is back-extrapolated to the y-axis as in Figure 4.4, the y-intercept can be presented by

$$\text{y-intercept} = \frac{F\,D\,k_a}{Vd\,(k_a - k)} \quad (4.12)$$

The area under the curve (AUC) after a single oral drug administration can be expressed in terms of the other pharmacokinetic parameters as in the case of intravenous (IV) drug administration. Here, the AUC from time zero to infinity can be expressed as

$$AUC_{oral}\Big|_{t=0}^{t=\infty} = \frac{F\,D}{k\,Vd} = \frac{F\,Dose}{CL_T} \quad (4.13)$$

where CL_T is the total body clearance.

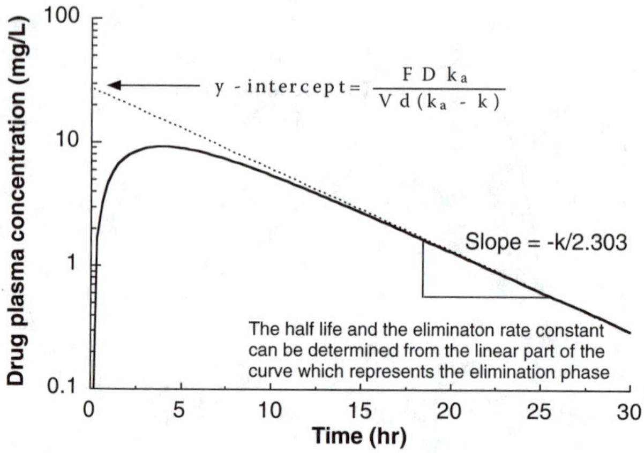

FIGURE 4.4 The plasma drug concentration–time profile after administration of a single oral dose of the drug plotted on the semilog scale. The half-life and the first-order elimination rate constant can be calculated during the elimination phase of the drug.

4.4 DETERMINATION OF ABSORPTION RATE CONSTANT

4.4.1 Method of Residuals

For the method of residuals, the assumptions are as follows:

1. The absorption rate constant is larger than the elimination rate constant, that is $k_a > k$.
2. Both drug absorption and elimination processes follow first-order kinetics.
3. The drug pharmacokinetics follow the one-compartment model.

The equation that describes the plasma drug concentration after oral administration (Equation 4.5) is the difference between two exponential terms, one of which vanishes faster than the other. After drug administration, as the time t gets bigger, the term $e^{-k_a t}$ approaches zero more rapidly than the other exponential term, e^{-kt}. After a long time, when the term $e^{-k_a t}$ is essentially equal to zero, Equation 4.5 can be reduced to

$$Cp = \frac{F\,D\,k_a}{Vd\,(k_a - k)}\,e^{-kt} \tag{4.14}$$

In other words, when the absorption process is completed (during the elimination phase), the plasma drug concentration declines at a rate dependent on the elimination rate constant. The half-life and the elimination rate constant can be calculated from this part of the curve as described before. This can be illustrated in Figure 4.5.

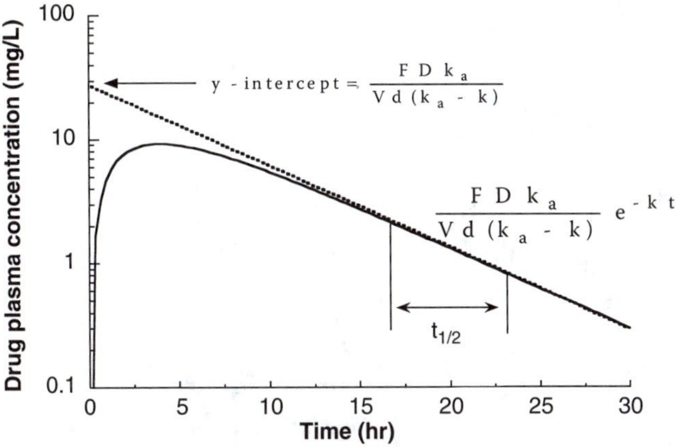

FIGURE 4.5 The plasma drug concentration during the elimination phase after administration of a single oral dose declines at a rate dependent on the first-order elimination rate constant.

When this linear part of the curve is extrapolated to time zero, the y-intercept is equal to

$$\text{y-intercept} = \frac{F\,D\,k_a}{Vd\,(k_a - k)}$$

as mentioned in Equation 4.12 and illustrated in Figure 4.5.

During the absorption phase, when the absorption and elimination processes occur simultaneously, the difference between the extrapolated line from the elimination phase and the measured drug concentration is equal to the residuals:

$$\text{Residuals} = \frac{F\,D\,k_a}{Vd\,(k_a - k)}\,e^{-kt} - Cp \tag{4.15}$$

$$\text{Residuals} = \frac{F\,D\,k_a}{Vd\,(k_a - k)}\,e^{-kt} - \frac{F\,D\,k_a}{Vd\,(k_a - k)}\left(e^{-kt} - e^{-k_a t}\right) \tag{4.16}$$

$$\text{Residuals} = \frac{F\,D\,k_a}{Vd\,(k_a - k)}\,e^{-k_a t} \tag{4.17}$$

The first-order absorption rate constant can be calculated using the method of residuals as illustrated in Figure 4.6 by the following procedure:

- Plot the plasma concentration–time profile on semilog graph paper.
- Calculate the slope of the terminal elimination phase and back-extrapolate the line representing the elimination phase to time zero.

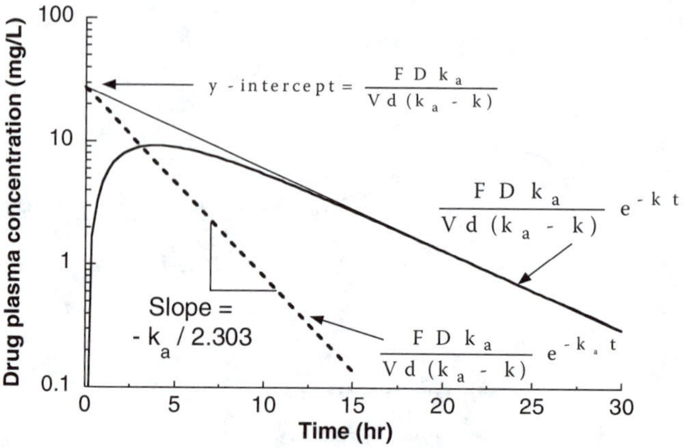

FIGURE 4.6 The method of residuals. The residuals-versus-time plot (the dashed line) declines at a rate dependent on the first-order absorption rate constant, and the first-order absorption rate constant is calculated from the slope of this plot.

- Take at least three points on the upper part of the extrapolated line and drop vertical lines to obtain the corresponding points on the plasma concentration–time curve.
- Calculate the difference between the values of the points on the extrapolated line and corresponding values on the curve (the residuals).
- Plot the values of the residuals versus the corresponding time (residuals versus time). A straight line will be obtained with a slope of $-k_a/2.303$.

4.4.1.1 Lag Time

In some individuals, the absorption of drug after an oral dose does not start immediately because of some physiological factors, such as stomach-emptying time and intestinal motility. This delay time before starting drug absorption is known as the *lag time for drug absorption*. The lag time for drug absorption is confirmed if the two lines obtained during residual calculations (the extrapolated line from the elimination phase and the line obtained from plotting the residuals versus time) intersect at a point after time zero on the x-axis as illustrated in Figure 4.7. The time at the point of intersection on the x-axis is the lag time. The lag time for drug absorption is different from the onset of the drug effect, which is the time required for the drug to reach the MEC at the site of action.

The method of residuals assumes first-order absorption. However, the absorption of drugs is not always first order. Other methods are available to determine the absorption rate constant when the absorption process is not first order.

4.4.1.2 Flip Flop of k_a and k

One of the assumptions of the method of residuals is that the absorption rate constant is larger than the elimination rate constant ($k_a > k$). In this case, the terminal

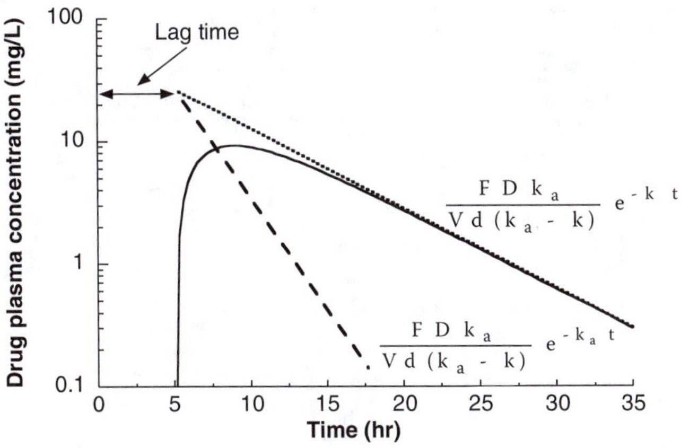

FIGURE 4.7 The method of residuals when there is lag time for the drug absorption after oral administration. The lag time is calculated from the x-coordinate of the point of intersection of the two lines.

elimination phase will represent the elimination process, and the residuals-versus-time plot will represent the absorption process. However, when the absorption rate constant is smaller than the elimination rate constant, the terminal elimination phase will represent the slower process (drug absorption). The residuals-versus-time plot will represent the elimination process. This behavior is known as flip flop of k_a and k.

Example

After oral administration of a single dose of an antibiotic, the following concentrations were measured:

Time (hr)	Drug Concentration (mg/L)
0	0
0.2	88
0.5	185
1.0	277
2.0	321
2.5	311
4.0	246
6.0	161
8.0	102

Calculate the first-order absorption rate constant

Answer

Plot the plasma concentration–time profile and follow the procedures for the method of residuals as in Figure 4.8.

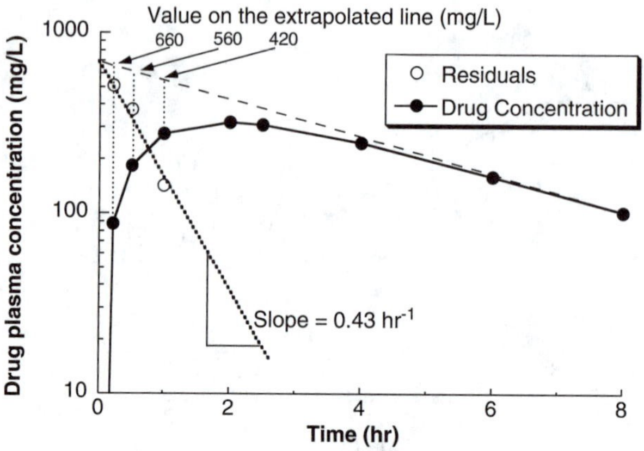

FIGURE 4.8 Application of the method of residuals to calculate the first-order absorption rate constant.

Calculate the residuals:

Time (hr)	Residuals (mg/L)
0.2	660 − 88 = 512
0.5	560 − 185 = 375
1.0	420 − 27 = 143

The line resulting from plotting the residuals versus time has a slope of $-0.43\ hr^{-1}$.

$$\text{Slope} = -\,0.43\ hr^{-1} = \frac{-\,k_a}{2.303}$$

$$k_a = 0.99\ hr^{-1}$$

4.4.2 Wagner–Nelson Method

The method of residuals assumes first-order absorption. However, absorption of drugs may not always be first order. The Wagner–Nelson method is useful in this situation. This method requires that the drug elimination follows first-order kinetics. A modification of this method can be used to assess the absorption process when the drug pharmacokinetics follows a two-compartment model.

The Wagner–Nelson method is a method that involves mathematical calculation of the cumulative amount of the drug absorbed at each time point A_a after drug administration and the total amount of the drug absorbed $A_{a\infty}$. The fraction $A_a/A_{a\infty}$ represents the fraction of the absorbed dose that is already absorbed at each time point. The fraction remaining to be absorbed can be examined to determine the nature of the absorption process.

$$\text{Fraction remaining to be absorbed} = 1 - \frac{A_a}{A_{a\infty}} \qquad (4.18)$$

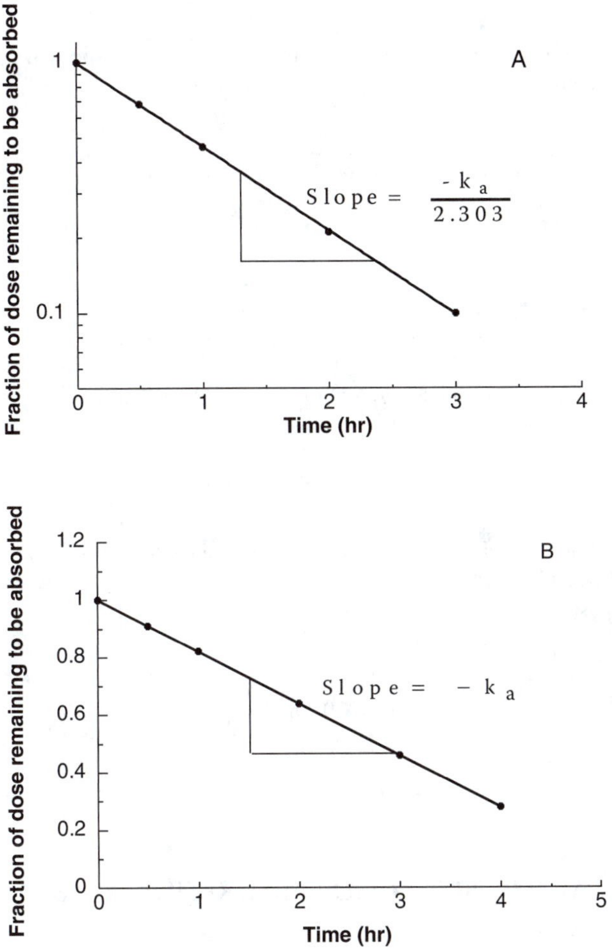

FIGURE 4.9 The fraction of dose remaining to be absorbed-versus-time plots (A) when the drug absorption follows first-order kinetics and (B) when the drug absorption follows zero-order kinetics.

A plot of the fraction of the drug remaining to be absorbed versus time can be used to determine the order of the absorption process and to calculate the absorption rate constant. If the absorption process is first order, then a plot of the fraction remaining to be absorbed versus time should give a straight line on semilog graph paper as in Figure 4.9A. The slope of this line is equal to $-k_a/2.303$. However, if the absorption process is zero order, then a plot of the fraction remaining to be absorbed versus time should give a straight line on Cartesian graph paper as in Figure 4.9B. The slope of this line is equal to $-k_a$. The fraction remaining to be absorbed can be expressed as percentage remaining to be absorbed by multiplying the fraction by 100.

Example

When applying the Wagner–Nelson method to determine the absorption rate constant for an oral hypoglycemic drug, the following data were obtained:

Time (hr)	Fraction Remaining to be Absorbed
1	0.63
2	0.40
3	0.25
5	0.10

1. What is the order of the absorption of this oral hypoglycemic drug?
2. Calculate the absorption rate constant.

Answer:

Plot the fraction remaining to be absorbed on Cartesian and semilog graph paper as in Figures 4.10A and 4.10B. The relationship is linear on semilog graph paper, indicating first-order absorption.

$$\text{Slope} = -\ 0.2\ \text{hr}^{-1} = \frac{-k_a}{2.303}$$

$$k_a = 0.46\ \text{hr}^{-1}$$

4.5 CLINICAL IMPORTANCE OF ABSORPTION RATE CONSTANT

The rate of drug absorption from different drug products for the same active drug may be different and is dependent on the formulation characteristics. The absorption rate constant determines the rate of drug absorption from the site of administration and the rate of the appearance of the drug in the systemic circulation. If the drug has to achieve a certain concentration to produce the pharmacological effect, then faster drug absorption results in faster onset of drug effect. So, faster drug absorption may be required when rapid therapeutic effect is needed to treat an acute condition.

On the other hand, sustained-release drug products are designed to release the active drug from the dosage form slowly, which results in slow drug absorption. The slow release and slow absorption of the active drug from the sustained-release products leads to maintaining an effective plasma drug concentration for a longer time after drug administration. This may result in prolongation of the therapeutic effect of the drug and a decrease in the fluctuation in the plasma drug concentration during multiple drug administrations.

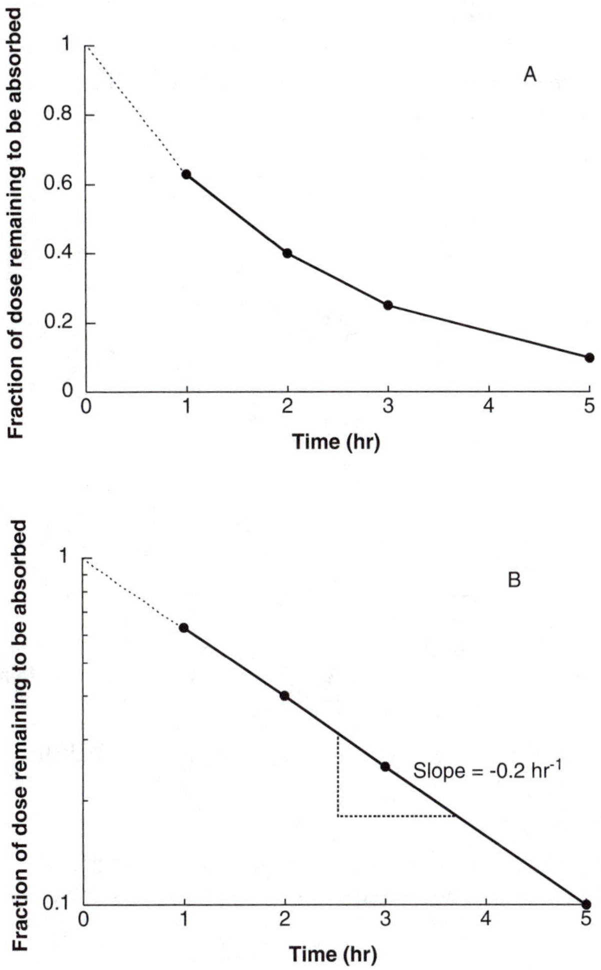

FIGURE 4.10 The fraction of dose remaining to be absorbed is (A) not linear on the Cartesian scale and (B) linear on the semilog scale, indicating a first-order absorption process.

4.6 SUMMARY

- The first-order absorption rate constant is the rate constant that determines the rate of drug absorption from the site of administration. A larger absorption rate constant results in a faster rate of drug absorption.
- The absorption rate constant determined after drug administration is an operative rate constant that accounts for all the necessary steps required for drug absorption into the systemic circulation, including disintegration, dissolution, and absorption.
- The first-order absorption rate constant has units of $time^{-1}$.

PRACTICE PROBLEMS

4.1. The plasma drug concentration in a patient who had received a single oral dose of a drug (10 mg/kg) was determined as follows:

Time (hr)	Drug Concentration (mg/L)
0	0
1	84
2	141
3	177
4	199
6	207
8	188
10	176
15	111
20	63
25	33.5
30	17.3

Plot the plasma concentration–time profile on a semilog graph paper and then find the following parameters directly from the graph (do not use the method of residuals):

a. The elimination rate constant and the elimination half-life
b. The t_{max}
c. The C_{max}

4.2. Two drugs have the following pharmacokinetic parameters after a single oral dose of 500 mg (both drugs are completely absorbed):

Drug	k_a (hr^{-1})	k (hr^{-1})	Vd (L)
A	1.0	0.2	10
B	0.2	1.0	20

a. Calculate t_{max} for each drug.
b. Calculate C_{max} for each drug.

4.3. The plasma concentration–time profile after a single oral dose can be expressed as

$$Cp = \frac{F\,D\,k_a}{Vd\,(k_a - k)}\,(e^{-kt} - e^{-k_a t})$$

After administration of a single 500-mg oral dose of a drug, the plasma concentration–time profile can be expressed as

$$Cp = 75\ \text{mg/L}\ (e^{-0.1t} - e^{-0.9t})$$

where Cp is in milligrams per liter, t is in hours, and

$$\frac{F\,D\,k_a}{Vd\,(k_a - k)} = 75\ \text{mg/L}$$

a. Calculate the t_{max} after administration of the 500-mg oral dose.
b. Calculate the C_{max} after administration of the 500-mg oral dose.
c. Do you expect t_{max} and C_{max} to be different if the dose was 100 mg?

4.4. A single dose of 500 mg of an antibiotic was given as an oral tablet to a 70-kg patient. The plasma concentration–time profile can be described by the following equation:

$$Cp = 21\ \text{mg/L}\ (e^{-0.115t} - e^{-0.624t})$$

where Cp is in milligrams per liter, and t is in hours. The drug has 100% bioavailability (F = 1).

a. Calculate the plasma concentration 6 hr after drug administration.
b. Calculate the elimination half-life of this drug.
c. Calculate the first-order absorption rate constant of this drug.
d. Calculate the volume of distribution of this drug.
e. Calculate t_{max}.
f. Calculate C_{max}.
g. What is the slope of the terminal elimination phase for the plasma concentration-time plot (on a semilog scale) after administration of the 500-mg dose?

4.5. A single dose of 500 mg of an antibiotic was given as an oral tablet to a 70-kg patient. The plasma concentration–time profile can be described by the following equation:

$$Cp = 10(e^{-0.154t} - e^{-0.954t})$$

where Cp is in milligrams per liter, t is in hours, and the drug is completely absorbed.

a. Calculate the elimination half-life of this drug.
b. Calculate the volume of distribution of this drug.
c. Calculate the total body clearance of this drug.
d. Calculate t_{max} and C_{max}.
e. Calculate the AUC after administration of a 500-mg oral dose.

4.6. A patient received a single 5-mg oral dose of a bronchodilator that is completely absorbed after oral administration. The following plasma concentration-time data were obtained:

Time (hr)	Concentration (ng/ml)	Time (hr)	Concentration (ng/ml)
0.0	0.00		
0.2	10.0	4.0	31.1
0.5	21.5	6.0	18.6
1.0	33.4	8.0	10.2
2.0	40.7	10.0	5.44
3.0	37.6	14.0	1.47

a. Plot the plasma concentration–time curve and determine the absorption rate constant using the method of residuals.
b. What is the equation that describes the plasma concentration–time profile of this drug after oral administration?
c. Calculate t_{max} and C_{max} for this drug after administration of a single 5-mg dose.

4.7. The following results were obtained when the Wagner–Nelson method was used to calculate the absorption rate constant after an oral administration:

Time (hr)	Fraction Remaining to be Absorbed
1	0.7
2	0.5
3	0.35
5	0.17

a. What is the order of absorption of this drug?
b. Calculate the absorption rate constant.

4.8. A 60-kg patient received a single 25-mg oral dose of an antibiotic that is completely absorbed after oral administration. Serial samples were drawn, and the drug plasma concentrations were determined using a sensitive analytical method. The plasma concentrations were as follows:

Time (hr)	Concentration (ng/ml)	Time (hr)	Concentration (ng/ml)
0.0	0.00	4.0	246.1
0.2	88.5	6.0	161.0
0.5	184.9	8.0	102.2
1.0	276.9	10.0	64.5
2.0	321.6	12.0	40.66
3.0	292.8	14.0	25.61

a. Calculate the absorption rate constant of this drug using the method of residuals.
b. Calculate the half-life and the volume of distribution of this drug.

5 Drug Pharmacokinetics Following Single Oral Drug Administration: Extent of Drug Absorption

OBJECTIVES

After completing this chapter you should be able to:

- Define the bioavailability and the bioequivalence of drug products
- Describe the different components of the first-pass effect after oral drug administration
- Determine the absolute bioavailability and the relative bioavailability of oral drug products
- Calculate the area under the curve (AUC) using the trapezoidal rule
- Describe the general principles for designing and evaluating bioavailability and bioequivalence studies
- Analyze the effect of changing the drug pharmacokinetic parameters on the plasma concentration–time profile after oral drug administration

5.1 INTRODUCTION

The availability of drug formulations from different pharmaceutical manufacturers with similar or identical labeling is increasingly common in clinical practice. The pioneering pharmacokinetic work in the early 1960s gave substantial evidence that the composition and the finished dosage form can affect the in vivo properties of the drug product and the observed therapeutic effect. This has been attributed to the effect of the drug excipients, the manufacturing procedures, and the properties of the final dosage form on the rate and extent of drug absorption from its site of administration. Variation in the therapeutic effect is observed after administration of drug products from different sources. This is because the fraction of the administered dose that has been released in vivo and is capable of reaching the bloodstream represents the effective dose rather than the labeled dose on the packaged form of the drug. This has added a new dimension to the issue of quality of drug products, namely, bioavailability and bioequivalence.

5.1.1 General Definitions

Bioavailability The rate and extent to which the active drug ingredient or therapeutic moiety is absorbed from the drug product and becomes available at the site of drug action.

Absolute bioavailability The fraction of the administered dose that reaches the systemic circulation after extravascular administration. It is a measure of the extent of absorption after extravascular drug administration. The absolute bioavailability is determined by comparing the amount of drug that reaches the systemic circulation after extravascular administration and after intravenous (IV) administration of the same amount of the same drug. This is because after intravenous administration, the entire dose reaches the systemic circulation.

Relative bioavailability The absolute bioavailability of a drug product relative to the absolute bioavailability of a second drug product that contains the same active drug moiety. The relative bioavailability is determined by comparing the amount of the drug that reaches the systemic circulation after administration of an oral drug product and an oral reference standard preparation of the same active drug moiety.

Equivalence A term that indicates that one drug is similar to another with respect to bioavailability, therapeutic response, or any set of established standards.

Pharmaceutical alternative Products contain the same active drug but different salts, esters, dosage forms, and strengths.

Pharmaceutical equivalence Drug products that contain the same active drug ingredient and are identical in strength, concentration, dosage form, and route of administration.

Bioequivalence The drug in two or more similar dosage forms reaches the systemic circulation at the same rate and to the same extent, that is, the plasma concentration–time profiles of the active moiety following the administration of the two different products are within expected standard variance.

Therapeutic equivalence Describes drug products that contain the same therapeutically active drug and have the same therapeutic effect and the same equal potential for adverse effects under the condition specified in the labeling.

The ultimate criterion for assessing the equivalence of "equivalent" drug products would appear to be the therapeutic equivalency, the degree to which the products provide an effect that controls a symptom or disease. However, this is not easy to do because many symptoms and disease processes are difficult to quantitate (e.g., anxiety, pain, bronchoconstriction, etc.). Because it is believed that the therapeutic effect of a drug is related to the blood levels the product produces in vivo, it is felt that blood level studies designed to assess the bioavailability of equivalent products represent a reasonable alternative to studies that assess therapeutic equivalence.

5.2 PURPOSE OF BIOAVAILABILITY AND BIOEQUIVALENCE STUDIES

The literature is full of examples in which the effectiveness of the drug can be altered by the composition and the manufacturing procedures of the finished formulation. Variations in the bioavailability of drug products have been recognized as responsible for possible therapeutic failures. The increasing number of drugs that can be obtained from different manufacturers and the phenomenal growth of the generic pharmaceutical industry have prompted regulatory agencies such as the Food and Drug Administration (FDA) to establish the bioavailability and the bioequivalence regulations put into effect in January 1977. These regulations included for the first time the requirement for submission of in vivo bioavailability and bioequivalence data and the criteria for waiving of such studies during the drug product approval process.

Product efficacy depends on how much of the drug is ultimately absorbed from its formulation and how rapidly the drug is absorbed. The extent and the rate at which the drug is absorbed form the basis of bioavailability and bioequivalence testing. Bioequivalence studies are investigations designed to compare the bioavailability of the drug from two or more drug products. If two preparations containing equivalent amounts of the same active ingredient produce similar concentrations of the drug entity in blood, then they are bioequivalent and therefore assumed to be therapeutically equivalent. Bioequivalent products can be substituted for one another with full expectation that the substituted products will provide the same therapeutic effect as the prescribed product.

5.3 CAUSES FOR VARIATION IN DRUG BIOAVAILABILITY

After extravascular administration, the drug bioavailability can vary significantly depending on the route of administration, the dosage form, the drug properties, and physiological and pathological factors that can affect the process of drug absorption into the systemic circulation.

5.3.1 Factors Related to Drug Formulation and Route of Administration

5.3.1.1 Route of Administration

Parenteral formulations in general are more bioavailable than oral or rectal preparations. IV administration allows direct administration of the drug into the systemic circulation, resulting in complete (100%) bioavailability. Intramuscular administration may be less bioavailable than IV administration but is usually results in more efficient absorption than subcutaneous and intradermal administration.

5.3.1.2 Dosage Form

For oral administration, preparation in the form of a solution is usually the most readily absorbed; however, stability and solubilization problems usually force the formulator to choose a tablet or capsule preparation. It has been well documented that the bioavailability of a drug can be different from different dosage forms.

5.3.1.3 Excipient

Drugs are rarely administered as a pure chemical entity. Usually, a number of excipients, depending on the type of dosage form, are added to be able to prepare the desired drug product. The type and the amount of these excipients in addition to their physicochemical characteristics can greatly affect the drug dissolution rate and bioavailability. Manufacturing and the processing conditions such as temperature, humidity, storage time, and timing and efficiency of each manufacturing step can result in variation in the properties of the final drug product and its bioavailability.

5.3.2 Factors Related to the Drug

5.3.2.1 Drug Solubility

The chemical structure of the drug substance usually determines the drug's major properties, which can influence its dissolution and bioavailability. The physical properties of the drug, such as the crystalline state and the particle size, are important in determining its solubility. Drugs that have low aqueous solubility are expected to possess bioavailability problems, and methods to improve their solubility should be considered. Minor modifications in the drug molecule (e.g., salt formation or esterification, micronization to decrease the drug particle size and to increase the effective surface area, and complexation with inert water-soluble materials) are strategies that have been used to enhance the aqueous solubility of these drugs.

5.3.2.2 Drug Partition Coefficient

Another important property related to the chemical structure of the drug molecule is its ability to cross the barrier of the cell membrane at the absorption site to enter the systemic circulation. In addition to the chemical structure, the permeability of the drug molecule depends on the molecular size, the presence or absence of electric charge, and the magnitude of this charge. The lipophilic/hydrophilic properties of the drug are good indicators for the potential to permeate a membrane, with lipophilic drugs crossing biological membranes more readily than hydrophilic drugs.

5.3.2.3 Stability and Drug Interaction

Drug stability at the site of administration can also play an important role in determining its bioavailability. The degradation of many acid-labile drugs in the acidic environment of the stomach leads to low systemic bioavailability when administered orally. Also, enzymatic hydrolysis of drugs at the site of administration can result in variation in their bioavailability. Coadministration of drugs can result in the interference of one drug with the absorption of another. Drug–drug interactions in the gastrointestinal tract, which can result in variation in drug bioavailability, may be caused by the formation of complexes that are incapable of crossing the gastrointestinal tract membrane, competing for similar mechanisms such as active transport or simply by modifying the stomach-emptying rate or gastrointestinal motility.

5.3.3 Factors Related to the Patient

5.3.3.1 Individual Variability

The human body is a complex and dynamic structure that constantly reacts and interacts with any foreign materials, such as drugs introduced within its boundaries. Therefore, from the time of its introduction and in vivo release until its final elimination from the body, the drug is continually subjected to numerous processes, including absorption, metabolism, and elimination. Intra- and intersubject variability in the rate and extent of each of these processes will greatly affect the drug bioavailability.

After oral administration of drugs, the pH at the absorption site is an important factor in facilitating and inhibiting the absorption process. This variability in the gastrointestinal pH can be a major source for intersubject variability in bioavailability. Other factors that can cause variation in the bioavailability of drugs are gastric emptying and gastrointestinal motility. This is because the small intestine is the major site of absorption of most drugs because of its large surface area, and the gastric-emptying rate will determine the rate of drug absorption. Food can also play an important role in the bioavailability of orally administered drugs.

5.3.3.2 Site of Administration

The absorption of drugs is most favorable from areas rich in capillaries, such as skeletal muscles. Absorption from intramuscular sites is significantly faster than absorption from subcutaneous areas. The reason for the high efficiency of absorption from the buccal and sublingual sites is their high degree of vascularity. The same is true for the intestinal mucosa. The blood flow to the site of administration will also affect the rate of drug absorption. A high flow rate maximizes the effect of concentration gradient across the biological membrane and helps keep the blood near the administration site as a perfect sink, thereby increasing the rate and probably the extent of drug absorption.

5.3.3.3 Diseases

Malabsorption is noticed with advanced age because of the natural changes in biological functions. This can be a source of decreased drug bioavailability in elderly patients. Also, drugs such as phenytoin and chemotherapeutic agents can affect the absorption of other drugs and decrease their bioavailability.

5.3.4 First-Pass Effect

After oral administration, the drug in the gut lumen may undergo chemical hydrolysis or enzymatic metabolism caused primarily by the gut flora. A fraction of the administered dose can be absorbed from the gut lumen, and the rest of the dose is excreted unchanged with the feces. During the absorption process, the drug can be metabolized in the gut wall. Only a fraction of the absorbed dose will reach the portal circulation. The drug absorbed into the portal vein will have to go through the liver before it reaches the systemic circulation. A fraction of the absorbed dose can be metabolized during this first pass through the liver before the drug reaches the systemic circulation.

The fraction of the dose that reaches the systemic circulation (bioavailable drug) is the fraction of the dose that escapes hydrolysis and metabolism in the gut lumen, metabolism in the gut wall, and metabolism during the first pass through the liver. Elimination of the drug before it reaches the systemic circulation is called *presystemic elimination* or the *first-pass effect*.

5.4 PHARMACOKINETIC BASIS OF DRUG BIOAVAILABILITY AND BIOEQUIVALENCE

After extravascular administration of a single dose of drug, it has to be absorbed into the bloodstream to produce the desired pharmacological effect. The shape and magnitude of the plasma concentration–time profile depend on the rate of drug absorption, the rate of drug elimination, and the amount of drug absorbed. In assessing drug bioavailability and bioequivalence, three parameters are usually measured to describe the plasma concentration–time profile of the administered drugs:

The maximum (peak) drug plasma concentration C_{max}: Represents the highest drug concentration in the systemic circulation achieved after extravascular drug administration. A higher C_{max} indicates a faster rate or higher extent of drug absorption. For drugs that have a direct relationship between the plasma concentration and the pharmacological response, C_{max} is an indication of the intensity of the therapeutic effect.

The time of maximum drug concentration t_{max}: Represents the length of time required to achieve the maximum concentration of the drug in the systemic circulation. A shorter t_{max} usually indicates a faster rate of drug absorption. The t_{max} is not affected by the extent of drug absorption.

The area under the plasma concentration–time curve (AUC): The value of the AUC is directly proportional to the amount of the administered drug that reaches the systemic circulation in the same individual (constant total body clearance). The AUC measured after administration of different products for the same active ingredient can be used to compare the extent of absorption of the drug from these formulations. The AUC is not affected by the rate of drug absorption.

5.5 DETERMINATION OF DRUG BIOAVAILABILITY

When the drug elimination follows first-order kinetics (most drugs do), then the area under the plasma concentration–time curve from zero time to infinity (i.e., until no further drug can be measured in the plasma) after an IV administration is given by

$$AUC_{IV} = \frac{\text{Dose}}{k\ Vd} \tag{5.1}$$

The AUC for a drug after oral (or intramuscular, subcutaneous, rectal, etc.) administration is given by

$$AUC_{oral} = \frac{F\ Dose}{k\ Vd} \tag{5.2}$$

where F is the absolute bioavailability of the oral dosage form or the fraction of the dose that actually reaches the systemic circulation. The absolute bioavailability can range from 0, when the drug is not absorbed at all from the administered formulation, to unity (1) when the drug is completely absorbed. The absolute bioavailability is determined in practice by comparing the AUC after oral and after IV administration of equal doses of the same drug to the same subjects. The bioavailability can also be expressed as percentage (e.g., bioavailability of 0.7 can be expressed as 70%).

$$\text{Absolute bioavailability} = \frac{AUC_{oral}}{AUC_{IV}} = \frac{F\ Dose_{oral}/k\ Vd}{Dose_{IV}/k\ Vd} = F \tag{5.3}$$

The relative bioavailability of a group of pharmaceutical equivalent dosage forms may be determined by comparing the AUCs measured after administration of these formulations to the same individuals. Pharmaceutical equivalence implies that the formulations contain the same amount of the same active drug.

The *relative bioavailability* is a term used to compare the relative extent to which different dosage forms of the same drug are absorbed. For example, the relative bioavailability of product A (250 mg of drug X) may be stated as 60% of that of product B (250 mg of drug X). This statement does not give information about the absolute bioavailability of product A or B. This means that the ratio of the absolute bioavailability of product A to that of product B is 60%. For example, the ratios of the amounts absorbed in milligrams from products A and B may be represented by any of the following ratios: 150/250, 120/200, 30/50, and so on. For two different formulations of the same drug (e.g., products A and B),

$$AUC_{oral\ A} = \frac{F_A\ Dose_A}{k\ Vd} \tag{5.4}$$

$$AUC_{oral\ B} = \frac{F_B\ Dose_B}{k\ Vd} \tag{5.5}$$

To determine the relative bioavailability of product A to product B, we can compare the AUC when equal doses of the two products are given to the same subject or group of subjects. Thus,

$$\text{Relative bioavailability} = \frac{AUC_{oral\ A}}{AUC_{oral\ B}} = \frac{F_A\ Dose/k\ Vd}{F_B\ Dose/k\ Vd} = \frac{F_A}{F_B} \tag{5.6}$$

where F_A/F_B is the bioavailability of product A relative to the bioavailability of product B. Note that this does not tell us anything about the individual values for F_A and F_B. The relative bioavailability is used to compare the extent of absorption of new formulations to the absorption of a standard formulation.

Bioequivalence of different formulations of the same drug substance indicates equivalence with respect to the rate and extent of drug absorption. Two formulations with rates and extents of absorption that differ by −20%/+25% or less are generally considered bioequivalent. The use of this rule is based on a medical decision that, for most drugs, a −20%/+25% difference in the concentration of the active ingredient in blood will not result in significantly different therapeutic effect.

5.5.1 Expected Values for Drug Bioavailability

The *bioavailability* is a measure of the fraction of the administered dose that reaches the systemic circulation. The *absolute bioavailability* is the fraction of the total dose that reaches the systemic circulation. It can have values between 0, if the drug is not absorbed at all, to 1 when all the administered dose reaches the systemic circulation. The absolute bioavailability can be expressed in terms of percentage (0–100%). On the other hand, the relative bioavailability is the bioavailability of a drug product relative to the bioavailability of another drug product (reference standard preparation). The relative bioavailability can have any value above 0. It can be more than 1 when the product under investigation has bioavailability higher than that of the reference standard.

5.5.2 Clinical Importance of Bioavailability and Bioequivalence

Single-dose administration: Drug absorption from different oral dosage forms may occur at different rates and to different extents. The drug plasma concentration achieved after administration of drug products with low bioavailability may not reach the concentration required to produce the pharmacological effect (therapeutic failure). The plasma concentration may exceed the concentration required to produce the pharmacological effect for a short period of time (short duration of effect) as illustrated in Figure 5.1.

Multiple drug administrations: Patients who take medication for a long time build up a steady state or a constant level in the body. When patients switch to drug products with different bioavailability during chronic oral dosing, this can lead to a significant change in the steady-state concentration of the drug. This change may lead to drug toxicity (if a product with a higher F is used) or subtherapeutic effect (if a product with a lower F is used).

Bioequivalence: When the different drug products for the same active drug moiety are proven to be bioequivalent, it will be possible to switch between drug products without affecting the resulting therapeutic effects. This will be beneficial for the physician, the pharmacist, and the patient. The physician can write the prescription using the generic name of the drugs without the need to know all the brand names for all the drug products. The pharmacist will stock fewer drug products, and it will be possible to switch

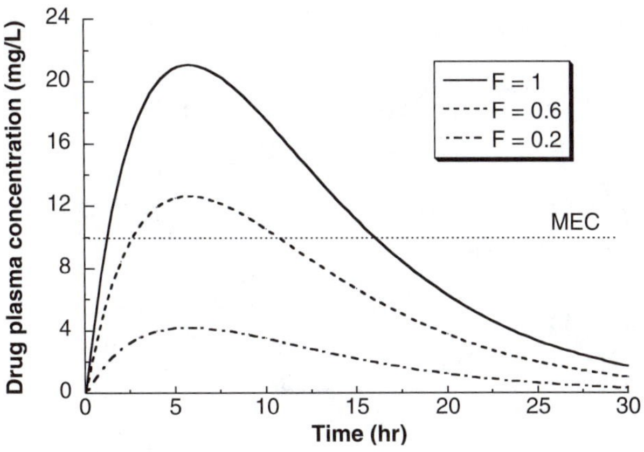

FIGURE 5.1 The drug plasma concentration–time profiles after a single administration of the same dose of a drug from different drug products with different bioavailability.

bioequivalent drug products of the same active drug in case of shortage of a specific product. Also, the patient can chose to use the cheaper drug products without any compromise in the therapeutic effect.

5.6 CALCULATION OF AREA UNDER THE CURVE (LINEAR TRAPEZOIDAL RULE)

The plasma drug concentration–time profile is divided into a number of trapezoids, and the total AUC can be approximated by the sum of the area of these trapezoids. The area of each trapezoid can be calculated as in Figure 5.2, and it is equal to

$$\text{Area} = \left(\frac{a + b}{2}\right).\ W$$

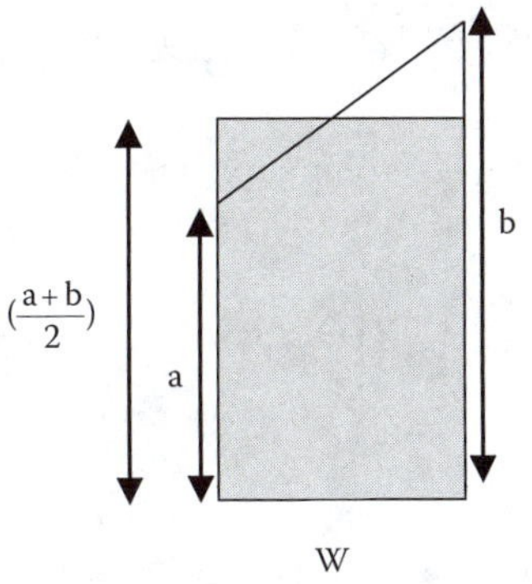

FIGURE 5.2 Calculation of the area of a trapezoid: Area of a trapezoid $= \left(\frac{a+b}{2}\right)$ (w).

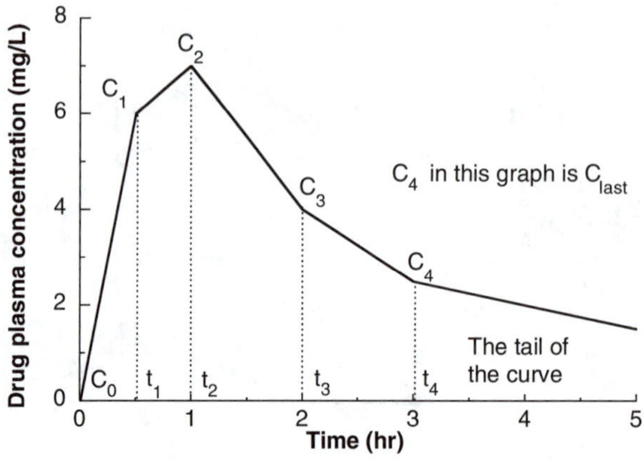

FIGURE 5.3 The AUC is the sum of the area of all trapezoids and the area under the tail of the curve.

The total AUC is found by summing all trapezoids and adding the area under the tail of the curve as in Figure 5.3.

The area of each trapezoid is calculated as

$$\text{Area} = \left(\frac{C_n + C_{n+1}}{2}\right) . \ (t_{n+1} - t_n) \tag{5.7}$$

and the area of the tail is

$$\text{Area of the tail} = \frac{C_{last}}{k} \tag{5.8}$$

or

$$\text{Area of the tail} = \frac{C_{last} \ t_{1/2}}{0.693} = 1.44 \ C_{last} \ t_{1/2} \tag{5.9}$$

where C_{last} is the last measured concentration, and k is the elimination rate constant. The total AUC is the sum of all trapezoids plus the area of the tail.

$$AUC = (1/2)(C_0 + C_1)(t_1 - t_0) + (1/2)(C_1 + C_2)(t_2 - t_1) + \ldots + \text{Area of tail} \tag{5.10}$$

Example

In a study to evaluate the bioavailability of an antibiotic, a patient received a single 250-mg intravenous bolus dose, a single 500-mg dose in the form of an oral suspension, and a single 500-mg dose in the form of an oral capsule on three separate occasions, and the following plasma concentrations were obtained:

Time (hr)	IV bolus (250 mg) Concentration (mg/L)	Oral Suspension (500 mg) Concentration (mg/L)	Oral Capsule (500 mg) Concentration (mg/L)
1	6.3	5.0	3.1
2	5.0	7.0	4.7
3	4.0	7.4	5.2
4	3.2	7.0	5.3
6	2.0	5.4	4.5
8	1.3	3.7	3.4
12	0.5	1.6	1.7

The half-life of this antibiotic is 3 hr, and the absorption process is complete after 12 hr of oral administration

1. Calculate the absolute bioavailability of the oral suspension and the oral capsule of this antibiotic.
2. Calculate the bioavailability of the oral capsule relative to the oral suspension of this antibiotic.

Answer

1. To calculate the absolute bioavailability of the oral suspension and the capsule, we need to calculate the AUC after administration of the IV and the oral formulations:
   Calculation of the AUC after administration of 250 mg IV: Plot the plasma concentration–time profile after IV administration on semilog graph paper and back-extrapolate the resulting line to calculate the initial plasma concentration Cp_0. The Cp_0 is 8 mg/l, and the elimination rate constant (k) is 0.693/3 hr = 0.231 hr^{-1}.

$$AUC_{IV} = \frac{Cp_0}{k} = \frac{8\ \text{mg/L}}{0.231\ \text{hr}^{-1}} = 34.63\ \text{mg-hr/L}$$

Calculation of the AUC after administration of 500-mg oral suspension by the trapezoidal rule:

$$\text{Area of a trapezoid} = \left(\frac{C_n + C_{n+1}}{2}\right) . (t_{n+1} - t_n)$$

Please note that after oral administration the drug concentration at time 0 is equal to 0, and this 0,0 point should be used in calculating the AUC after oral administration.

$$\text{Area of trapezoid 1} = \left(\frac{0+5}{2}\right) . (1-0) = 2.5\ \text{mg-hr/L}$$

$$\text{Area of trapezoid 2} = \left(\frac{5+7}{2}\right) . (2-1) = 6\ \text{mg-hr/L}$$

$$\text{Area of trapezoid 3} = \left(\frac{7+7.4}{2}\right) . (3-2) = 7.2\ \text{mg-hr/L}$$

$$\text{Area of trapezoid } 4 = \left(\frac{7.4+7}{2}\right).(4-3) = 7.2 \text{ mg-hr/L}$$

$$\text{Area of trapezoid } 5 = \left(\frac{7+5.4}{2}\right).(6-4) = 12.4 \text{ mg-hr/L}$$

$$\text{Area of trapezoid } 6 = \left(\frac{5.4+3.7}{2}\right).(8-6) = 9.1 \text{ mg-hr/L}$$

$$\text{Area of trapezoid } 7 = \left(\frac{3.7+1.6}{2}\right).(12-8) = 10.6 \text{ mg-hr/L}$$

$$\text{Area of the tail} = \frac{C_{last}}{k} = \frac{1.6 \text{ mg/L}}{0.231 \text{ hr}^{-1}} = 6.93 \text{ mg-hr/L}$$

$$\text{Total AUC} = 2.5+6.0+7.2+7.2+12.4+9.1+10.6+6.93 = 61.93 \text{ mg-hr/L}$$

Calculation of the AUC after administration of 500-mg oral capsule by the trapezoidal rule:

$$\text{Area of trapezoid } 1 = \left(\frac{0+3.1}{2}\right).(1-0) = 1.55 \text{ mg-hr/L}$$

$$\text{Area of trapezoid } 2 = \left(\frac{3.1+4.7}{2}\right).(2-1) = 3.9 \text{ mg-hr/L}$$

$$\text{Area of trapezoid } 3 = \left(\frac{4.7+5.2}{2}\right).(3-2) = 4.95 \text{ mg-hr/L}$$

$$\text{Area of trapezoid } 4 = \left(\frac{5.2+5.3}{2}\right).(4-3) = 5.25 \text{ mg-hr/L}$$

$$\text{Area of trapezoid } 5 = \left(\frac{5.3+4.5}{2}\right).(6-4) = 9.8 \text{ mg-hr/L}$$

$$\text{Area of trapezoid } 6 = \left(\frac{4.5+3.4}{2}\right).(8-6) = 7.9 \text{ mg-hr/L}$$

$$\text{Area of trapezoid } 7 = \left(\frac{3.4+1.7}{2}\right).(12-8) = 10.2 \text{ mg-hr/L}$$

$$\text{Area of the tail} = \frac{C_{last}}{k} = \frac{1.7 \text{ mg/L}}{0.231 \text{ hr}^{-1}} = 7.36 \text{ mg-hr/L}$$

$$\text{Total AUC} = 1.55+3.9+4.95+5.25+9.8+7.9+10.2+7.36 = 50.9 \text{ mg-hr/L}$$

The absolute bioavailability of the suspension (note that the doses for the IV and the oral suspension are different):

$$F_{suspension} = \frac{AUC_{suspension}}{AUC_{IV}} \times \frac{Dose_{IV}}{Dose_{suspension}} = \frac{61.93\ \text{mg-hr/L}}{34.63\ \text{mg-hr/L}} \times \frac{250\ \text{mg}}{500\ \text{mg}} = 0.89$$

The absolute bioavailability of the capsule (note that the doses for the IV and the oral capsule are different):

$$F_{capsule} = \frac{AUC_{capsule}}{AUC_{IV}} \times \frac{Dose_{IV}}{Dose_{capsule}} = \frac{50.9\ \text{mg-hr/L}}{34.63\ \text{mg-hr/L}} \times \frac{250\ \text{mg}}{500\ \text{mg}} = 0.73$$

2. The bioavailability of the capsule relative to the suspension (the dose is similar):

$$F_{relative} = \frac{AUC_{capsule}}{AUC_{suspension}} \times \frac{Dose_{suspension}}{Dose_{capsule}} = \frac{50.9\ \text{mg-hr/L}}{61.93\ \text{mg-hr/L}} \times \frac{500\ \text{mg}}{500\ \text{mg}} = 0.82$$

The relative bioavailability can also be determined from the ratio of the absolute bioavailability of the two oral products:

$$F_{relative} = \frac{F_{capsule}}{F_{suspension}} = \frac{0.73}{0.89} = 0.82$$

5.7 REGULATORY REQUIREMENTS FOR BIOAVAILABILITY AND BIOEQUIVALENCE

Bioavailability studies are required for drugs that are not approved for marketing and for approved drugs under certain conditions. For new drugs not fully approved for marketing, regulatory agencies require that in vivo bioavailability studies should be performed on the dosage form proposed for marketing. Also, the pharmacokinetic parameters of the active drug ingredient must be characterized. These parameters, including the rate and extent of systemic absorption and the rate of drug elimination and metabolism, should be determined after single-dose and multiple-dose drug administration. The data from these studies are important to establish the recommended dosage and to support drug labeling.

Also, in vivo bioavailability studies are required for new formulations of the active drug ingredient that are approved for marketing. The purpose of these studies is to determine the bioavailability and characterize the pharmacokinetics of the new formulation, new dosage form, or new salt relative to a reference standard.

For approved drugs, the bioequivalence studies are performed to compare the performance of different drug products of the same active ingredient. Abbreviated new drug applications are permitted for duplicates of drugs (i.e., drug products that are the same as already approved drug products in dosage form, route of administration, kind and amount of active ingredient, and indication) on the condition that the new drug product is shown to be bioequivalent to the originally approved drug product. For establishing bioequivalence, the fraction of the dose that reaches the systemic circulation after administration of the new drug product and the innovator drug product (the reference standard product) should not be significantly different. Also, the absorption rate of the drug should be close enough so that similar plasma drug concentration–time profiles are obtained after administration of the two drug products.

5.7.1 Design and Evaluation of Bioequivalence Studies

The primary objective of the bioequivalence study is to compare in healthy normal volunteers the rate and extent of drug absorption from the new drug product and from a reference standard product that contain the same active drug moiety.

The volunteers: It is recommended that 24 subjects are used in the bioequivalence study. The volunteers should be free of any condition that can affect the absorption, distribution, and elimination of the drug under investigation. This should be assessed from the volunteer history, laboratory tests, and physical examination.

The reference standard product: The reference standard product should contain the same active ingredient as the test drug product under investigation. The reference standard for a drug is usually a formulation currently approved and marketed that is well accepted by the medical profession and has a long history of clinical use. The reference standard is usually the innovator's or the original manufacturer's product.

Study design: A balanced crossover experimental design. Volunteers participating in the study are divided into groups I and II. Volunteers in group I receive the test drug product, and volunteers in group II receive the reference standard product. After leaving a period of time to make sure that all the drug is eliminated from the body (washout period), volunteers in group I receive the reference drug product, and volunteers in group II receive the test drug product. This is the balanced crossover experimental design in which each volunteer acts as his or her own control. Evaluation of the bioequivalence of modified release formulations may require multiple drug administrations, and the bioequivalence study is performed at steady state. A parallel experimental design in which the test and the reference drug products are administered to two different groups of volunteers may be used for drugs with long half-lives.

Sampling schedule: The sampling schedule after each drug administration should be designed to include at least three samples before the expected t_{max}. Samples should continue for two to three half-lives after the expected t_{max}.

Sample analysis: The plasma samples should be analyzed utilizing validated analytical procedures.

Pharmacokinetic parameters: The pharmacokinetic parameters AUC, t_{max}, and C_{max} are calculated for each volunteer after administration of the test drug product and after the reference standard product.

Statistical analysis: Each of the calculated parameters are compared using:

- Analysis of variance (ANOVA): This test determines the contribution of treatment (the different products), the sequence, the period, and the subjects to the difference in the calculated pharmacokinetic parameters. This statistical analysis examines if any of these factors is significant.
- The two one-sided test: This test examines if the pharmacokinetic parameters (AUC and C_{max}) after the test and the reference products are comparable. The test drug product is considered bioequivalent to the reference drug product if the 90% confidence interval for the difference between the log-transformed value for AUC and C_{max} for the test and reference products fall within 80–125% of the mean for the reference product for each parameter.

5.7.2 Criteria for Waiver of Bioavailability Requirements

The in vivo bioavailability of certain drug products may be self-evident or not important for the achievement of the product's desired effect. The in vivo bioavailability requirements are waived by regulatory agencies if the drug product meets one of the following criteria:

- Preparations intended for IV use or topical preparation intended for local effect
- Oral dosage forms not intended for systemic absorption, such as antacids and radiopaque media or products administered by inhalation as a gas or vapor
- Oral solution, elixir, syrup, tincture, or other solubilized forms that contain a previously approved active ingredient and have no added inactive ingredient that is known to affect drug absorption
- Orally administered drugs that have been proven to be highly soluble and highly permeable

5.8 FACTORS AFFECTING THE BLOOD CONCENTRATION–TIME PROFILE AFTER A SINGLE ORAL DOSE

After a single oral drug administration, the plasma concentration–time profile depends on the dose, bioavailability, total body clearance, volume of distribution, and the absorption rate constant of the drug. It is important to note that the total body clearance and the volume of distribution are constants for a given drug in a given patient and are independent of the route of administration and the formulation characteristics. However, the drug bioavailability and absorption rate constant are dependent on the characteristics of the formulation, and different products for the same drug can have different bioavailability and different rates of absorption.

5.8.1 Dose

Administration of increasing doses of the same drug to the same individual should produce proportional increases in C_{max} and AUC without affecting CL_T, Vd, and k (when drug elimination follows first-order kinetics).

5.8.2 Bioavailability

Administration of the same dose of the same drug in the form of drug products that have different bioavailability but similar rates of drug absorption should produce different C_{max} and AUC. Products with higher bioavailability should produce proportionally higher C_{max} and AUC without affecting CL_T, Vd, k_a, and k.

5.8.3 Total Body Clearance

Administration of the same dose of a drug in the form of the same product to a group of individuals who have different CL_T results in different AUC and different rates of decline of the drug blood concentration during the elimination phase if the Vd of the drug is similar in this group of individuals. Individuals with the higher CL_T eliminate the drug at a faster rate (larger k and shorter $t_{1/2}$) and will have lower AUC.

5.8.4 Volume of Distribution

Administration of the same dose of the same drug to a group of individuals will result in a slower rate of drug elimination without affecting the AUC (if the CL_T is similar in these individuals). Note that the same drug can have different Vd in individuals with different body weights. Administration of the same dose of a drug to individuals with different Vd will produce different drug concentration–time profiles depending on Vd and CL_T.

5.8.5 Absorption Rate Constant

A larger absorption rate constant results in faster drug absorption. The change in the absorption rate constant does not usually affect CL_T, Vd, F, AUC, and k.

PRACTICE PROBLEMS

5.1. Explain why an ampicillin 500-mg capsule that is rapidly and completely absorbed is not considered bioequivalent to an amoxicillin 500-mg capsule that is also rapidly and completely absorbed.

5.2. Explain why a sustained-release tablet of theophylline with bioavailability of 94% is not bioequivalent to a conventional (immediate-release) theophylline tablet that has bioavailability of 92%.

5.3. After administration of a single-dose IV bolus of 300 mg acyclovir to a patient, the total AUC was 16 mg-hr/L, and the elimination half-life was 2.4 hr; after oral administration of a 300-mg tablet to the same patient, the following plasma concentrations were obtained:

Time (hr)	Drug Concentration (mg/L)
0	0
1	0.364
3	0.716
5	0.787
7	0.730
10	0.569
15	0.318
20	0.162

a. Calculate the absolute bioavailability of acyclovir in this patient.

5.4. Different formulations of the same drug were administered to the same individuals, and the following data were obtained:

- After IV bolus administration of 10 mg, the AUC was 5 mg-hr/L.
- After intramuscular administration of 20 mg, the AUC was 9 mg-hr/L.
- After oral administration of a 50-mg capsule, the AUC was 10 mg-hr/L.
- After oral administration of a 20-mg oral suspension, the AUC was 5 mg-hr/L.

a. Calculate the absolute bioavailability of the drug from the capsules.
b. Calculate the absolute bioavailability of the drug after intramuscular administration.
c. Calculate the bioavailability of the oral suspension relative to the capsules.
d. Which formulation has the highest absolute bioavailability?
e. Do you think the intravenous and the intramuscular formulations are bioequivalent? Why?

5.5. A group of volunteers received a single oral dose of two different formulations of an oral hypoglycemic drug. Each tablet from the two formulations contains 500 mg of the drug. The average plasma drug concentrations obtained at different time points after administration of the two formulations are tabulated next:

Time (hr)	Formulation A Concentration (mg/L)	Formulation B Concentration (mg/L)
0	0	0
1	12.9	6.89
2	18.6	11.9
4	20.9	17.7
6	18.8	19.8
8	15.9	19.8
10	13.2	18.6
12	10.8	16.8
20	4.87	9.36
30	1.79	3.78

a. Which formulation is absorbed faster? Why?
b. What is the bioavailability of formulation A relative to the bioavailability of formulation B? How can you interpret this result?

5.6. Different formulations of the same drug were administered to a group of individuals, and the plasma concentrations were measured after administration of each formulation. The results are tabulated next:

Time (hr)	Concentration (mg/L), 200-mg IV	Concentration (mg/L), 500-mg Syrup	Concentration (mg/L), 500-mg Capsule	Concentration (mg/L), 500-mg Tablet
0		0	0	0
1	7.40	9.22	6.0	4.22
2	5.5	11.9	8.14	5.99
3	4.56	11.6	8.25	6.32
5	2.23	8.32	6.35	5.27
7	1.22	5.16	4.15	3.70
10	0.50	2.27	1.94	1.89
15	0.111	0.527	0.475	0.518
20	0.0245	0.119	0.11	0.129

a. Calculate the half-life and volume of distribution of this drug.
b. Which oral formulation has the fastest absorption rate?
c. Calculate the absolute bioavailability of the three oral formulations.
d. Calculate the bioavailability of the oral capsule relative to that of the syrup.
e. Calculate the bioavailability of the tablet relative to the bioavailability of the capsule.

5.7. The following plasma concentrations were obtained after administration of a single 500-mg tablet of an antihypertensive drug to a patient:

Time (hr)	Concentration (mg/L)
1	3.75
3	6.1
6	5.2
10	3.14
15	1.32
20	0.56
26	0.197

When a single IV bolus dose of 250 mg was administered to the same patient, the total AUC was 60 mg-hr/L.

a. What is the half-life of this drug in this patient?
b. What is the total AUC of the drug after administration of a 500-mg oral dose in this patient?
c. What is the bioavailability of the oral tablet in this patient?
d. What are the CL_T and the Vd of this drug in this patient?

5.8. A patient received a single 300-mg IV bolus dose and a single 500-mg oral dose of an antibiotic on two separate occasions, and the following plasma concentrations were obtained:

IV Administration		Oral Administration	
Time (hr)	Concentration (mg/L)	Time (hr)	Concentration (mg/L)
2	12.86	0	0
6	9.45	1	2.24
12	5.95	3	4.69
24	2.36	5	5.54
		7	5.58
		10	5.0
		15	3.68
		20	2.57
		30	1.20

a. Calculate the half-life and volume of distribution of this drug in this patient.
b. Calculate the fraction of the drug absorbed after oral administration.

5.9. After oral administration of a single 500-mg tablet of an antihypertensive drug to a normal volunteer, the total calculated AUC was 70 mg-hr/L. After an IV bolus administration of the same drug to the same volunteer, the drug half-life was 3 hr, and the volume of distribution was 25 L.

a. Calculate the bioavailability of the oral tablet in this volunteer.
b. What is the expected AUC after administration of a single IV bolus dose of 250 mg of this drug to the same volunteer?

6 Steady-State Principle and Drug Pharmacokinetics during Constant-Rate Intravenous Infusion

OBJECTIVES

After completing this chapter you should be able to:

- Define the steady-state condition during constant-rate intravenous (IV) infusion
- Identify the factors that affect the steady-state plasma concentration during constant-rate IV infusion
- Determine the steady-state drug concentrations and the pharmacokinetic parameters during constant-rate IV infusion
- Analyze the effect of changing one or more of the pharmacokinetic parameters on the steady-state plasma concentration during constant-rate IV infusion
- Recommend an appropriate IV loading dose and IV infusion rate to achieve specific steady-state plasma concentrations
- Evaluate the appropriateness of certain infusion rates in specific patients

6.1 INTRODUCTION

The *steady-state principle* during continuous/repeated drug administration is defined as the condition when the rate of drug administration is equal to the rate of drug elimination. At steady state, the amount of the drug in the body and the drug plasma concentration are constant. The amount of the drug in the body will reach steady state as long as the rate of drug administration is constant and the drug elimination pathways follow first-order kinetics.

Continuous drug administration usually involves either drug administration by constant rate IV infusion or repeated administration of a fixed dose of the drug every fixed dosing interval. Drug administration by constant rate IV infusion will achieve one steady-state concentration as long as the rate of drug administration and the total body clearance do not change. However, drug administration by repeated IV or oral doses will achieve drug concentration–time profiles that are identical during each of the dosing intervals τ at steady state if the same dose is administered at equally spaced dosing intervals. This means that the maximum drug concentration, the minimum drug concentration, and the average drug concentrations during each dosing interval will be similar at steady state.

6.2 Plasma Concentration during Continuous Constant-Rate IV Drug Administration

Initially, there is no drug in the body before starting the infusion. Once the constant-rate intravenous infusion starts, the amount of the drug in the body will increase. If the drug elimination follows first-order kinetics, the rate of drug elimination will increase with time because the amount of the drug in the body is increasing.

$$\text{Drug elimination rate} = kA \tag{6.1}$$

where k is the first-order elimination rate constant, and A is the amount of the drug in the body. As the constant-rate infusion continues, the rate of administration remains constant, and the rate of drug elimination increases. When the rate of drug administration becomes equal to the rate of drug elimination, the amount of the drug in the body and the plasma drug concentration will be constant despite the continued drug administration (Figure 6.1). This is the steady state. At steady state,

$$\text{Rate of drug administration} = \text{Rate of drug elimination}$$

$$K_0 = kA_{ss} \tag{6.2}$$

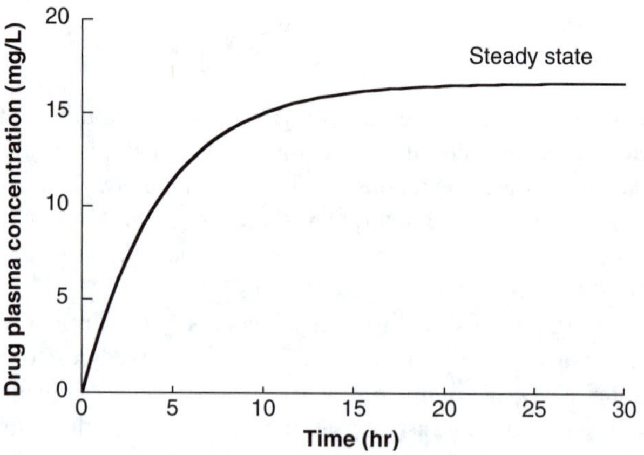

FIGURE 6.1 The drug plasma concentration–time profile after the start of the continuous constant-rate IV drug infusion.

where K_0 is the rate of drug infusion, k is the first-order elimination rate constant, and A_{ss} is the amount of drug in the body at steady state. The amount of drug in the body at steady state is given by

$$A_{ss} = \frac{K_0}{k} \tag{6.3}$$

The steady-state drug plasma concentration can be obtained by dividing the amount of the drug by the volume of distribution:

$$Cp_{ss} = \frac{K_0}{k\,Vd} \tag{6.4}$$

where Cp_{ss} is the steady-state plasma concentration of the drug, K_0 is the rate of drug infusion, k is the first-order elimination rate constant, and Vd is the volume of distribution. The drug plasma concentration at steady state is directly proportional to the rate of the IV infusion (i.e., the higher the rate of infusion, the higher will be the steady-state drug plasma concentration) and inversely proportional to the drug total body clearance (i.e., the higher the drug clearance, the lower will be the steady-state drug plasma concentration).

6.3 TIME REQUIRED TO REACH STEADY STATE

The time required to reach steady state is dependent on the half-life of the drug. Generally, it takes five or six half-lives of continuous IV infusion to reach steady state. The longer the drug half-life, the longer it takes to reach steady state. Figure 6.2 shows the time required to achieve steady state during administration of different drugs that have different half-lives. Administration of the same drug at different infusion rates to a group of individuals who have the same CL_T and the same Vd will achieve

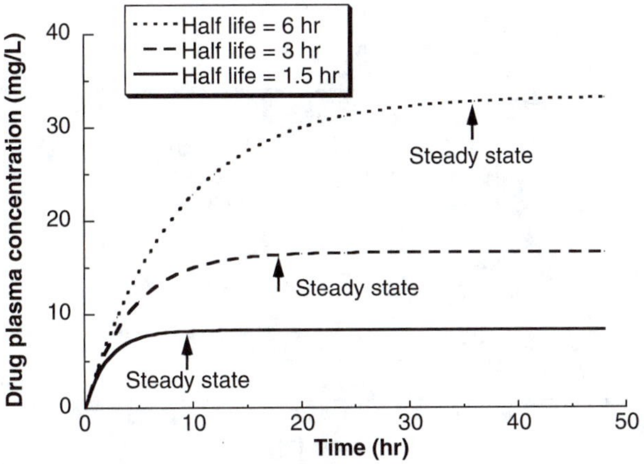

FIGURE 6.2 The time required to achieve steady state during continuous IV infusion is dependent on the half-life of the drug. The longer the half-life, the longer it takes to achieve steady state.

steady-state concentrations that are proportional to the IV infusion rate. However, the time to achieve the steady state will be the same because the assumption is that the drug half-life is similar in all individuals.

6.4 LOADING DOSE

During constant-rate IV drug administration, the drug accumulates until steady state is achieved after five or six half-lives. If rapid drug effect is required, such as in emergency situations, then immediate achievement of therapeutic drug concentrations will be required. In this case, administration of a loading dose will be necessary. The loading dose is an IV bolus dose administered at the time of starting the IV infusion to achieve a faster approach to steady state.

Rapid achievement of a therapeutic drug concentration can be accomplished by administration of an IV bolus dose (loading dose) and starting the constant-rate IV infusion simultaneously. The loading dose is chosen to achieve a plasma concentration similar or close to the desired plasma concentration that will be achieved by the IV infusion at steady state. In this case, the drug concentration at any time will be the sum of the drug concentration resulting from the IV infusion, which increases with time, and the drug concentration resulting from the IV bolus dose, which decreases with time as illustrated Figure 6.3.

$$\text{Cp total} = \text{Cp from infusion} + \text{Cp from IV bolus} \tag{6.5}$$

It is important to notice that the steady-state drug plasma concentration is dependent only on the infusion rate and the drug total body clearance as indicated from Equation 6.4. So, the loading dose does not have any effect on the steady-state concentration. If the loading dose achieves an initial plasma concentration higher than the steady-state drug concentration that should be achieved by the infusion, then the drug concentration will decline slowly to reach the steady state. If the

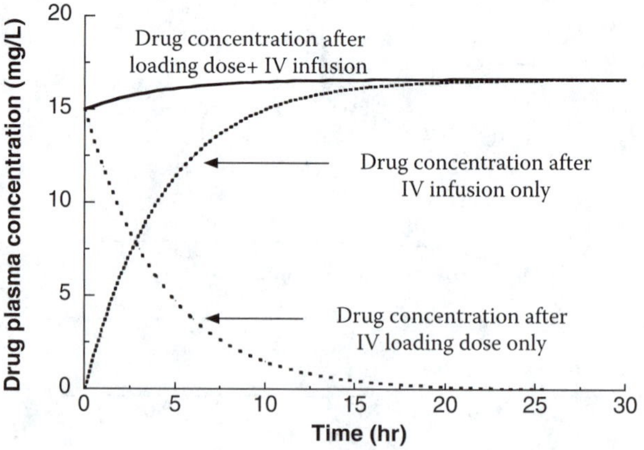

FIGURE 6.3 The drug plasma concentration–time profile after administration of a bolus IV dose (loading dose) and continuous constant-rate IV infusion simultaneously.

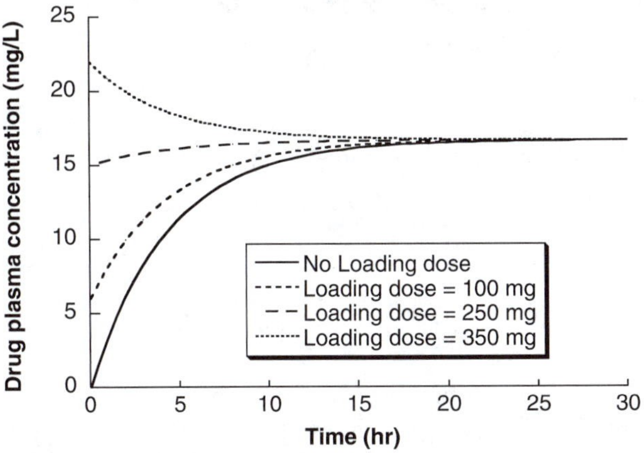

FIGURE 6.4 The drug plasma concentration–time profile after administration of different loading doses followed immediately by the same continuous IV infusion rate of the drug.

loading dose achieves an initial plasma concentration lower than the steady-state drug concentration that should be achieved by the infusion, then the drug concentration will increase slowly to reach the steady state. It takes five or six half lives for the initial drug concentration to reach steady state after administration of the loading dose. However, the initial plasma concentration is usually closer to steady state after administration of the loading dose, as shown in Figure 6.4.

Drug administration by constant-rate IV infusion results in increasing the drug concentration until steady state is achieved. Termination of the IV infusion at any time leads to decline in the drug concentration. The decline in drug concentration is dependent on the elimination rate constant of the drug as illustrated in Figure 6.5.

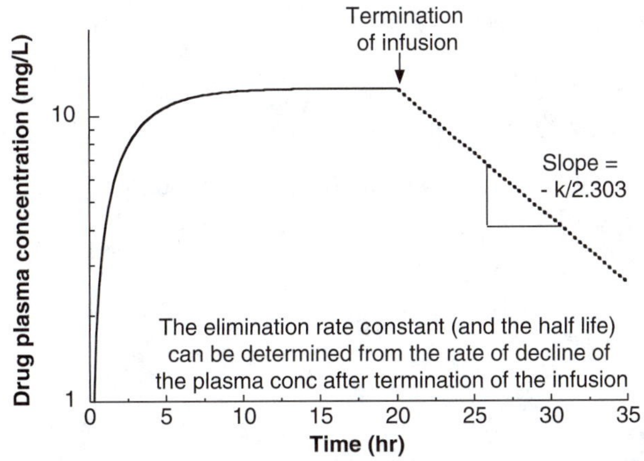

FIGURE 6.5 The drug plasma concentration–time profile during and after termination of the continuous IV infusion of the drug.

6.5 DETERMINATION OF THE PHARMACOKINETIC PARAMETERS

6.5.1 Total Body Clearance

The total body clearance can be determined from the IV infusion rate and the steady-state concentration:

$$CL_T = \frac{K_0}{Cp_{ss}} \tag{6.6}$$

The steady-state plasma concentration can be determined by measuring the plasma concentration during the IV infusion at steady state or from the plasma concentrations obtained after termination of the IV infusion. In this case, the plasma concentrations after termination of the IV infusion are drawn on semilog graph paper. The postinfusion drug plasma concentration–time profile is back-extrapolated to obtain the plasma concentration at the time of termination of the IV infusion, which is equal to the steady-state drug concentration.

6.5.2 Elimination Rate Constant

The elimination rate constant can be determined from the slope of the drug plasma concentration–time profile after termination of the IV infusion on semilog graph paper:

$$\text{Slope} = \frac{-k}{2.303} \tag{6.7}$$

The drug half-life can be determined from the elimination rate constant (Half-life = 0.693/k). Also, the half-life can be determined graphically from the drug profile after termination of the IV infusion, and k can be calculated from the half-life.

6.5.3 Volume of Distribution

The volume of distribution is determined from the total body clearance and the elimination rate constant:

$$Vd = \frac{CL_T}{k} \tag{6.8}$$

Example

A patient is receiving an antiarrhythmic drug as a constant rate IV infusion of 24 mg/h. After 3 days, the drug infusion was terminated, and three plasma samples were obtained.

Time After the End of Infusion (hr)	Concentration (mg/L)
1	3.3
3	2.2
6	1.2

1. Calculate the CL_T and Vd of this drug in this patient.
2. The patient experienced irregular heart rhythm again, and the physician wanted to restart this antiarrhythmic drug. Recommend an IV loading dose and a constant-rate IV infusion that should achieve a steady state of 10 mg/L.

Answer

The steady-state drug plasma concentration and the half-life (or the elimination rate constant) can be estimated from the plot of the drug plasma concentrations obtained after termination of the infusion versus time on a semilog scale as in Figure 6.6.

Time zero represents the time when the infusion was terminated, so the y-intercept will be equal to the steady-state drug concentration.

1.

$$Cp_{ss} = 4 \text{ mg/L}$$

$$Cp_{ss} = \frac{K_0}{CL_T}$$

$$CL_T = \frac{24 \text{ mg/hr}}{4 \text{ mg/L}} = 6 \text{ L/hr}$$

$$t_{1/2} = 3.5 \text{ hr} \quad k = 0.198 \text{ hr}^{-1}$$

$$Vd = \frac{CL_T}{k} = \frac{6 \text{ L/hr}}{0.198 \text{ hr}^{-1}} = 30.3 \text{ L}$$

2.

$$LD = Cp \times Vd = 10 \text{ mg/L} \times 30.3 \text{ L} = 303 \text{ mg}$$

$$K_0 = Cp_{ss} \times CL_T = 10 \text{ mg/L} \times 6 \text{ L/hr} = 60 \text{ mg/hr}$$

The recommendation is 303 mg administered as an IV bolus dose followed immediately by 60 mg/hr as a constant-rate IV infusion. This regimen should achieve a steady-state concentration of 10 mg/L.

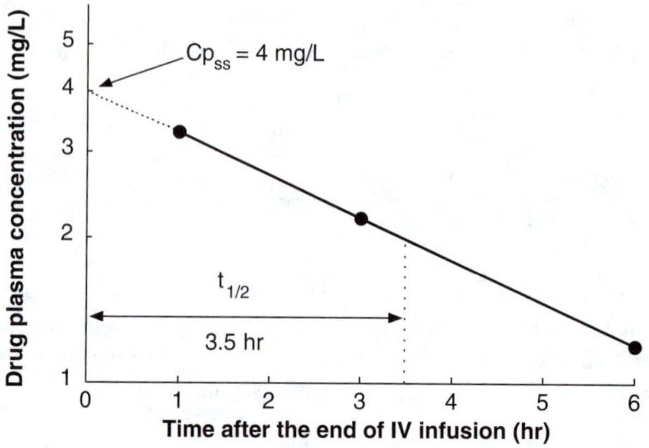

FIGURE 6.6 A plot of the drug plasma concentrations obtained after termination of the infusion versus time on the semilog scale. The y-intercept is equal to the steady-state concentration, and the half-life can be calculated graphically.

6.6 EFFECT OF CHANGING THE PHARMACOKINETIC PARAMETERS ON STEADY-STATE PLASMA CONCENTRATION DURING CONSTANT-RATE IV INFUSION

6.6.1 Infusion Rate

The steady-state plasma concentration is proportional to the infusion rate of the drug. Increasing the infusion rate of the drug causes a proportional increase in the steady-state drug concentration if the total body clearance of the drug remains constant.

6.6.2 Volume of Distribution

The volume of distribution does not affect the steady-state concentration. The steady-state drug concentration is only dependent on the total body clearance and the infusion rate K_0. When the volume of distribution is different in patients with similar total body clearance, the half-life and k (the dependent parameters) will be different in these individuals. This will result in a faster approach to the same steady state for the drugs with the larger CL_T/Vd ratio (larger k and shorter half-life).

6.6.3 Total Body Clearance

The steady-state drug concentration is inversely proportional to the total body clearance. Lower CL_T results in higher steady-state concentration when the infusion rate is kept constant. The same drug can have different CL_T in different individuals because of differences in the function of the eliminating organs. Administration of the same infusion rate of the drug to patients with different CL_T will produce a higher steady-state drug concentration in patients with lower CL_T.

PRACTICE PROBLEMS

6.1. A physician asks you to recommend a loading dose and a constant rate IV infusion of a drug to rapidly achieve a steady-state concentration of 15 mg/L. The half-life of this drug is 6 hr, and the volume of distribution is 30 L. What is your recommendation?

6.2. A patient received an antiasthmatic medication as a 200-mg IV loading dose followed immediately by a constant-rate IV infusion of 70 mg/hr. The IV infusion continued for 5 days, and after termination of the infusion the half-life was 3 hr, and the volume of distribution was 30 L.

a. What is the elimination rate of this drug during the infusion at steady state?
b. What is the steady-state concentration during the infusion?
c. What is the elimination rate constant of this drug?
d. What is the steady-state concentration if a loading dose of 400 mg was administered followed by the 70-mg/hr infusion?
e. What is the time to reach steady state if no loading dose was administered?
f. What is the steady-state concentration if an infusion rate of 140 mg/hr was administered?

6.3. A patient was admitted to the hospital because of cardiac arrhythmia. He received an antiarrhythmic drug as an IV loading dose injection followed by a constant-rate infusion of 30 mg/hr. The infusion continued for 3 days, and then the physician decided to stop the infusion. Samples were obtained after the end of infusion. A plot of the plasma concentrations obtained after stopping the infusion versus time is linear on semilog graph paper and has a slope of $-0.043\ hr^{-1}$ and an intercept of 7.5 mg/L.

a. Calculate the half-life and the volume of distribution of the antiarrhythmic drug in this patient.
b. Recommend an IV loading dose and a constant-rate infusion that can achieve a steady-state plasma concentration of 12 mg/L.

6.4. A patient received an antiasthmatic medication as a 300-mg IV loading dose followed immediately by a constant-rate IV infusion of 100 mg/hr. The IV infusion continued for 5 days, and after termination of the infusion, three plasma samples were obtained. A plot of the plasma concentrations obtained after termination (stopping) of the infusion has a y-intercept of 16 mg/L and a slope of $-0.06\ hr^{-1}$.

a. What is the half-life of this drug?
b. What is the volume of distribution of this drug?
c. What is the steady-state concentration if no loading dose was administered?
d. What is the steady-state drug concentration if the infusion rate was 200 mg/hr?

6.5. A patient received an antiasthmatic medication as a 300-mg IV loading dose followed immediately by a constant-rate IV infusion of 100 mg/hr. The IV infusion continued for 5 days, and after termination (stopping) of the infusion, three plasma samples were obtained.

Time After Termination of the Infusion (hr)	Plasma Drug Concentration (mg/L)
3	10.6
6	7.0
12	3.0

a. Calculate the plasma drug concentration at steady state graphically.
b. What is the elimination rate of the drug at steady state?
c. What is the half-life of this drug?
d. What is the steady-state concentration if the loading dose was changed to 600 mg?
e. What is the steady-state drug concentration if the infusion rate was 200 mg/hr?

6.6. A 60-kg male was admitted to the hospital with a chief complaint of shortness of breath. He was diagnosed as having acute bronchial asthma. He received a single IV loading dose of theophylline, followed by a constant-rate IV infusion of 60 mg/hr of the same drug. On the fourth day after starting the IV infusion, the patient complained of nausea and vomiting, which are the most common adverse effects of this drug. For this reason, the continuous IV infusion was stopped, and three plasma samples were obtained 1, 3, and 9 hr after termination of the IV infusion.

Time After Termination of the IV Infusion (hr)	Concentration (mg/L)
1	18.3
3	15.0
9	8.3

a. What is the rate of elimination of this antiasthmatic drug during the constant-rate IV infusion at steady state?
b. Calculate the half-life of this drug graphically.
c. Calculate the volume of distribution of this drug.
d. Recommend an IV loading dose and an IV infusion rate that should achieve a steady-state theophylline concentration of 15 mg/L in this patient.

6.7. A patient received an anticancer drug by a constant-rate IV infusion of 20 mg/hr. The IV infusion continued for 3 days, and after termination of the infusion, the half-life was 6 hr, and the volume of distribution was 35 L.

a. What is the elimination rate of this drug during the infusion at steady state?
b. What is the steady-state concentration during the infusion?
c. What is the elimination rate constant of this drug?
d. What is the steady-state concentration if a loading dose of 200 mg was administered followed by the 20-mg/hr infusion?
e. What is the time to reach steady state if the loading dose was not administered?
f. What is the steady-state concentration if the infusion rate was 40 mg/hr?

7 Steady State during Multiple Drug Administrations

OBJECTIVES

After completing this chapter, you should be able to:

- Define the steady state during multiple drug administrations
- Identify the factors that affect the steady-state plasma concentration during multiple drug administrations
- Determine the steady-state drug concentrations and patients' pharmacokinetic parameters during multiple drug administrations
- Analyze the effect of changing one or more of the pharmacokinetic parameters on the steady-state plasma concentration during multiple drug administrations
- Recommend the dosing regimen to achieve specific plasma concentrations in patients
- Evaluate the appropriateness of certain dosing regimens for patients

7.1 INTRODUCTION

Treatment of chronic diseases involves repeated administration of the same maintenance dose D every fixed dosing interval τ for a certain period of time. During repeated drug administration, the dose of the drug is administered before the previous dose is completely eliminated. This will cause drug accumulation in the body. If the drug elimination follows first-order kinetics, then the rate of drug elimination will be increasing because of the increase in the amount of drug in the body. When the rate of drug elimination is equal to the rate of drug administration, the amount of drug in the body will be constant, and steady state will be achieved. At steady state, the amount of the drug eliminated during one dosing interval is equal to the dose during repeated drug administrations. The amount of the drug in the body will reach steady state as long as the dosing rate is constant and the drug elimination pathways follow first-order kinetics.

7.2 DRUG PLASMA CONCENTRATION-TIME PROFILE DURING MULTIPLE DRUG ADMINISTRATIONS

The plasma drug concentration during repeated intravenous (IV) bolus administration changes during each dosing interval. However, the drug concentration–time profile during each dosing interval will be identical at steady state if a constant dose is administered at equally spaced intervals. At steady state, the maximum plasma drug concentration Cp_{max} achieved right after drug administration and the minimum plasma concentration Cp_{min}, which is the plasma concentration immediately before drug administration, are similar during multiple drug administrations as illustrated in Figure 7.1.

The maximum amount of the drug at steady state ($A_{ss\ max}$) during multiple IV bolus administrations is equal to:

$$A_{ss.\ max} = \frac{D}{(1 - e^{-k\tau})} \tag{7.1}$$

where D is the dose, k is the elimination rate constant, and τ is the dosing interval.

Also,

$$A_{ss.\ min} = A_{ss.\ max}\ e^{-k\tau} \tag{7.2}$$

where $A_{ss.min}$ is the minimum drug amount present in the body at steady state, that is, the drug amount in the body just before administration of the new dose. It is also true that

$$A_{ss.\ max} - A_{ss.\ min} = \text{Dose} \tag{7.3}$$

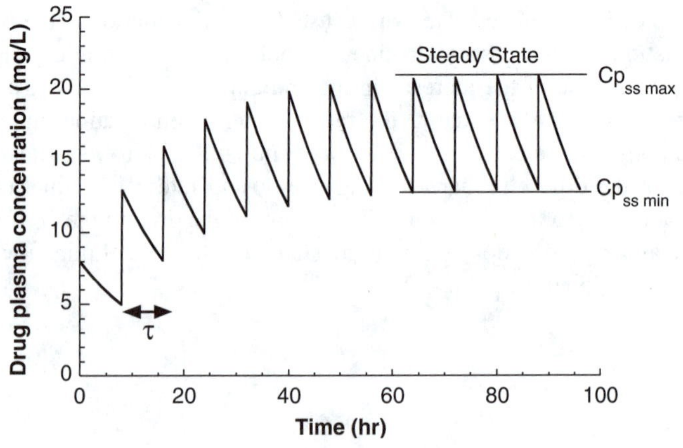

FIGURE 7.1 The drug plasma concentration–time profile during multiple IV administrations of a fixed dose of the drug every fixed dosing interval.

The maximum and minimum plasma concentrations at steady state can be determined by dividing the amounts of the drug by the volume of distribution Vd, that is,

$$Cp_{ss.\,max} = \frac{D}{Vd\,(1 - e^{-k\tau})} \tag{7.4}$$

and

$$Cp_{ss.\,min} = Cp_{ss.\,max}\; e^{-k\tau} \tag{7.5}$$

and

$$Cp_{ss.\,max} - Cp_{ss.\,min} = \frac{Dose}{Vd} \tag{7.6}$$

These relationships are derived assuming that a constant dose of the drug D is administered repeatedly by IV bolus injections every fixed dosing interval τ. When the drug is given by extravascular administration and the rate of drug absorption to the systemic circulation is rapid, the same relationships can be applied to approximate the relationship between the maximum and the minimum drug concentrations at steady state. Rapid drug absorption allows most of the absorbed drug to reach the systemic circulation before a significant amount of the drug is eliminated, and the time difference between Cp_{max} and Cp_{min} is approximately equal to the dosing interval. So, the drug profile during repeated oral drug administration with rapid absorption approximates the profile after repeated IV bolus administration. However, during oral drug administration, the bioavailability of the drug F has to be considered because rapid absorption does not mean complete absorption. So, for repeated oral administration when the drug absorption is rapid, the following equations can be used to determine the drug plasma concentration at steady state:

$$Cp_{ss.\,max} = \frac{F\;D}{Vd\,(1 - e^{-k\tau})} \tag{7.7}$$

and

$$Cp_{ss.\,min} = Cp_{ss.\,max}\; e^{-k\tau}$$

similar to Equation 7.5, and

$$Cp_{ss.\,max} - Cp_{ss.\,min} = \frac{F\;Dose}{Vd} \tag{7.8}$$

When the drug is not rapidly absorbed, these equations cannot be used because a significant amount of the drug is eliminated during the absorption phase. Also, the time between Cp_{max} and Cp_{min} is not equal to τ.

7.3 AVERAGE PLASMA CONCENTRATION AT STEADY STATE

During multiple drug administrations, the plasma drug concentrations at steady state and the Cp_{max} and Cp_{min} fluctuate around an average drug concentration as in Figure 7.2. The average plasma concentration at steady state is dependent on the dosing rate FD/τ and the total body clearance CL_T.

$$Cp_{ss\ average} = \frac{F\,D}{CL_T\ \tau} \tag{7.9}$$

Different dosing regimens can have the same dosing rate if the bioavailability is constant. For example, consider the following dosing regimens:

100 mg every 4 hr
150 mg every 6 hr
200 mg every 8 hr
300 mg every 12 hr

All these dosing regimens have the same dosing rate. So, the average steady-state concentration achieved at steady state after administration of these regimens should be similar if the total body clearance remains constant. However, the fluctuations in plasma concentration around this average concentration will be different after

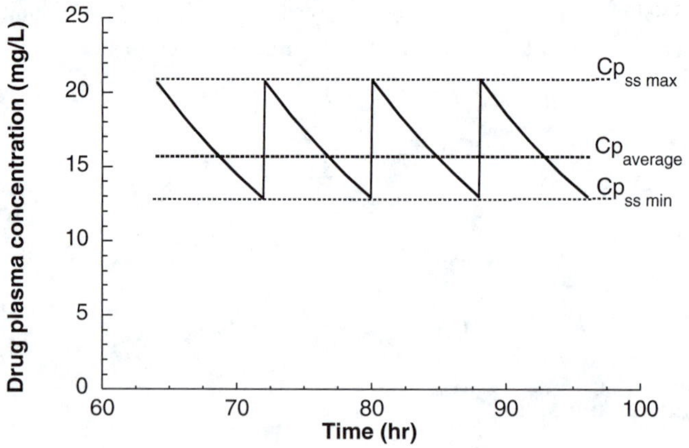

FIGURE 7.2 During multiple drug administrations, the drug plasma concentrations fluctuate around the average drug plasma concentration.

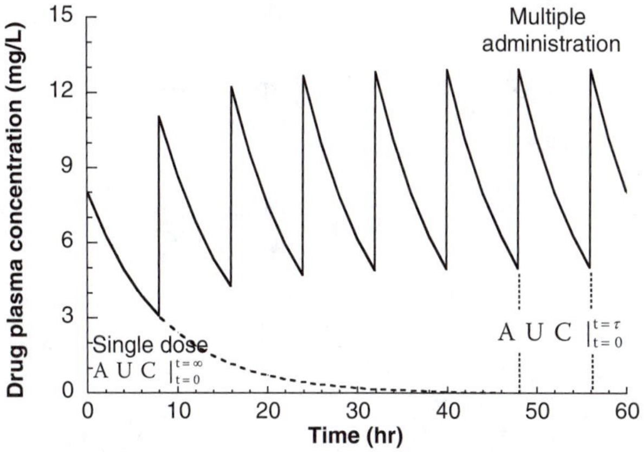

FIGURE 7.3 The AUC from time zero to ∞ after a single dose is equal to the AUC from time zero to τ at steady state during multiple administrations of the same dose.

administration of these different dosing regimens. This means that the maximum and the minimum concentrations will be different, but the average concentration will be the same. The regimen with the longest dosing interval will have the largest fluctuations in the plasma concentration. It is important to note that the average concentration is not the mean value of the maximum and the minimum plasma concentrations. The area under the curve (AUC) from time zero to ∞ after a single dose is equal to the AUC from time zero to τ at steady state during multiple administrations of the same dose as shown in Figure 7.3. The AUC is equal to

$$AUC = \frac{F\,D}{k\ Vd} \tag{7.10}$$

Therefore,

$$Cp_{ss\ \text{average}} = \frac{AUC}{\tau} \tag{7.11}$$

This means that the average plasma concentration at steady state can be calculated by calculating the AUC after a single dose and dividing it by the dosing interval.

Example

A patient is receiving 1000 mg of an antibiotic as repeated IV bolus doses every 12 hours to treat her lung infection. The maximum and minimum steady state plasma concentrations of this antibiotic are 48 mg/L and 5 mg/L, respectively.

1. Calculate the volume of distribution and the total body clearance of this antibiotic.
2. Calculate the average plasma concentration of this antibiotic at steady state while receiving 1000 mg every 12 hr.

Answer

$$Cp_{ss.\,max} - Cp_{ss.\,min} = \frac{Dose}{Vd}$$

$$48\ mg/L - 5\ mg/L = \frac{1000\ mg}{Vd}$$

$$Vd = \frac{1000\ mg}{43\ mg/L} = 23.3\ L$$

$$Cp_{ss.min} = Cp_{ss.\,max}\ e^{-k\,\tau}$$

$$5\ mg/L = 48\ mg/L\ e^{-k\ 12\,hr}$$

$$\ln\ \frac{5\ mg/L}{48\ mg/L} = -k\ \ 12\ hr$$

$$-2.262 = -k\ \ 12\ hr$$

$$k = 0.188\ hr^{-1}$$

$$CL_T = 0.188\ hr^{-1}\ 23.3\ L = 4.38\ L/hr$$

2.

$$Cp_{ss\ average} = \frac{F\,D}{k\ \ Vd\ \ \tau}$$

$$Cp_{ss\ average} = \frac{1000\ mg}{0.188\ hr^{-1}\ 23.3\ L\ \ 12\ hr} = 19\ mg/L$$

7.4 TIME REQUIRED TO REACH STEADY STATE

The time required to reach steady state depends on the half-life of the drug. Generally, it takes five to six elimination half-lives to reach steady state. This means that the drug has to be administered repeatedly for a period equal to five to six elimination half-lives of the drug to achieve steady state. The longer the drug half-life, the longer it takes to reach steady state.

Administration of different doses of the same drug to a group of individuals who have the same half-life and volume of distribution for the drug will achieve steady-state concentrations that are proportional to the dose. However, the time to achieve the steady state will be the same because we assume that the drug half-life is similar in all individuals.

7.5 LOADING DOSE

The loading dose is a dose larger than the maintenance dose administered at the initiation of therapy to achieve a faster approach to steady state. Administration of a loading dose is required when rapid therapeutic effect is necessary, such as in emergency situations. In these cases, waiting for five to six half-lives to achieve steady state may not be appropriate. The loading dose should be chosen to achieve a therapeutic drug concentration immediately. Then, the maintenance dose is chosen to maintain this therapeutic concentration at steady state.

7.5.1 Intravenous Drug Administration

$$\text{Loading dose} = Cp_{\text{desired}} \times Vd \tag{7.12}$$

7.5.2 Extravascular Drug Administration

$$\text{Loading dose} = \frac{Cp_{\text{desired}}\ Vd}{F} \tag{7.13}$$

It is important to note that the steady-state plasma concentration is dependent on the dosing rate FD/τ and the total body clearance. The loading dose does not affect the steady-state concentration.

7.6 DRUG ACCUMULATION

Repeated drug administration involves administration of the new doses before the drug from the previous doses is completely eliminated. This results in drug accumulation until steady state is achieved. Drugs are accumulated in the body to different degrees depending on the drug characteristics. The accumulation ratio Raccum is defined as the amount of drug in the body at steady state relative to the dose of the drug.

$$R_{\text{accum}} = \frac{A_{\text{ss average}}}{F\,D} \tag{7.14}$$

$$R_{\text{accum}} = \frac{F\,D/k\,\tau}{F\,D} = \frac{1}{k\,\tau} \tag{7.15}$$

A higher accumulation ratio means that the average amount of the drug in the body at steady state is much higher than the single dose of the drug and indicates a higher degree of drug accumulation.

7.7 CONTROLLED-RELEASE FORMULATIONS

Controlled-released formulations are specially designed to slowly release the drug from the dosage form over a long period of time. The rate of drug absorption will depend on the rate of its release from the formulation. This means that if the formulation is prepared such that it releases the drug at a constant rate over a long time, the rate of drug absorption will be constant, and this decreases the fluctuation in the drug plasma concentration during the dosing interval. Controlled-release formulations allow administration of larger doses of the drug less frequently without increasing the fluctuations in the drug concentration during the dosing interval. Also, the smaller fluctuations in the plasma drug concentrations at steady state can produce a relatively constant therapeutic effect when there is a direct relation between the drug concentration and the pharmacological effect.

After administration of the immediate release formulation, the drug is absorbed rapidly. Then, the plasma drug concentration declines until the time for the following dose. This results in large fluctuations in the plasma drug concentration during the dosing interval. However, after administration of the same dose of a controlled-release formulation, the drug is absorbed slowly, and this will produce much less fluctuation in the plasma concentrations during the dosing interval, as illustrated in Figure 7.4.

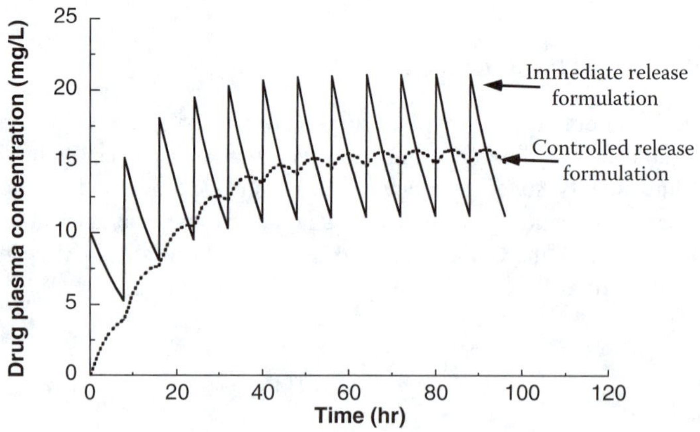

FIGURE 7.4 The plasma concentration–time profile after multiple administrations of the same dose of immediate-release and controlled-release oral formulations.

7.8 EFFECT OF CHANGING THE PHARMACOKINETIC PARAMETERS ON STEADY-STATE PLASMA CONCENTRATION DURING REPEATED DRUG ADMINISTRATION

7.8.1 Dosing Rate

The average steady-state plasma concentration is directly proportional to the dosing rate FD/τ. Increasing the dosing rate causes a proportional increase in the average steady-state concentration if the total body clearance remains constant. The dosing rate is increased by using a larger dose, a product with higher bioavailability, or administering the drug more frequently.

7.8.2 Total Body Clearance

The steady-state plasma concentration is inversely proportional to the total body clearance of the drug. Lower CL_T results in higher steady-state concentration when the dosing rate is kept constant. The same drug can have a different CL_T in different individuals because of differences in the function of the eliminating organs. Administration of a drug at the same dosing rate to patients with different CL_T will produce higher steady-state drug concentration in patients with lower CL_T.

7.8.3 Volume of Distribution

The volume of distribution does not affect the steady-state concentration if the total body clearance and the dosing rate are constant. The steady-state concentration is only dependent on the total body clearance and the dosing rate FD/τ. When the volume of distribution is different in patients with similar total body clearance, the half-life and k (the dependent parameters) will be different in these individuals. In these individuals, the steady state will be the same (same CL_T and FD/τ); however, the approach to steady state will be faster in the individuals with larger CL_T/Vd ratios (larger k and shorter half-life).

7.8.4 Absorption Rate Constant

The absorption rate of the drug does not affect the average steady-state drug concentration. However, administration of products that have a faster rate of drug absorption produces larger fluctuations in drug concentration during the dosing interval.

7.9 DOSAGE REGIMEN DESIGN

7.9.1 Factors to Be Considered

7.9.1.1 Therapeutic Range of the Drug

Drugs with a well-defined therapeutic range will have to be administered in doses that can maintain the plasma drug concentration within the therapeutic range all the time at steady state. Selection of the dosing regimens for drugs with a wide therapeutic range is easy because a wide range of doses can maintain the plasma concentration within the therapeutic range at steady state. However, drugs with a narrow therapeutic range require accurate selection of the appropriate dosing regimen.

7.9.1.2 Required Onset of Effect

When immediate drug effect is required, an appropriate loading dose should be administered to achieve the steady state faster. For the treatment of a chronic condition, administration of a loading dose may not be necessary.

7.9.1.3 Drug Formulation

Sustained-release formulations produce little fluctuations in drug concentration within each dosing interval; formulations that rapidly release the drug produce large fluctuations in drug concentration during multiple administrations. Formulations that release the drug rapidly may need to be administered more frequently in smaller doses.

7.9.1.4 Patient Disease State

Periodic evaluation of the dosing regimen and the therapeutic effects is necessary when the patient disease state is not stable and when the response of the body to the drug changes with time.

7.9.2 Estimation of Patient Pharmacokinetic Parameters

The selection of a drug dosing regimen to achieve steady-state concentration within the therapeutic range requires knowledge of the patient-specific pharmacokinetic parameters. Estimates for the drug pharmacokinetic parameters in a particular patient depend on the available information about the patient.

7.9.2.1 Lack of the Patient's Medical History

The average values for the drug pharmacokinetic parameters in the general population can be used as an estimate for the patient pharmacokinetic parameters when absolutely no information is known about the patient's medical history.

7.9.2.2 Information Available about the Patient's Medical History

The drug pharmacokinetic parameters can be estimated based on the patient's medical history by identifying any condition that might alter the drug pharmacokinetics. For example, the pharmacokinetic parameters of an aminoglycoside antibiotic (eliminated mainly by the kidney) in a particular patient can be estimated depending on the kidney function of the patient.

7.9.2.3 Patient with History of Using the Drug

When the patient has a history of using the drug under consideration, this information should be used to estimate the drug pharmacokinetic parameters. Consider any new changes in the patient's condition that may alter the drug pharmacokinetics. When the drug under consideration has a narrow therapeutic index, attempts should be made to determine the patient-specific pharmacokinetic parameters after starting drug therapy. These specific parameter estimates can be useful for individualization of drug therapy.

7.9.3 Selection of Dose and Dosing Interval

The selection of dose and dosing interval depends on the drug pharmacokinetic parameters and the characteristics of the drug formulation.

7.9.3.1 Controlled-Release Oral Formulation

The dose and dosing interval should be chosen to achieve average plasma concentration within the therapeutic range according to

$$Cp_{ss\ average} = \frac{F\,D}{k\ Vd\ \tau}$$

The choice of the dosing interval for sustained-release formulations usually depends on the formulation characteristics. This is usually recommended by the manufacturer.

7.9.3.2 Fast-Release Oral Formulations and IV Bolus Administration

During repeated administration of IV bolus and fast-release oral formulations, large fluctuation in the plasma concentrations is observed. The steady-state maximum and minimum plasma concentrations have to be within the therapeutic range.

7.9.3.2.1 Selection of the Dosing Interval

The desired maximum and minimum plasma concentrations are selected based on the therapeutic range of the drug. Then, the dosing interval is determined as the time period required for the maximum plasma concentration to decline to the minimum plasma concentration. The desired maximum and minimum concentrations and the elimination rate constant k are substituted in the following equation, which is solved for the dosing interval:

$$Cp_{ss.\ min} = Cp_{ss.\ max}\ e^{-k\tau}$$

The selected dosing interval should be rounded to the nearest practical dosing interval (6, 8, 12, 18, 24 hr, etc.).

7.9.3.2.2 Selection of Dose

The dose required to achieve the desired maximum steady-state drug concentration when given every τ can be determined from

$$Cp_{ss.\ max} = \frac{F\ D}{Vd\ (1 - e^{-k\tau})}$$

Again, it may be necessary to round the selected dose to the nearest practical dose.

7.9.4 Selection of Loading Dose

When a loading dose is required, the loading dose is selected based on the desired plasma concentration and the drug volume of distribution:

$$\text{Loading dose} = \frac{Cp_{\text{desired}}\ Vd}{F}$$

Example

A patient was admitted to the hospital after experiencing an episode of ventricular arrhythmia. The physician decided to start the patient on an IV regimen of an antiarrhythmic drug. The volume of distribution of this antiarrhythmic drug is 45 L, the half-life is 7 hr, and the therapeutic range is 4–12 mg/L.

1. Recommend an IV loading dose and the IV dosing regimen (dose and dosing interval) that should maintain the drug concentration within the therapeutic range all the time.
2. The patient was stabilized on the regimen you recommended and is ready to go home. The physician wanted to shift the patient to an oral formulation of the same drug. What will be the dosing regimen (dose and dosing interval) from the oral formulation if the oral formulation of this drug is rapidly absorbed and has a bioavailability of 75%?

Answer

1. The loading dose is the dose that should achieve the maximum plasma concentration:

$$\text{Loading dose} = Cp_{\text{desired}}\ Vd$$

$$\text{LD} = 12\ \text{mg/L} \times 45\ \text{L} = 540\ \text{mg}$$

Dosing interval:

$$4\ \text{mg/L} = 12\ \text{mg/L}\ e^{-0.099\ \text{hr}^{-1}\ \tau}$$

$$\ln \frac{4\ \text{mg/L}}{12\ \text{mg/L}} = -\ 0.099\ \text{hr}^{-1}\ \tau$$

$$-1.0986 = -0.099\ \text{hr}^{-1}\ \tau$$

$$\tau = 11\ \text{hr}$$

So, an appropriate dosing interval will be 12 hr.

Selection of dose:

$$Cp_{ss.\,max} = \frac{D}{Vd\,(1 - e^{-k\tau})}$$

$$12\ \text{mg/L} = \frac{D}{45\ \text{L}\,(1 - e^{-0.099\ \text{hr}^{-1}\ 12\ \text{hr}})}$$

$$\text{Dose} = 375\ \text{mg}$$

The recommendation is that the patient should receive an IV loading dose of 540 mg and then 375 mg administered as IV bolus doses every 12 hr.

2. For the dosing regimen for the oral formulation, the dosing interval is dependent on the rate of elimination of the drug, so this rapidly absorbed oral formulation should also be administered every 12 hr. However, the dose will be different because of the incomplete bioavailability.

$$Cp_{ss.\,max} = \frac{F\,D}{Vd\,(1 - e^{-k\tau})}$$

$$12\ \text{mg/L} = \frac{0.75\ D}{45\ \text{l}\,(1 - e^{-0.099\ \text{hr}^{-1}\ 12\ \text{hr}})}$$

Dose = 500 mg

The recommendation is for 500 mg of the oral formulation every 12 hr.

PRACTICE PROBLEMS

7.1. An antibiotic has a volume of distribution of 20 L and an elimination rate constant of 0.1 hr^{-1}. This antibiotic is administered by repeated IV bolus doses of 200 mg every 8 hr.

a. Calculate the maximum and the minimum plasma drug concentration at steady state.
b. Calculate the average steady-state concentration of this antibiotic.
c. What is the dose that should be given every 8 hr to achieve a steady-state average plasma drug concentration of 25 mg/L?

7.2. A 72-year-old, 85-kg male patient was admitted to the hospital for the treatment of severe lung infection. His dosing regimen of the antibiotic was 500 mg daily given at 8 a.m. by IV bolus administration. At steady state, the maximum and the minimum plasma concentration of this antibiotic were 35 mg/L and 10 mg/L, respectively.

a. Calculate the half-life of this antibiotic in this patient.
b. Calculate the volume of distribution of this antibiotic in this patient.
c. Calculate the average steady-state plasma concentration of the drug.

7.3. After a single oral dose of 200 mg theophylline to a 10-year-old patient, the total AUC was 100 mg-h/L. (Assume that theophylline is completely absorbed.)

a. Calculate the average theophylline plasma concentration at steady state if this patient is taking 200 mg theophylline every 6 hr.
b. Calculate the average theophylline plasma concentration at steady state if this patient is shifted to 400 mg every 12 hr from a controlled-release formulation.
c. Calculate the dose of the controlled-release formulation that can achieve an average steady-state concentration of 10 mg/L in this patient if the dose is administered every 12 hr.

7.4. An antihypertensive drug is administered as 200 mg daily for a controlled-release formulation that is known to have 75% bioavailability. The drug has a half-life of 24 hr and a volume of distribution of 24 L.

a. Calculate the average steady-state concentration of this drug.
b. What is the dose required to achieve an average steady-state concentration of 20 mg/L using the same formulation?
c. What is the daily IV dose required from an IV formulation of the drug to achieve an average steady-state concentration of 20 mg/L?
d. Calculate the maximum and the minimum plasma drug concentration at steady state while taking the regimen you recommended in answer to question 7.4c.

7.5. A patient is receiving antihypertensive medication as 500 mg every 8 hr in the form of an oral capsule. After administration of this oral capsule, only 80% of the active ingredient in the capsule reaches the systemic circulation. The CL_T of this drug in this patient was 2.5 L/hr.

a. What is the average steady-state plasma concentration of this drug in this patient?
b. What will be the average steady-state plasma concentration if the patient was taking 1000 mg every 8 hr from the same oral drug product?
c. What will be the CL_T of the drug in this patient while taking the 1000 mg every 8 hr orally?
d. What will be the oral dose required to achieve an average plasma concentration of 30 mg/L from this drug in this patient?
e. Because the patient had problems swallowing the oral capsules, he was shifted to 500 mg IV every 8 hr. What will be the average steady-state concentration of this drug in this patient?

7.6. A patient received a single IV bolus dose of 300 mg of an antibiotic, and the following plasma concentrations were obtained:

Time (hr)	Drug Concentration (mg/L)
2	12.86
6	9.45
12	5.95
24	2.36

a. What are the maximum and the minimum steady-state drug concentrations in a patient who was taking 250 mg every 12 hr from a rapidly absorbed oral formulation with a bioavailability of 80%?
b. What is the average steady-state concentration of this drug in the patient while taking the regimen in question 7.6a?
c. What will be the maximum and the minimum steady state drug concentrations if the dose was increased to 500 mg every 12 hr from this oral formulation?

7.7. A patient is taking 450 mg of an antibiotic every 12 hr as IV bolus doses. At steady state, the maximum and minimum plasma antibiotic concentrations were 40 mg/L and 10 mg/L, respectively.

a. Calculate the half-life of this antibiotic in this patient.
b. Calculate the volume of distribution of this antibiotic in this patient.
c. Calculate the average steady-state plasma concentration of the drug.
d. What is the approximate time for this drug to achieve steady state?
e. What is the amount of the drug eliminated from this antibiotic during one dosing interval at steady state?

7.8. A patient is receiving IV theophylline to control an acute episode of bronchial asthma. The maintenance dose is a 320-mg IV bolus of theophylline every 8 hr. At steady state, the maximum and minimum theophylline plasma concentrations were 18 mg/L and 10 mg/L, respectively.

a. What are the half-life and the volume of distribution of theophylline in this patient?
b. What is the daily dose of an oral theophylline preparation that is required to achieve an average plasma theophylline concentration of 18 mg/L? (The bioavailability of the oral preparation is 100%.)

7.9. A patient was admitted to the hospital because of severe ventricular arrhythmia. The patient's acute condition was treated, and the physician wanted to start the patient on multiple IV bolus administrations of an antiarrhythmic drug. The physician asks you to recommend a loading dose and the dosing regimen that should maintain the maximum and the minimum steady state drug concentrations of approximately 20 mg/L and 10 mg/L, respectively. This drug has an elimination rate constant of 0.06 hr^{-1} and a volume of distribution of 30 L.

a. What is your recommendation for the IV loading dose that should immediately achieve 20 mg/L?
b. What is the most appropriate dosing interval for this drug?
c. What is the appropriate maintenance dose for this drug?
d. What is the average steady-state concentration of this drug achieved from the regimen you recommended?
e. The patient was stabilized on the regimen you recommended and is ready to go home. The physician asks you to recommend the dosing

regimen of the oral formulation of the same drug to achieve the same average steady-state concentration if this oral formulation is known to have bioavailability of 75%. What is your recommendation?

7.10. The therapeutic range of an antihypertensive drug is 8–25 mg/L. The drug has a half-life of 7 hr and volume of distribution of 30 L. After oral administration, this drug is rapidly absorbed, and only 85% of the dose reaches the systemic circulation.

a. What is the most appropriate dosing interval for this drug?
b. What is the appropriate maintenance dose for this drug?
c. What is the average steady-state concentration achieved from the regimen you recommended?

8 Renal Drug Elimination

OBJECTIVES

After completing this chapter you should be able to:

- Discuss the mechanisms of renal drug excretion
- Determine the drug pharmacokinetic parameters from the urinary excretion rate data
- Calculate the renal clearance of drugs from the urinary excretion rate data
- Analyze the effect of changing the dose, total body clearance, and renal clearance on the urinary excretion of drugs
- Predict the change in the overall elimination rate of drugs caused by the change in their renal excretion

8.1 INTRODUCTION

Elimination of drugs from the body can occur by one or more pathways. The major elimination pathways include renal excretion, metabolism, biliary excretion, and lung excretion. The rate of the overall elimination process is governed by the elimination rate constant k. When the drug elimination pathways follow first-order kinetics, the overall elimination rate constant is the sum of the rate constants associated with each of the individual pathways. For example, if a drug is excreted by renal excretion, metabolism, and biliary excretion, the overall elimination rate constant k will be equal to

$$k = k_e + k_m + k_b \tag{8.1}$$

where k_e is the renal excretion rate constant, k_m is the metabolic rate constant, and k_b is the biliary excretion rate constant. Also, by multiplying both sides of Equation 8.1 by the volume of distribution Vd,

$$kVd = k_eVd + k_mVd + k_bVd \tag{8.2}$$

which means that

Total body clearance = Renal clearance + Metabolic clearance + Biliary clearance

that is, the total body clearance is the sum of the individual organ clearances.

It is important to study the kinetics of the individual elimination pathways of the drug in addition to studying the kinetics of the overall elimination process to determine the contribution of each pathway to the overall elimination process. This also allows study of the effect of changing the function of one of the eliminating organs on the drug pharmacokinetics and studying drug interactions that involve a specific elimination pathway. The renal excretion of drugs can be studied by collecting urine samples and measuring the amount of drug excreted over a certain period of time.

8.2 MECHANISMS OF RENAL EXCRETION OF DRUGS

The three processes involved in the renal excretion of drugs are the glomerular filtration, tubular secretion, and tubular reabsorption.

8.2.1 Glomerular Filtration

The blood is filtered in the glomeruli at a rate of 120 ml/min, and the rate of this process is called the *glomerular filtration rate* (GFR). All small molecules with molecular weight below 2000 g/mol can be filtered freely in the glomeruli. Larger molecules can be filtered through the glomeruli depending on their molecular size. However, large protein molecules such as albumin cannot be filtered. So, drug molecules that are bound to plasma protein cannot be filtered, and only free drug molecules are filtered. The rate of drug filtration in the glomeruli is the product of the free (unbound) drug concentration in plasma and the GFR (i.e., Free drug concentration × GFR). Reduced kidney function can lead to a lower GFR. Also, some diseases (e.g., nephrotic syndrome) can affect the glomerular filtration process and allow the filtration of larger protein molecules such as albumin and globulins.

8.2.2 Tubular Secretion

Drug molecules can be actively secreted in the proximal tubules. There are specific transport systems for anions, cations, and quaternary amines in the renal tubules. These transport systems actively secrete the drug molecules from the plasma to the lumen of the nephron. These transport systems are not specific; however, they can transport compounds with similar characteristics. So, drugs can compete with each other for the same transport system, and drugs with higher affinity for the transport system can inhibit the secretion of other drugs with lower affinity (e.g., probenecid inhibits the active secretion of penicillins in the renal tubules). Because most of the water filtered in the glomeruli is reabsorbed in the renal tubules, the drug concentration in the nephron lumen is always higher than the plasma drug concentration. So, the drug cannot be passively secreted in the renal tubules.

8.2.3 Tubular Reabsorption

Drugs and solutes filtered in the glomeruli or actively secreted in the proximal tubules can be reabsorbed throughout the tubules. This reabsorption process can be passive or active. Because of the water reabsorption in the renal tubules, solutes become concentrated and can be reabsorbed passively to the bloodstream. Lipophilic molecules can cross the tubular membrane and can be reabsorbed easier than hydrophilic molecules.

Ionizable molecules can be reabsorbed better when they are in their un-ionized form compared to their ionized form. So, the reabsorption and urinary secretion of ionizable molecules can be manipulated by changing the urinary pH. Some vitamins, amino acids, and glucose can be reabsorbed by an active saturable transport system.

The rate of renal excretion of a drug is the sum of the rates of filtration and active secretion minus the rate of reabsorption from the renal tubules:

Renal excretion rate = Rate of filtration + Rate of active secretion − Rate of reabsorption

8.3 DETERMINATION OF RENAL EXCRETION RATE

The drug present in a collected urine sample represents the amount of the drug excreted during the period of time during which the urine was formed. Because the renal excretion of most drugs follows first-order kinetics, the renal excretion rate at any time is equal to

$$\frac{dA_e}{dt} = k_e\ A \qquad (8.3)$$

where A_e is the amount of the drug excreted in urine, k_e is the first-order renal excretion rate constant, and A is the amount of the drug in the body. However, urine samples are usually collected over certain time intervals.

$$\frac{\Delta A_e}{\Delta t} = k_e\ A_{average} \qquad (8.4)$$

where ΔA_e is the amount of the drug excreted in urine over a certain urine collection interval Δt, $\Delta A_e/\Delta t$ is the renal excretion rate, k_e is the first-order renal excretion rate constant, and $A_{average}$ is the average amount of the drug in the body during the urine collection interval.

8.3.1 Experimental Determination of Renal Excretion Rate

- Select the length of time for each of the urine collection intervals.
- Collect urine samples at the end of each urine collection interval.
- Measure the volume of each urine sample.
- Determine the drug concentration in each urine sample.
- Calculate the amount of the drug excreted during each urine collection interval.

  Amount excreted = Drug concentration in urine × Sample volume

- Calculate the renal excretion rate.

$$\text{Renal excretion rate} = \frac{\text{Amount excreted}}{\text{Time of urine collection}} \qquad (8.5)$$

The calculated renal excretion rate is the average renal excretion rate during each of the urine collection intervals.

8.3.2 Renal Excretion Rate–Time Profile

The renal excretion rate is dependent on the renal excretion rate constant and the amount of the drug in the body, assuming that the renal excretion process follows first-order kinetics. Because the amount of the drug in the body decreases with time because of drug elimination, the renal excretion rate will always be decreasing. The renal excretion rate after a single intravenous (IV) administration can be described by

$$\frac{\Delta A_e}{\Delta t} = k_e \; A_0 \; e^{-kt} \tag{8.6}$$

where k_e is the renal excretion rate constant, A_0 is the initial amount of the drug in the body that is equal to the dose, and k is the (overall) elimination rate constant. This is because the amount of the drug in the body decreases at a rate dependent on the overall elimination rate constant. A plot of the renal excretion rate versus time on semilog graph paper will be a straight line with the y-intercept equal to k_eA_0 (or k_e Dose) and a slope of $-k/2.303$. This means that the elimination half-life, the elimination rate constant, and the renal excretion rate constant of the drug can be determined from the plot of the renal excretion rate versus time as in Figure 8.1.

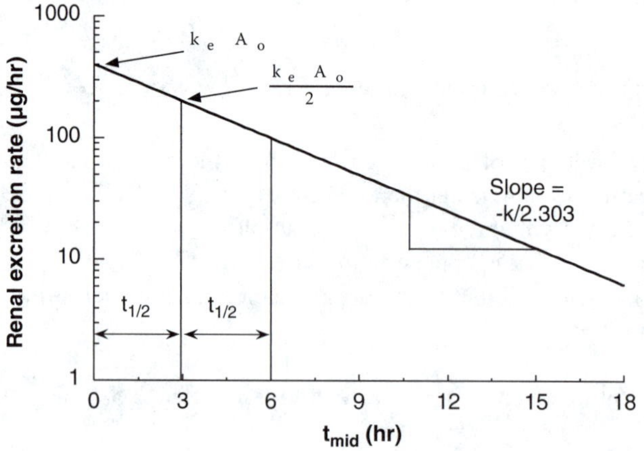

FIGURE 8.1 The half-life and the renal excretion rate constant can be determined from the plot of the renal excretion rate versus time on the semilog scale.

8.4 RENAL CLEARANCE

The *renal clearance* is defined as the volume of the blood or plasma that is completely cleared of the drug per unit time by the kidney.

The renal excretion rate is determined by

$$\frac{\Delta A_e}{\Delta t} = k_e \ A_{t-mid} \tag{8.7}$$

where $A_{t\text{-mid}}$ is the amount of drug in the body at the midpoint of the urine collection interval, which is approximately equal to the average amount of the drug during the urine collection interval. Because the amount of the drug is equal to the drug concentration times the volume of distribution,

$$\frac{\Delta A_e}{\Delta t} = k_e \ Vd \ Cp_{t-mid} \tag{8.8}$$

and

$$\frac{\frac{\Delta A_e}{\Delta t}}{Cp_{t-mid}} = \text{Renal clearance} \tag{8.9}$$

where $Cp_{t\text{-mid}}$ is the drug plasma concentration at the midpoint of the urine collection interval. A plot of the renal excretion rate versus the plasma concentration at the middle of the urine collection interval on the Cartesian scale will be a straight line going through the origin, and the slope of the line is equal to the renal clearance as in Figure 8.2.

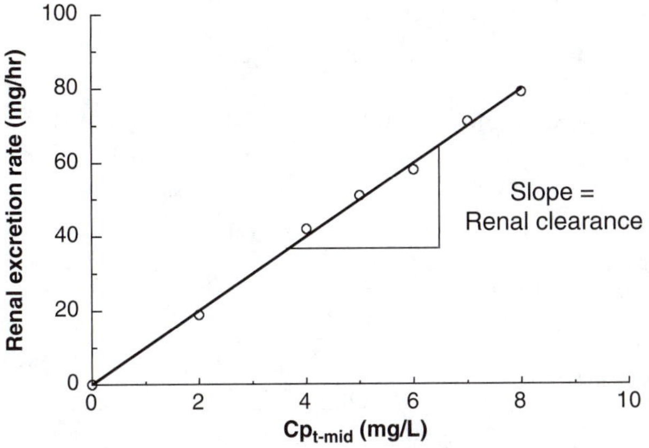

FIGURE 8.2 The renal excretion rate versus plasma concentration at the middle of the urine collection interval plot. The renal clearance is equal to the slope of the line.

So, the renal clearance can be determined experimentally by collecting urine samples over short time intervals after drug administration. The amount of drug excreted during each urine collection interval is determined, and the rate of drug excretion is calculated by dividing the amount excreted by the time interval of the urine collection. The plasma concentration at the middle of each urine collection interval is also determined. The relationship in Equation 8.9 can be used to determine the renal clearance during each urine collection. Also, the renal excretion rate is plotted versus the plasma concentration obtained in the middle of each urine collection interval. The slope of the resulting line is equal to the renal clearance.

Drugs with renal clearance larger than the GFR are actively secreted in the renal tubules. When the renal clearance is lower than the GFR, this means that the drug undergoes glomerular filtration and then reabsorption, or the drug undergoes glomerular filtration, tubular secretion, and then reabsorption.

8.4.1 Creatinine Clearance as a Measure of Kidney Function

Creatinine is an endogenous compound that is completely eliminated from the body by the kidney. It is filtered in the glomeruli and neither secreted nor reabsorbed to any significant extent. So, the renal clearance of creatinine represents an accurate measure of the GFR. The creatinine clearance is used as a diagnostic test to evaluate kidney function.

The creatinine clearance is determined as follows:

- Collect all the urine excreted by the patient over a period of 24 hr.
- Obtain a plasma sample and determine the plasma creatinine concentration. Because creatinine plasma concentration is relatively constant, this sample represents the average creatinine plasma concentration during the urine collection period.
- Determine the total volume of the urine collected and the creatinine concentration in the urine sample.
- Calculate the total amount of creatinine excreted (Amount = Volume × Concentration).
- Calculate the renal excretion rate.

$$\text{Renal excretion rate} = \frac{\text{Amount excreted}}{\text{Time of urine collection}}$$

- Calculate the creatinine clearance

$$\text{Creatinine clearance} = \frac{\text{Creatinine excretion rate}}{\text{Creatinine plasma concentration}} \qquad (8.10)$$

Example

The physician asked a patient to collect urine over a period of 24 hr for the determination of creatinine clearance. By the end of the 24 hr, the total volume of urine collected was 2200 ml. Aliquots of the urine sample together with 1 ml serum were sent to the lab for creatinine determination. The creatinine concentration in urine was 0.2 mg/ml, and the serum creatinine was 3.0 mg/dl (3.0 mg/100 ml).

Calculate the creatinine clearance in this patient.

Answer

$$\text{Total amount of creatinine excreted in 24 hr} = \text{Urine volume} \times \text{Urine concentration}$$
$$= 2200 \text{ ml} \times 0.2 \text{ mg/ml} = 440 \text{ mg}$$

$$\text{Renal excretion rate} = \frac{440 \text{ mg}}{24 \text{ hr } 60 \text{ min/hr}} = 0.3055 \text{ mg/min}$$

$$\text{Creatinine clearance} = \frac{\text{Renal excretion rate}}{\text{Serum creatinine concentration}} = \frac{0.3055 \text{ mg/min}}{3 \text{ mg/100 ml}} = 10.2 \text{ ml/min}$$

8.5 CUMULATIVE AMOUNT OF THE DRUG EXCRETED IN URINE

After a single intravenous dose of the drug, the rate of the renal excretion is determined by Equation 8.6. This means that the cumulative amount of the drug excreted in urine increases exponentially until it reaches a plateau as in Figure 8.3. The total cumulative amount of the drug excreted in urine is determined by integrating Equation 8.6 and substituting for time by infinity.

$$A_{e\infty} = \frac{k_e}{k} A_0 = \frac{k_e}{k} \text{ Dose} \tag{8.11}$$

This means that the fraction of the administered IV dose excreted unchanged in urine is equal to the ratio of the renal excretion rate constant to the elimination rate constant. Similarly, the fraction of the administered IV dose excreted unchanged in urine is equal to the ratio of the renal clearance to the total body clearance.

$$A_{e\infty} = \frac{k_e \text{ Vd}}{k \text{ Vd}} \text{ Dose} = \frac{\text{Renal clearance}}{\text{Total body clearance}} \text{ Dose} \tag{8.12}$$

When the entire dose of the drug is excreted unchanged in urine, the total body clearance will be equal to the renal clearance, and k_e is equal to k. When no drug is excreted unchanged in urine, the renal clearance and the renal excretion rate constant will be equal to zero.

The same principle can be applied for extravascular drug administration; however, in this case the fraction of the bioavailable dose excreted unchanged in urine

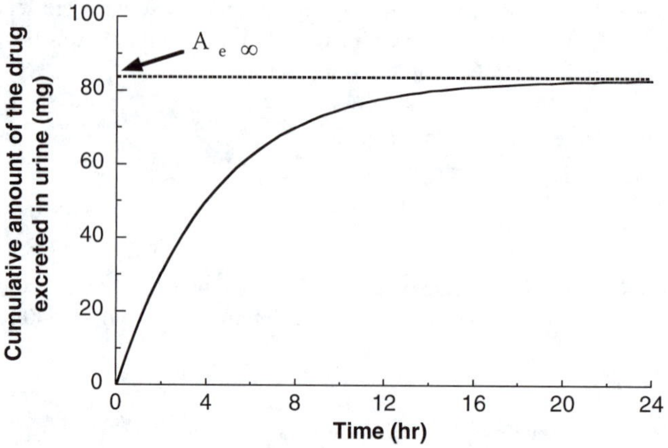

FIGURE 8.3 The cumulative amount of the drug excreted in urine after a single IV dose increases exponentially until it reaches a plateau.

is equal to the ratio of the renal excretion rate constant to the elimination rate constant. Also, the fraction of the bioavailable dose excreted unchanged in urine is equal to the ratio of the renal clearance to the total body clearance.

$$\frac{A_{e\infty}}{F\ D} = \frac{k_e}{k} = \frac{\text{Renal clearance}}{\text{Total body clearance}} \tag{8.13}$$

The fraction of the bioavailable dose excreted unchanged in urine is constant for the same drug in the same patient. This means that the higher the amount of the drug that reaches the systemic circulation, the higher will be the cumulative amount of the drug excreted in urine after administration of different products of the same drug to the same patient.

8.5.1 Determination of Renal Clearance from the Cumulative Amount Excreted in Urine

The fraction of the administered dose excreted unchanged in urine is determined from the ratio of the renal clearance to the total body clearance.

$$\frac{A_{e\infty}}{F\ D} = \frac{k_e\ Vd}{k\ Vd} \tag{8.14}$$

Because FD/kVd is equal to the area under the curve (AUC), the renal clearance can be determined from the amount of the drug excreted unchanged in urine and the drug AUC.

$$\text{Renal clearance} = k_e\ Vd = k\ Vd\ \frac{A_{e\infty}}{FD} = \frac{A_{e\infty}}{AUC|_0^\infty} \tag{8.15}$$

This relationship can be applied for both IV and oral administration because the bioavailability will affect the amount excreted unchanged in urine and the AUC to the same extent. The renal clearance can also be calculated by plotting the renal excretion rate versus the partial plasma AUCs (i.e., the AUC during each urine collection interval) on Cartesian graph paper. The slope of this plot is equal to the renal clearance.

8.6 DETERMINATION OF PHARMACOKINETIC PARAMETERS FROM RENAL EXCRETION RATE DATA

8.6.1 Elimination Rate Constant and Half-Life (k and $t_{1/2}$)

- A plot of the renal excretion rate versus time on semilog graph paper will be a straight line with a slope of –k/2.303.
- Also, the half-life can be determined graphically from the plot by determining the time required for the renal excretion rate to decrease by 50%.

8.6.2 Renal Excretion Rate Constant k_e

- The y-intercept in the plot of renal excretion rate versus time is equal to k_eA_0. Because A_0 is equal to the dose, the renal excretion rate constant can be determined from the y-intercept value.
- The renal excretion rate constant can be determined if the renal clearance and the Vd are known (Renal clearance = k_eVd).
- The renal excretion rate constant can be determined if the fraction of dose excreted unchanged in urine and the elimination rate constant are known (Fraction = k_e/k).

8.6.3 Volume of Distribution V_d

- The volume of distribution cannot be determined from the plot of renal excretion rate versus time.
- Plasma samples after drug administration are required to estimate the volume of distribution.
- The volume of distribution can be determined if the renal clearance and the renal excretion rate constant are known (Renal clearance = k_eVd)

8.6.4 Renal Clearance CL_R

- The renal clearance can be determined from the renal excretion rate constant and the volume of distribution (Renal clearance = k_eVd).
- The renal clearance during each urine collection interval is determined from the ratio of the renal excretion rate and the average plasma concentration during the urine collection interval.
- When serial urine and plasma samples are obtained, the renal clearance can be determined from the slope of the plot of the renal excretion rate versus the plasma concentration at the midpoint of the urine collection interval.

- The renal clearance can be determined from the total amount of the drug excreted unchanged in urine and the drug AUC (Renal clearance = $A_{e\infty}$/AUC).
- The renal clearance can be calculated if the fraction of dose excreted unchanged in urine and the CL_T are known (Fraction = CL_R/CL_T).

8.6.5 Fraction of Dose Excreted Unchanged in Urine

The fraction of the bioavailable dose excreted unchanged in urine is determined from the ratios of k_e/k or CL_R/CL_T.

8.6.6 Bioavailability

- The fraction of the bioavailable dose excreted unchanged in urine is constant for the same drug in the same patient. Based on this principle, the bioavailability of orally administered drug can be determined from the cumulative amount of the drug excreted in urine if a reasonable fraction of the dose is excreted unchanged in urine.
- The absolute bioavailability is determined from the ratio of the cumulative amount of the drug excreted unchanged in urine after oral and after IV administration of the same dose of the drug.

$$F_{\text{absolute}} = \frac{A_{e\infty\ \text{oral}}}{A_{e\infty\ \text{IV}}} \tag{8.16}$$

- The relative bioavailability is determined from the ratio of the cumulative amount of the drug excreted unchanged in urine after administration of the formulation under investigation and after administration of the reference standard formulation.

$$F_{\text{relative}} = \frac{A_{e\infty\ \text{test}}}{A_{e\infty\ \text{standard}}} \tag{8.17}$$

Example

After an IV injection of 500 mg of a new drug to a patient, the following data were obtained:

Collection Interval (hr)	Urine Volume (ml)	Urine Concentration (mg/ml)	$Cp_{t\text{-mid}}$ (mg/mL)
0–2	119	0.60	22.3
2–4	81	0.70	17.7
4–8	160	0.50	12.5
8–12	220	0.23	7.88
12–18	284	0.15	4.42
18–24	212	0.10	2.21

1. Estimate the biological half-life of this drug in this patient using the urinary excretion data.
2. Estimate the renal clearance of this drug in this patient.
3. Calculate the fraction of the administered dose excreted unchanged in the urine from the available data.

Answer

Use the available information to calculate the renal excretion rate as follows:

Collection Interval (hr)	Urine Volume (ml)	Urine Concentration (mg/ml)	Amount Excreted (mg)	Renal Excretion Rate (mg/hr)	$Cp_{t\text{-mid}}$ (mg/L)
0–2	119	0.60	71.4	35.7	22.3
2–4	81	0.70	56.7	28.35	17.7
4–8	160	0.50	80.0	20.00	12.5
8–12	220	0.23	50.6	12.65	7.88
12–18	284	0.15	42.6	7.10	4.42
18–24	212	0.10	21.2	3.53	2.21

1. The half-life can be estimated from the plot of the renal excretion rate versus time as in Figure 8.4.

$$\text{Half-life} = 6\ \text{hr},\ k = 0.1155\ \text{hr}^{-1}$$

The elimination rate constant can also be determined from the slope of the line.

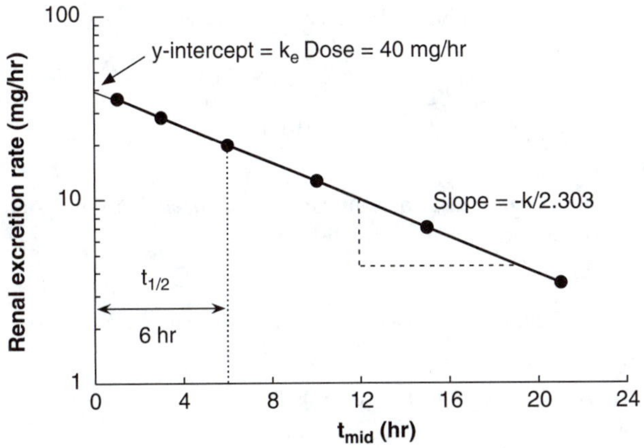

FIGURE 8.4 The plot of the renal excretion rate versus time on the semilog scale.

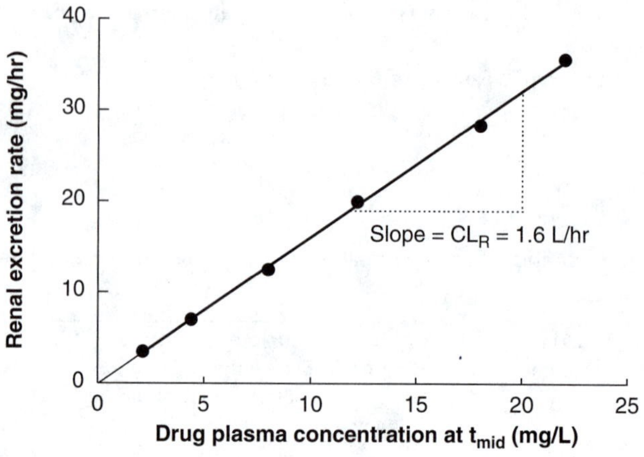

FIGURE 8.5 The renal excretion rate versus drug plasma concentration at the middle of the urine collection interval plot on the Cartesian scale.

2. The renal clearance can be estimated from the slope of the plot of the renal excretion rate versus plasma concentration as in Figure 8.5.

$$\text{Renal clearance} = 1.6\ \text{L/hr}$$

3. The fraction excreted unchanged in urine can be calculated from the ratio k_e/k or CL_R/CL_T. The plasma concentration-time data can be used to determine the total body clearance. Plot the plasma concentration-time data and calculate the Vd, k, and CL_T.

$$\text{Total body clearance} = 2.31\ \text{L/hr}$$

$$\text{Fraction} = \frac{CL_R}{CL_T} = \frac{1.6\ \text{L/hr}}{2.31\ \text{L/hr}} = 0.69$$

Also, the renal excretion rate constant can be calculated from the y-intercept of the renal excretion rate–time profile.

$$\text{y-intercept} = k_e\,\text{Dose} = k_e\,500\ \text{mg} = 40\ \text{mg/hr}$$

$$k_e = 0.08\ \text{hr}^{-1}$$

$$\text{Fraction} = \frac{k_e}{k} = \frac{0.08\ \text{hr}^{-1}}{0.1155\ \text{hr}^{-1}} = 0.69$$

8.7 EFFECT OF CHANGING THE PHARMACOKINETIC PARAMETERS ON URINARY EXCRETION OF DRUGS

8.7.1 Dose

Administration of increasing doses of the drug results in a proportional increase in the cumulative (total) amount of the drug excreted unchanged in urine if k_e and k remain constant (the fraction of the dose excreted unchanged in urine is constant).

The renal excretion rate-time plot after administration of increasing doses on the semilog scale is linear with the same slope because the elimination rate constant is constant. However, the initial renal excretion rate (Intercept = k_e Dose) after administration of the different doses is proportional to the administered dose because k_e is constant.

8.7.2 Total Body Clearance

The total body clearance may decrease without affecting the renal clearance, such as when a patient develops liver failure, which can affect the metabolic drug clearance without affecting the renal clearance. In this case, if the volume of distribution does not change, then the rate of decline of the renal excretion rate versus time plot will be slower because the slope of this plot depends on the overall elimination rate constant k ($k = CL_T/Vd$). Also, enzyme induction can result in increasing the total body clearance without affecting the renal clearance of the drug. In this case, if the volume of distribution is not affected, then the rate of decline of the renal excretion rate versus time plot will be faster because the overall elimination rate constant k will be larger.

The fraction of the administered dose excreted unchanged in urine is determined from the ratio of CL_R/CL_T. After administration of the same dose, the amount of the drug excreted unchanged in urine will be larger in patients with liver failure if the drug is eliminated unchanged in the urine and metabolized by the liver. However, in cases of enzyme induction, there is a decrease in the ratio of CL_R/CL_T, which will result in a smaller fraction of dose excreted unchanged in urine.

8.7.3 Renal Clearance

When the renal clearance changes, this will usually be accompanied by a decrease in the total body clearance. For example, when a patient develops kidney dysfunction, this will decrease the renal clearance and the total body clearance of the drug because the total body clearance is the sum of all organ clearances. However, the decrease in the renal clearance, for example, is usually accompanied by a less-than-proportional decrease in the total body clearance because in most cases the nonrenal clearance is not affected by the decrease in kidney function. If the decrease in kidney function does not affect the volume of distribution of the drug, then the rate of decline of the renal excretion rate versus time plot will be slower because the slope of this plot depends on the overall elimination rate constant k ($k = CL_T/Vd$).

The fraction of the administered dose excreted unchanged in urine is determined from the ratio of CL_R/CL_T. As mentioned, the decrease in renal clearance is usually accompanied by a less-than-proportional decrease in the total body clearance, so the ratio of the renal clearance to the total body clearance usually decreases in patients with renal dysfunction. So, after administration of the same dose, the amount of the drug excreted unchanged in urine will be smaller in patients with renal dysfunction.

PRACTICE PROBLEMS

8.1. Urine was collected from a patient over a 24-hr period to determine the creatinine clearance. The total volume of urine collected was 1800 ml, and the creatinine concentration in urine was 0.4 mg/ml. If the serum creatinine determined in this patient was 1 mg/dl (1 mg/100 ml), do the following:

a. Calculate the amount of creatinine excreted (eliminated) during the 24-hr period.
b. Calculate the average renal excretion rate of creatinine during the 24-hr period.
c. Calculate the creatinine clearance in this patient.
d. Calculate the renal clearance of creatinine in this patient.

8.2. A patient received a single 1000-mg IV dose of an antibiotic. Urine and plasma samples were collected, and the following results were obtained:

Interval (hr)	Urine Volume (ml)	Urine Concentration (μg/ml)	Plasma Concentration (μg/ml) ($Cp_{t\text{-}mid}$)
0–1	67	2.1	Not determined
1–2	70	1.01	Not determined
2–4	100	0.5	0.5 μg/ml at time 3 hr
4–8	250	0.05	Very low

a. Calculate the average renal excretion rate of the drug during the first urine collection interval (0–1 hr).
b. Calculate the average renal excretion rate of the drug during the third urine collection interval (2–4 hr).
c. Calculate the renal clearance of this drug in this patient.
d. What is the slope of the plot of the renal excretion rate versus time on semilog graph paper?

8.3. A new antihypertensive drug is rapidly but incompletely absorbed. When 800 mg is given intravenously to normal volunteers, 800 mg is recovered in urine unchanged from time 0 to ∞, and the AUC obtained from time 0 to infinity is 400 mg-hr/L. When 400 mg is given orally, only 350 mg of the drug is recovered unchanged in urine from time 0 to ∞, and the elimination half-life is 8 hr.

a. What is the bioavailability of this drug after oral administration?

8.4. After an IV injection of 10 mg of a new drug to a patient, the following data were obtained:

Collection Interval (day)	Urine Volume (ml)	Urinary Drug Concentration (μg/ml)	$Cp_{t\text{-mid}}$ (μg/L)
0–1	1250	1.8	16.0
1–2	1500	0.984	10.4
2–3	1750	0.544	6.8
3–4	1380	0.448	4.4
4–5	1630	0.248	2.9
5–7	3130	0.136	1.5

a. Using a graphical method, estimate the biological half-life of this drug in this patient.
b. Calculate the renal clearance and the total body clearance of this drug in this patient.
c. Calculate the fraction of the administered dose excreted unchanged in the urine from these data.
d. Estimate how much drug is in the body 5 days after the dose was administered.
e. Assuming that the unexcreted portion of this drug is metabolized, determine its metabolic rate constant k_m in this patient.

8.5. After an intravenous injection of 1000 mg of a new drug to a patient, the following data were obtained:

Collection Interval (hr)	Urine Volume (ml)	Urinary Concentration (mg/ml)	$Cp_{t\text{-mid}}$ (mg/L)
0–2	125	1.776	15.9
2–4	150	0.933	10.0
4–6	175	0.504	6.3
6–8	138	0.403	3.97
8–10	163	0.215	2.51
10–14	313	0.112	1.24

a. Using a graphical method, estimate the biological half-life of this drug in this patient.
b. Calculate the renal clearance of this drug in this patient.
c. Calculate the fraction of the administered dose excreted unchanged in the urine from these data.
d. Assuming that the unexcreted portion of this drug is metabolized, determine its metabolic rate constant k_m in this patient.

9 Metabolite Pharmacokinetics

OBJECTIVES

After completing this chapter you should be able to:

- Describe the pharmacokinetic processes involved in the formation and elimination of the metabolites after parent drug administration
- Describe the models that describe the formation of metabolites after administration of the parent drug
- Define the mathematical expressions that describe the plasma concentration–time profiles of the drug and its metabolite at any time after intravenous (IV) drug administration
- Identify the factors that affect the metabolite formation after administration of the parent drug
- Calculate the different metabolite pharmacokinetic parameters after IV administration of the parent drug
- Analyze the effect of changing each of the drug and metabolite pharmacokinetic parameters on the drug and metabolite profiles after a single drug administration
- Analyze the effect of changing each of the drug and metabolite pharmacokinetic parameters on the drug and metabolite profiles at steady state during multiple drug administrations

9.1 INTRODUCTION

Drugs are usually eliminated from the body by metabolism or excretion through a number of pathways. Drug metabolism occurs by enzymatic or chemical modification of the chemical structure of a parent drug to form a new chemical entity called a *metabolite*. Study of the metabolite pharmacokinetics is important because some metabolites possess pharmacological activity, and some metabolites are responsible for the adverse effects of the parent drug.

Procainamide is an antiarrhythmic drug metabolized to *n*-acetyl procainamide (NAPA), which also possesses antiarrhythmic activity. Cocaethylene, which is a cocaine metabolite formed only when cocaine is abused simultaneously with alcohol, was found to be more lethal than cocaine and as potent as cocaine regarding its central nervous system stimulant activity. Also, the antiepileptic drug carbamazepine is metabolized to carbamazepine epioxide, which is responsible for most of the parent drug's toxicity.

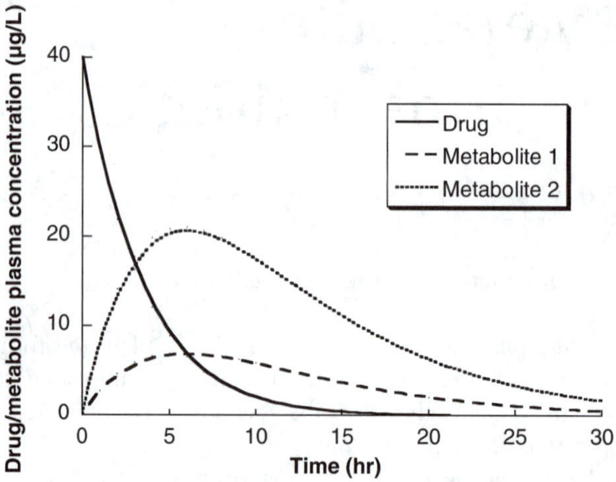

FIGURE 9.1 The drug and metabolite plasma concentration–time profiles after IV administration of a drug that is metabolized to two different metabolites.

Drugs and chemicals can be metabolized through a number of metabolic pathways: oxidation, reduction, hydrolysis, conjugation, and so on. So after administration of the drug, more than one metabolite can be detected simultaneously in the body as in Figure 9.1. Also, drugs can be metabolized and eliminated unchanged (e.g., in urine or in bile) simultaneously. A drug can be metabolized to different metabolites through parallel pathways, and the formed metabolites are eliminated from the body (parallel metabolism). Sometimes, the formed metabolite is further metabolized to another metabolite, which is then excreted from the body (sequential metabolism) as illustrated in Figure 9.2.

When a drug or a chemical is eliminated via parallel pathways, the amount of the drug eliminated through each pathway is proportional to the clearance (and the rate constant) associated with each of the pathways (assuming first-order elimination)

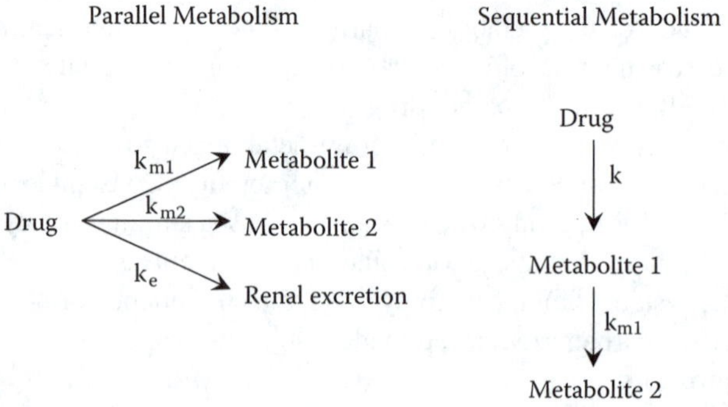

FIGURE 9.2 Schematic presentation of parallel and sequential drug metabolism.

as presented in Figure 9.2. The overall elimination rate constant for the drug k is the sum of the rate constants associated with the three pathways, that is,

$$k = k_{m1} + k_{m2} + k_e \tag{9.1}$$

Because the rate of any first-order process is the product of the first-order rate constant for the process and the amount of the compound available for the process A, the rate of each of the three parallel processes presented in Figure 9.2 can be determined as follows:

$$\text{Rate of formation of metabolite 1} = Ak_{m1}$$

$$\text{Rate of formation of metabolite 2} = Ak_{m2}$$

$$\text{Rate of urinary excretion} = Ak_e$$

The fraction of the dose of the drug that is metabolized to metabolite 1 is

$$\text{Fraction} = \frac{k_{m1}}{k_{m1} + k_{m2} + k_e} = \frac{k_{m1}}{k}$$

and the fraction of dose that is metabolized to metabolite 2 is

$$= \frac{k_{m2}}{k_{m1} + k_{m2} + k_e} = \frac{k_{m2}}{k}$$

and the fraction of dose excreted unchanged in urine is

$$= \frac{k_e}{k_{m1} + k_{m2} + k_e} = \frac{k_e}{k}$$

So, the fraction of dose excreted by any pathway can be determined as follows:

$$\text{Fraction} = \frac{\text{Rate constant for the pathway}}{\text{Elimination rate constant (k)}} \tag{9.2}$$

9.2 SIMPLE MODEL FOR METABOLITE KINETICS

The simple model for drug metabolism can be described by the scheme in Figure 9.3, and the model has the following assumptions:

- The drug is administered intravenously.
- The drug is 100% metabolized to one metabolite by a first-order process.
- The metabolite is excreted in urine by a first-order process.
- The metabolite cannot be converted back to the parent drug.

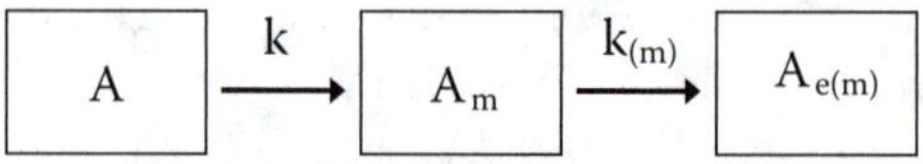

FIGURE 9.3 Schematic presentation of a simple model for drug metabolism, where A is the amount of drug in the body; k is the first-order rate constant for drug elimination; $A_{(m)}$ is the amount of metabolite in the body; $k_{(m)}$ is the first-order elimination rate constant for the metabolite; and $A_{e(m)}$ is the amount of metabolite eliminated from the body.

- The metabolite and the parent drug follow a one-compartment pharmacokinetic model.
- Molar amounts and concentrations are used.

The rate of change of the amount of metabolite in the body is equal to the difference between the rate of metabolite formation and the rate of metabolite elimination. The rate of drug elimination is equal to the rate of formation of the metabolite because the drug is eliminated by a single pathway. The rate of metabolite formation that occurs by a first-order process can be determined as follows:

$$\text{Rate of metabolite formation} = Ak$$

$$\text{Rate of metabolite elimination} = A_{(m)}k_{(m)}$$

$$\frac{dA_{(m)}}{dt} = Ak - A_{(m)}k_{(m)} \tag{9.3}$$

by integration of Equation 9.3:

$$A_{(m)} = \frac{kD}{k_{(m)} - k}\left(e^{-kt} - e^{-k_{(m)}t}\right) \tag{9.4}$$

To obtain an expression that describes the time course for the metabolite concentration in the body, Equation 9.4 can be divided by the volume of distribution of the metabolite $V_{(m)}$.

$$Cp_{(m)} = \frac{kD}{Vd_{(m)}(k_{(m)} - k)}\left(e^{-kt} - e^{-k_{(m)}t}\right) \tag{9.5}$$

Equation 9.5 describes the time course for the metabolite plasma concentration at any time t. This expression is biexponential because it describes two different processes: the formation and the elimination of the metabolite. At time zero, there is no metabolite in the body, and $Cp_{(m)}$ is equal to zero. After drug administration,

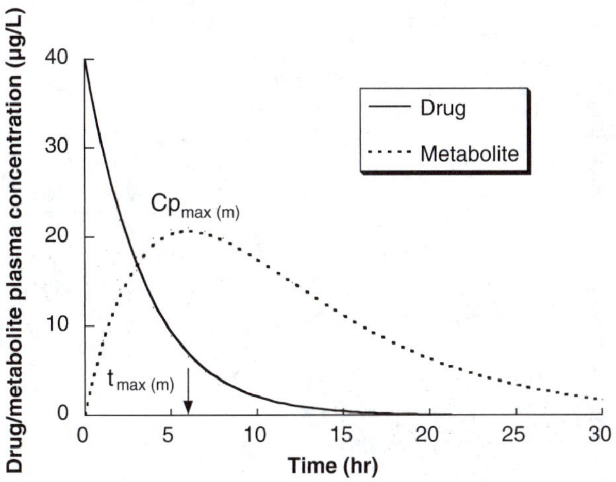

FIGURE 9.4 The drug and metabolite concentration–time profiles after IV administration of a single dose of the drug.

the amount of metabolite in the body starts to increase because the rate of metabolite formation is more than the rate of its elimination. As time proceeds, the rate of metabolite formation decreases, and the rate of metabolite elimination increases. When the metabolite formation rate becomes equal to the metabolite elimination rate, the metabolite plasma concentration reaches a maximum value $Cp_{max(m)}$. The time when the metabolite plasma concentration is at its maximum value is called $t_{max(m)}$. After $t_{max(m)}$, the rate of metabolite elimination is larger than the rate of metabolite formation, and the metabolite plasma concentration decreases. The drug and metabolite plasma concentration–time profile after IV administration of a single dose of the drug is illustrated in Figure 9.4.

It is important to note that when a metabolite is formed from the parent drug, this metabolite is a new chemical entity that has pharmacokinetic behavior different from the parent drug, that is, the half-life, Vd, and clearance of the metabolite are different from the parameters of the parent drug.

9.2.1 Elimination Rate Limitation

When $k_{(m)} < k$, that is, the half-life of the metabolite is longer than the half-life of the parent drug, the slope of the terminal phase of the metabolite plasma profile will reflect the elimination rate of the metabolite as in Figure 9.5.

The plasma profile of the metabolite in this case can be described as elimination rate limited. Usually, the decline of the metabolite concentration-versus-time curve reflects the metabolite elimination rate after about five elimination half-lives for the parent drug. Notice that the plasma concentration of the metabolite can be lower or higher than the plasma concentration of the parent drug.

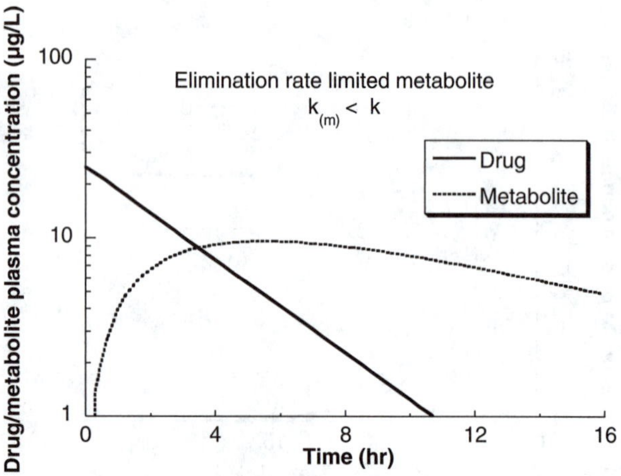

FIGURE 9.5 The drug and metabolite concentration–time profiles after IV administration of a single dose of the drug when the metabolite elimination rate constant is smaller than the drug elimination rate constant.

9.2.2 Formation Rate Limitation

When $k_{(m)} > k$, that is, the half-life of the metabolite is shorter than the half-life of the parent drug, the rate of decline (the slope) of the terminal phase/plasma profile of the metabolite concentration will be the same as that of the parent drug as in Figure 9.6. The slope of the metabolite plasma profile does not reflect the rate of metabolite elimination but the rate of formation of the metabolite, which is also

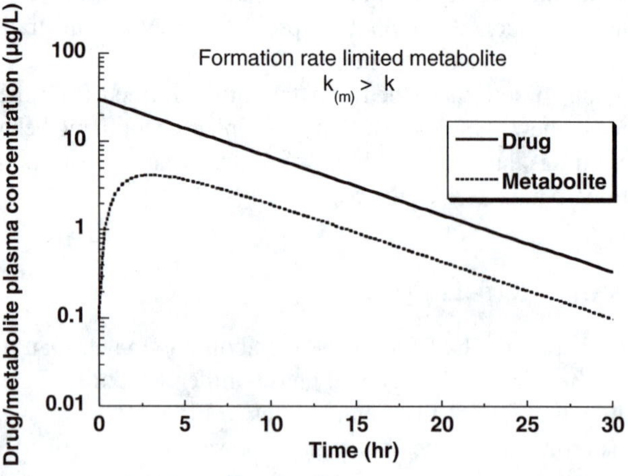

FIGURE 9.6 The drug and metabolite concentration–time profiles after IV administration of a single dose of the drug when the metabolite elimination rate constant is larger than the drug elimination rate constant.

equal to the rate of elimination of the parent drug. The profile of the metabolite in this case can be described as formation rate limited.

9.2.3 Mathematical Description of Elimination Rate- and Formation Rate-Limited Metabolites

The metabolite plasma concentration–time profile after administration of the parent drug can be described by Equation 9.5:

$$Cp_{(m)} = \frac{k\,D}{Vd_{(m)}\,(k_{(m)} - k)}\,(e^{-kt} - e^{-k_{(m)}t})$$

- If $k_{(m)} < k$ (elimination rate-limited metabolites), then the term e^{-kt} approaches zero faster than the term $e^{-k_{(m)}t}$. So, as time gets longer, Equation 9.5 can be reduced to

$$Cp_{(m)} = \frac{k\,D}{Vd_{(m)}\,(k_{(m)} - k)}\,e^{-k_{(m)}t} \tag{9.6}$$

  So, the decline in metabolite concentration depends on the elimination rate of the metabolite.

- If $k_{(m)} > k$ (formation rate-limited metabolites), then the term $e^{-k_{(m)}t}$ approaches zero faster than the term e^{-kt}. So, as time gets longer, Equation 9.5 can be reduced to

$$Cp_{(m)} = \frac{k\,D}{Vd_{(m)}\,(k_{(m)} - k)}\,e^{-kt} \tag{9.7}$$

  So, the decline in metabolite concentration will be parallel to the decline of the parent drug.

9.2.4 Time to Achieve Maximum Metabolite Concentration

The time required to reach the maximum metabolite concentration can be determined by differentiation of the equation that describes the metabolite concentration–time profile (Equation 9.5). At $t_{max(m)}$, the rate of change of the metabolite concentration is equal to zero, that is, the result of the differentiation is equal to zero. So, $t_{max(m)}$ can be calculated:

$$t_{max\,(m)} = \frac{\ln\,(k_{(m)}/k)}{k_{(m)} - k} \tag{9.8}$$

The maximum metabolite concentration $Cp_{max(m)}$ can be determined by substitution for $t_{max(m)}$ in Equation 9.5. As $(k_{(m)}/k)$ increases (i.e., the rate of metabolite elimination is faster than the rate of parent drug elimination), the $t_{max(m)}$ increases, and $Cp_{max(m)}$ decreases.

9.3 GENERAL MODEL FOR METABOLITE KINETICS

A general model for drug metabolism is described by the scheme in Figure 9.7, and the model has the following assumptions:

- The drug is administered intravenously.
- A fraction of the drug dose f_m is metabolized to one metabolite by a first-order process.
- The metabolite is eliminated by a first-order process.
- The metabolite cannot be converted back to the parent drug.
- The metabolite and the parent drug follow a one-compartment pharmacokinetic model.
- Molar amounts and concentrations are used.

The general model differs from the simple model described by allowing for other elimination pathways that may represent another metabolic or nonmetabolic pathway. In this general model, the rate of metabolite formation is not equal to the rate of drug elimination because of the presence of other elimination pathways. The rate of metabolite formation is only a fraction f_m of the total elimination of the parent drug.

$$\text{Rate of metabolite formation} = f_m A k$$

$$\text{Rate of metabolite elimination} = A_{(m)} k_{(m)}$$

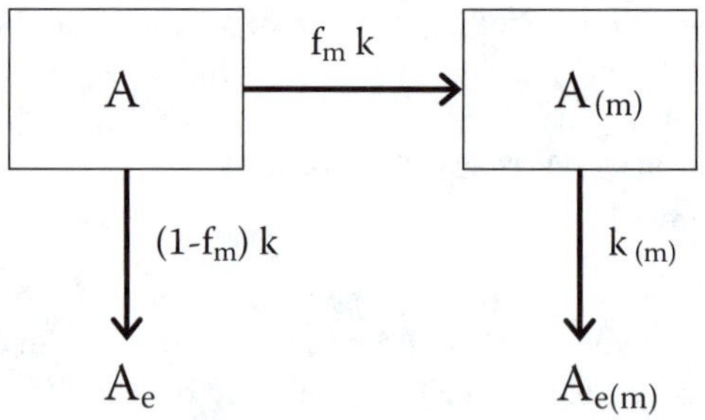

FIGURE 9.7 Schematic presentation of the general model for drug metabolism. A and $A_{(m)}$ are the amount of parent drug and metabolite in the body, respectively; k is the parent drug first-order elimination rate constant; $k_{(m)}$ is the metabolite first-order elimination rate constant; f_m is the fraction of the drug dose that is metabolized to the metabolite of interest; $(1 - f_m)$ is the fraction of the drug dose that is excreted by other pathways; A_e is the amount of the parent drug excreted by pathways other than metabolism; and $A_{e(m)}$ is the amount of metabolite excreted.

At any time, the rate of change of the metabolite in the body is the difference between the rate of formation and the rate of elimination, that is,

$$\frac{dA_{(m)}}{dt} = f_m A k - A_{(m)} k_{(m)} \tag{9.9}$$

By integration, we can get the expression that describes the amount of the metabolite in the body at any time.

$$A_{(m)} = \frac{f_m k D}{k_{(m)} - k} \left(e^{-kt} - e^{-k_{(m)} t}\right) \tag{9.10}$$

To obtain an expression that describes the time course for the metabolite concentration in the body, Equation 9.10 can be divided by the volume of distribution of the metabolite $Vd_{(m)}$.

$$Cp_{(m)} = \frac{f_m k D}{Vd_{(m)} (k_{(m)} - k)} \left(e^{-kt} - e^{-k_{(m)} t}\right) \tag{9.11}$$

This is the general expression for metabolite concentration. This general expression describes the plasma concentration–time profile of the metabolite when only a fraction f_m of the administered dose of the parent drug is metabolized and the rest of the dose is excreted by another pathway. Equation 9.5 is a special case of the general expression when all the dose of the parent drug is converted to one metabolite (i.e., $f_m = 1$). In the general model, only a fraction of the parent drug's total body clearance becomes responsible for the formation of the metabolite ($f_m CL_T$). This is also called the formation clearance of the metabolite. The formed metabolite can have a longer or shorter half-life compared to the parent drug. The formed metabolite follows the formation rate limitation or elimination rate limitation as described previously.

Integration of the equation that describes the metabolite concentration from time zero to time infinity, the metabolite area under the plasma concentration–time curve (AUC) can be determined. The $AUC_{(m)}$ is dependent on the amount of the metabolite formed and the total body clearance of the metabolite. The larger the amount of metabolite formed in vivo, the larger the metabolite AUC will be; the higher the metabolite clearance, the smaller the metabolite AUC will be, that is,

$$AUC_{(m)} = \frac{f_m D}{CL_{T(m)}} \tag{9.12}$$

The parent drug's AUC after IV administration of the parent drug is determined from the dose and the total body clearance of the drug as in Equation 9.13.

$$AUC = \frac{D}{CL_T} \tag{9.13}$$

The ratio of the AUC for the metabolite to that of the parent drug can give the ratio of the formation clearance to the elimination clearance of the metabolite as follows:

$$\frac{AUC_{(m)}}{AUC} = \frac{f_m \, CL_T}{CL_{T(m)}} \tag{9.14}$$

If the metabolite's AUC is larger than the parent drug's AUC, then this indicates that the metabolite clearance is smaller than the clearance of the parent drug.

9.4 ESTIMATION OF METABOLITE PHARMACOKINETIC PARAMETERS

When the drug metabolite is pharmacologically active or is responsible for any adverse effect, determination of the metabolite pharmacokinetic parameters becomes important. Parameters such as the metabolite elimination rate constant, the amount of the metabolite formed, metabolite clearance, and metabolite accumulation during repeated drug administrations are important for characterization of the metabolite kinetics. Some metabolite parameters can be determined from administration of the parent drug. However, determination of some of these parameters requires the administration of the preformed purified metabolite.

9.4.1 Metabolite Elimination Rate Constant

9.4.1.1 Elimination Rate-Limited Metabolites

The half-life of the elimination rate-limited metabolites is longer than the parent drug's half-life. So, when the parent drug is completely eliminated, the decline in the metabolite profile is dependent on the metabolite elimination rate constant. The metabolite elimination rate constant $k_{(m)}$ can be determined from the slope of the linear part of the metabolite concentration–time profile after drug administration on a semilog scale. Also, the metabolite half-life can be determined graphically from the same plot.

$$\text{Slope} = \frac{-k_{(m)}}{2.303}$$

9.4.1.2 Formation Rate-Limited Metabolites

The half-life of the formation rate-limited metabolites is shorter than the parent drug's half-life. So, the decline in the metabolite profile after administration of the parent drug does not reflect the elimination rate of the metabolite, and the metabolite elimination rate constant cannot be determined from the elimination phase of the metabolite after drug administration. Indirect methods can be used to determine the metabolite elimination rate constant after drug administration. The metabolite elimination rate constant and half-life can also be determined after administration of the preformed metabolite. This is possible if the metabolite is available in sufficient quantities, and it is safe to administer the preformed metabolite.

9.4.2 Fraction of the Parent Drug Converted to a Specific Metabolite (or Amount of Metabolite Formed)

After IV administration of the parent drug, the observed metabolite AUC is dependent on the amount of the metabolite formed in vivo and the CL_T of the metabolite as in Equation 9.12.

$$AUC_{(m)} = \frac{f_m D}{CL_{T(m)}}$$

where $AUC_{(m)}$ is the observed metabolite AUC after parent drug administration, f_m is the fraction of the drug intravenous dose that is converted to that particular metabolite, D is the drug dose, and $CL_{T(m)}$ is the clearance of the metabolite. Because both f_m and $CL_{T(m)}$ are unknown, the amount of metabolite formed after administration of the parent drug cannot be determined just from the information obtained from administration of the parent drug. For this reason, determination of the amount of metabolite formed after administration of the parent drug or the fraction of parent drug dose converted to a certain metabolite will require the administration of the preformed purified metabolite. The observed metabolite AUC after IV administration of the metabolite is equal to

$$AUC'_{(m)} = \frac{M}{CL'_{T(m)}} \tag{9.15}$$

where $AUC'_{(m)}$ is the observed metabolite AUC after metabolite administration, M is the dose of the metabolite, and $CL'_{T(m)}$ is the total body clearance of the metabolite after metabolite administration. If equal doses (equimolar) of the parent drug and the metabolite are administered (i.e., D = M) and because the metabolite clearance should be the same after parent drug administration and metabolite administration (i.e., $CL'_{T(m)} = CL_{T(m)}$), the fraction of the parent drug dose converted to the metabolite can be determined from the ratio of the metabolite AUC after administration of the parent drug and after administration of the preformed metabolite.

$$\frac{AUC_{(m)}}{AUC'_{(m)}} = \frac{f_m\ D\ CL'_{T(m)}}{M\ CL_{T(m)}} = f_m \tag{9.16}$$

The amount of metabolite formed in vivo can be determined from the dose of the parent drug and f_m. If different doses of the metabolite and the parent drug are administered, the observed metabolite AUCs can be corrected for the doses to determine the expected metabolite AUCs for equal doses of the parent drug and the metabolite.

Urinary recovery of the metabolite can be used to determine the fraction of parent drug dose converted to a particular metabolite under certain conditions. This can be used when the formed metabolite is excreted unchanged in urine without undergoing sequential metabolism, the metabolite is stable in the urine after excretion, and urine is collected until all drug and metabolites are completely eliminated.

9.4.3 Metabolite Clearance

The total body clearance of the metabolite can be obtained after parent drug administration only if f_m is known. This is determined by administration of a known dose of the parent drug and calculation of the observed $AUC_{(m)}$; then, $CL_{T(m)}$ can be calculated using Equation 9.12.

If f_m is not known, then administration of the preformed metabolite will be necessary for the determination of $CL_{T(m)}$. This can be determined from Equation 9.15.

9.4.4 Metabolite Volume of Distribution

Determination of the metabolite volume of distribution requires IV administration of the preformed metabolite. The metabolite volume of distribution can be determined as follows:

$$Vd_{(m)} = \frac{M}{Cp_{0\,(m)}} \tag{9.17}$$

where $Vd_{(m)}$ is the metabolite volume of distribution, M is the dose of the metabolite, and $Cp_{0(m)}$ is the initial metabolite concentration at time zero.

Also, $Vd_{(m)}$ can be determined if the metabolite clearance and the metabolite elimination rate constant are known.

$$Vd_{(m)} = \frac{CL_{T(m)}}{k_{(m)}} \tag{9.18}$$

9.4.5 Metabolite Formation Clearance

The metabolite formation clearance is the fraction of the CL_T of the parent drug that is responsible for the formation of this particular metabolite. This can be determined from the CL_T of the parent drug and the fraction of parent drug dose converted to the metabolite as follows:

$$\text{Metabolite formation clearance} = f_m\, CL_T \tag{9.19}$$

EXAMPLE

When cocaine (Coc) is administered to human or experimental animals, it is metabolized to two major metabolites, benzoylecgonine (BE) and ecgonine methylester (EME), in addition to several minor metabolites. After concurrent abuse of cocaine and ethanol, cocaethylene (CE), which is a pharmacologically active and more toxic metabolite, is formed in addition to the metabolites mentioned. Concurrent abuse of cocaine and alcohol has been associated with high incidence of sudden death. This has been attributed to the effect of ethanol on the rate of cocaine metabolism and the formation of the pharmacologically active and more toxic metabolite CE.

In an experiment to study the pharmacokinetic interactions between cocaine and ethanol in experimental animals, a group of rats received cocaine, cocaine plus ethanol, BE, BE plus ethanol, and CE plus ethanol by intraperitoneal administration in a crossover experimental design. The following results were obtained:

Treatment	Dose	AUC
Coc	100 μmol/kg	Coc 4.2 μmol-hr/L
		BE 8.15 μmol-hr/L
		CE 0.0 μmol-hr/L
BE	50 μmol/kg	BE 9.32 μmol-hr/L
Coc + ethanol	100 μmol/kg	Coc 6.78 μmol-hr/L
		BE 4.12 μmol-hr/L
		CE 0.432 μmol-hr/L
BE + ethanol	50 μmol/kg	BE 9.93 μmol-hr/L
CE + ethanol	50 μmol/kg	CE 1.02 μmol-hr/L

Assuming that the bioavailability of cocaine and its metabolites after intraperitoneal administration are equal to 100% and are not affected by alcohol administration, answer the following questions:

1. What is the effect of ethanol administration on cocaine CL_T?
2. What is the fraction of cocaine dose that is metabolized to BE when cocaine is administered alone and in combination with ethanol?
3. What is the fraction of cocaine dose that is metabolized to CE when cocaine is administered with alcohol?
4. What is the formation clearance of BE and CE when cocaine is administered alone and in combination with ethanol?
5. Comment on the effect of ethanol on cocaine's metabolic profile.

Answer

1. When cocaine was given alone,

$$CL_{T\ coc} = \frac{F\ Dose}{AUC} = \frac{100\ \mu mol}{4.2\ \mu mol\text{-}hr/L} = 23.8\ L/hr$$

When cocaine was given with ethanol,

$$CL_{T\ coc} = \frac{F\ Dose}{AUC} = \frac{100\ \mu mol}{6.78\ \mu mol\text{-}hr/L} = 14.7\ L/hr$$

Ethanol decreased the CL_T of cocaine by approximately 40%.

2. When BE was administered alone,

$$CL_{T\ BE} = \frac{F\ Dose}{AUC} = \frac{50\ \mu mol}{9.32\ \mu mol\text{-}hr/L} = 5.36\ L/hr$$

After cocaine administration,

$$AUC_{BE} = \frac{BE\ (amount)}{CL_{T\ BE}}$$

$$8.15\ \mu mol\text{-}hr/L = \frac{BE\ (amount)}{5.36\ L/hr}$$

BE amount = 43.7 μmol = 43.7% of the cocaine dose

The total body clearance when BE was administered with ethanol was as follows:

$$CL_{T\ BE} = \frac{F\ Dose}{AUC} = \frac{50\ \mu mol}{9.93\ \mu mol\text{-}hr/L} = 5.035\ L/hr$$

After cocaine administration with ethanol,

$$AUC_{BE} = \frac{BE\ (amount)}{CL_{T\ BE}}$$

$$4.12\ \mu mol\text{-}hr/L = \frac{BE\ (amount)}{5.035\ L/hr}$$

BE amount = 20.7 μmol = 20.7% of cocaine dose when given with ethanol

3. $$CL_{T\ CE} = \frac{F\ Dose}{AUC} = \frac{50\ \mu mol}{1.02\ \mu mol\text{-}hr/L} = 49\ L/hr$$

After cocaine administration with ethanol,

$$AUC_{CE} = \frac{CE\ (amount)}{CL_{T\ CE}}$$

$$0.432\ \mu mol\text{-}hr/L = \frac{CE\ (amount)}{49\ L/hr}$$

CE amount = 21.2 μmol = 21.2% of cocaine dose when given with ethanol

4. When cocaine is administered alone,

$$\text{Formation clearance of BE} = f_{mBE} \times CL_{T\,Coc} = (0.437)\ 23.8\ \text{L/hr} = 10.4\ \text{L/hr}$$

$$\text{Formation clearance of CE} = f_{mCE} \times CL_{T\,Coc} = (0)\ 23.8\ \text{L/hr} = 0\ \text{L/hr}$$

When cocaine is administered with ethanol,

$$\text{Formation clearance of BE} = f_{mBE} \times CL_{T\,Coc} = (0.207)\ 14.7\ \text{L/hr} = 3.04\ \text{L/hr}$$

$$\text{Formation clearance of CE} = f_{mCE} \times CL_{T\,Coc} = (0.212)\ 14.7\ \text{L/hr} = 3.12\ \text{L/hr}$$

5. Ethanol inhibits the CL_T of cocaine by approximately 40% and results in the formation of a new metabolite, cocaethylene. Also, when cocaine is administered with ethanol, the amount of BE formed will be lower than when cocaine is administered alone.

9.5 EFFECT OF CHANGING PHARMACOKINETIC PARAMETERS ON DRUG AND METABOLITE CONCENTRATION–TIME PROFILES AFTER A SINGLE IV DRUG ADMINISTRATION

The following discussion deals with the effect of changing one pharmacokinetic parameter on the drug and metabolite plasma concentration–time profiles. This discussion is intended to illustrate how each of the drug and metabolite pharmacokinetic parameters affects the drug/metabolite concentration–time profile. However, in reality the change in one pharmacokinetic parameter will be accompanied by a change in other parameters. For example, the change in the rate of drug metabolism caused by liver dysfunction will be accompanied by a change in the rate of metabolite elimination if the metabolite is further metabolized to a second metabolite by the liver. Also, the change in the drug volume of distribution caused by different body weight will be accompanied by a change in the metabolite volume of distribution.

9.5.1 Drug Dose

Administration of a higher dose of the drug results in the formation of a larger amount of the metabolite because f_m is constant.

- Increasing the drug dose results in a proportional increase in the drug AUC.
- Increasing the drug dose leads to a proportional increase in the amount of metabolite formed in vivo. This is because the fraction of the drug converted to the metabolite f_m is constant.
- The increase in metabolite formation will cause a proportional increase in the metabolite AUC.
- The metabolite/drug AUC ratio after administration of increasing doses of the drug remains constant.

9.5.2 Drug Total Body Clearance CL_T

Higher drug clearance results in a faster rate of metabolite formation. The total amount of metabolite formed does not change because the dose and f_m are constant.

- Drugs with larger CL_T are eliminated faster (if Vd is similar) and will have smaller AUCs (if the administered dose is similar).
- Administration of the same dose of different drugs results in the formation of the same amount of metabolite if the fraction of the drug converted to the metabolite f_m is constant. However, the metabolite formation rate will be faster for the drugs with higher clearance.
- Because the metabolite pharmacokinetic parameters are similar and the same amount of metabolite is formed in vivo, the metabolite AUC will be the same regardless of the parent drug AUC.

9.5.3 Drug Volume of Distribution Vd

The change in drug Vd affects the drug profile; however, the amount of metabolite formed will be the same.

- Administration of the same IV dose of drugs with different Vd will result in lower initial concentration and slower rate of elimination for the drugs with larger Vd (if CL_T is constant). Slower drug elimination results in a slower rate of metabolite formation.
- Administration of the same dose of drugs with different Vd leads to the formation of the same amount of the metabolite if the fraction of the drug converted to the metabolite f_m and the drug CL_T are constant.
- Because the metabolite parameters are similar and the same amount of metabolite is formed in vivo, the metabolite AUC will be similar regardless of the parent drug Vd and CL_T.

9.5.4 Fraction of Drug Dose Converted to Metabolite f_m

Larger f_m results in the formation of a larger amount of the metabolite after administration of the same dose of drug.

- Administration of the same dose of different drugs that have similar CL_T and Vd but different f_m will produce a similar drug concentration–time profile and AUC.
- Administration of the same dose of drugs with increasing f_m will result in a proportional increase in the amount of metabolite formed in vivo.
- Because the metabolite parameters are similar and the amount of metabolite formed in vivo increases proportional to f_m, the metabolite AUC will increase proportional to the increase in f_m.

9.5.5 Metabolite Total Body Clearance $CL_{T(m)}$

The metabolite declines at a rate dependent on $k_{(m)}$ when $k_{(m)}$ is less than k and declines at a rate dependent on k when $k_{(m)}$ is greater than k.

- Administration of the same dose of drugs with similar CL_T, Vd, and f_m will result in a similar drug concentration–time profile, AUC, and formation of similar amounts of the metabolites. Metabolites with higher clearance will be eliminated faster [if $Vd_{(m)}$ is constant] and will have a smaller metabolite AUC.
- When $k_{(m)}$ is less than k, the metabolite concentration–time profile declines at a rate dependent on $k_{(m)}$ (elimination rate limited). When $k_{(m)}$ is greater than k, the metabolite concentration–time profile declines at a rate dependent on k (formation rate limited).

9.5.6 Metabolite Volume of Distribution $Vd_{(m)}$

Larger metabolite volume of distribution results in a slower rate of metabolite elimination if $CL_{T(m)}$ is similar.

- Administration of the same dose of drugs with similar CL_T and Vd will produce a similar drug concentration–time profile and AUC.
- Administration of the same dose of different drugs that have similar f_m will result in the formation of a similar amount of metabolites.
- Larger metabolite volume of distribution will lead to a slower metabolite elimination [if $CL_{T(m)}$ is similar].
- The metabolite AUC will be the same because the amount of the metabolites formed in vivo is similar, and the $CL_{T(m)}$ is the same.

9.6 STEADY-STATE METABOLITE CONCENTRATION DURING REPEATED ADMINISTRATIONS OF PARENT DRUG

It is important to determine the steady-state metabolite concentration during repeated drug administrations for metabolites that have pharmacological or toxic effects. At steady state, the rate of metabolite formation is equal to the rate of metabolite elimination.

$$f_m \, CL_T \, Cp_{ss} = CL_{T(m)} \, Cp_{ss\,(m)} \quad (9.20)$$

where Cp_{ss} and $Cp_{ss(m)}$ are the steady-state parent drug and metabolite concentrations, respectively. By rearrangement,

$$\frac{Cp_{ss(m)}}{Cp_{ss}} = \frac{f_m \, CL_T}{CL_{T\,(m)}} \quad (9.21)$$

After administration of a single IV dose of the parent drug, the ratio of the AUC of the metabolite to that of the parent drug (Equation 9.14) was determined by dividing Equation 9.12 by Equation 9.13:

$$\frac{AUC_{(m)}}{AUC} = \frac{f_m\ CL_T}{CL_{T\ (m)}}$$

From Equation 9.14 and Equation 9.21, the following expression can be obtained:

$$\frac{Cp_{ss(m)}}{Cp_{ss}} = \frac{f_m\ CL_T}{CL_{T\ (m)}} = \frac{AUC_{(m)}}{AUC} \tag{9.22}$$

This relationship suggests that the ratio of the metabolite concentration to the parent drug concentration at steady state during constant-rate IV infusion of the parent drug can be predicted from the ratio of metabolite AUC to the parent drug AUC measured after a single IV bolus dose of the parent drug. Also, during repeated IV administrations, the ratio of the average metabolite concentration to the average parent drug concentration at steady state is the ratio of metabolite AUC to the parent drug AUC observed after a single IV bolus dose of the parent drug.

Example

After administration of a drug to humans, it is eliminated by renal excretion and metabolism to a pharmacologically active metabolite. This metabolite is eliminated in the urine or metabolized to a second metabolite that is completely excreted in urine according to the scheme in Figure 9.8.

After administration of 100 μmol of the parent drug to a normal volunteer, the total amounts of the parent drug, metabolite 1, and metabolite 2 recovered in the urine were 20, 30, and 50 μmol, respectively. The half-life of the parent drug is 4 hr, and its volume of distribution is 25 L.

1. Calculate the CL_T and the AUC of the parent drug after administration of the 100 -μmol dose.
2. What is the renal clearance of the parent drug?

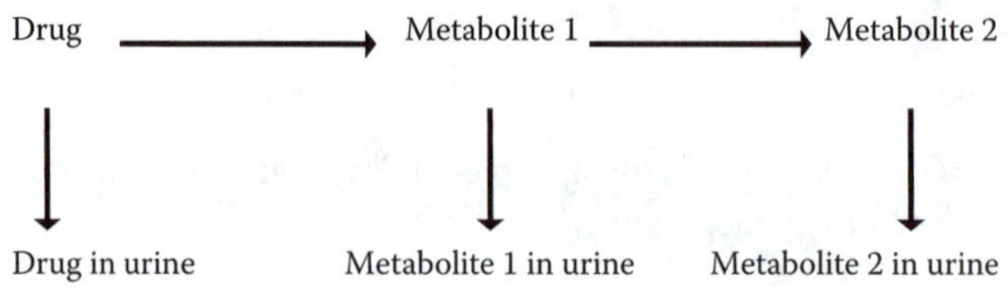

FIGURE 9.8 Schematic presentation of the different pathways involved in the elimination of the parent drug and its two metabolites.

3. What is the fraction of the administered dose of the parent drug that is metabolized to metabolite 1?
4. If the observed AUC of metabolite 1 was 10 μmol-hr/L, what is the CL_T of metabolite 1?
5. What is the renal clearance of metabolite 1?
6. What is the formation clearance of metabolites 1 and 2?
7. If a dose of 300 μmol of the parent drug is administered to the same volunteer, then what are the expected AUCs of the parent drug and metabolite 1?
8. If 100 μmol of metabolite 1 is administered to the same volunteer, then what are the total amounts of metabolites 1 and 2 that will be excreted in urine?
9. If a constant-rate IV infusion of the parent drug is administered to this volunteer, then what is the expected ratio of the metabolite concentration to that of the parent drug at steady state?
10. From the information provided above, can you determine whether metabolites 1 and 2 follow a formation rate-limited or an elimination rate-limited profile?

Answer

The fraction of the parent drug dose excreted in urine:

$$\text{Fraction (parent drug)} = \frac{\text{Amount excreted in urine}}{\text{Dose of parent drug}} = \frac{20\ \mu\text{mol}}{100\ \mu\text{mol}} = 0.2$$

1.

$$CL_T = k\ Vd = \frac{0.693}{4\ \text{hr}}\ 25\ \text{L} = 4.33\ \text{l/hr}$$

$$AUC = \frac{100\ \mu\text{mol}}{4.33\ \text{L/hr}} = 23\ \mu\text{mol-hr/L}$$

2. Renal clearance = Fraction excreted unchanged in urine × CL_T

$$CL_R = (0.2)4.33\ \text{L/hr} = 0.866\ \text{L/hr}$$

3. Fraction metabolized to metabolite 1 = 1 – 0.2 = 0.8
4.

$$CL_{T\,(m\,1)} = \frac{80\ \mu\text{mol}}{10\ \mu\text{mol-hr/L}} = 8\ \text{L/hr}$$

5.

$$\text{Fraction excreted in urine of metabolite 1} = \frac{\text{Amount of metabolite 1 excreted in urine}}{\text{Total amount of metabolite 1 formed}}$$

$$\text{Fraction}_{\ (m\,1)} = \frac{30\ \mu\text{mol}}{80\ \mu\text{mol}} = 0.375$$

Renal clearance of metabolite 1 = Fraction excreted in urine × CL_T of metabolite 1

$$CL_{R\,(m1)} = 0.375 \times 8 \text{ L/hr} = 3 \text{ L/hr}$$

6. Formation clearance (metabolite 1) = $f_{m\,(\text{metabolite 1})} \times CL_{T\,(\text{parent drug})}$

$$= 0.8 \times 4.33 \text{ L/hr} = 3.46 \text{ L/hr}$$

Formation clearance (metabolite 2) = $f_{m\,(\text{metabolite 2})} \times CL_{T\,(\text{metabolite 1})}$

= (1 − Fraction excreted in urine of metabolite 1) × $CL_{T\,(\text{metabolite 1})}$

$$= (1 - 0.375) \times 8 \text{ L/hr} = 3.46 \text{ L/hr}$$

7. Increasing the dose of the parent drug will cause a proportional increase in the drug AUC and the metabolite AUC:

$$AUC_{\text{parent drug}} = 3 \times 23\ \mu\text{mol-hr/L} = 69\ \mu\text{mol-hr/L}$$

$$AUC_{(m1)} = 3 \times 10\ \mu\text{mol-hr/L} = 30\ \mu\text{mol-hr/L}$$

8. After administration of 100 μmol of metabolite 1,

   Amount of metabolite 1 excreted in urine = (30/80) 100 μmol = 37.5 μmol

   Amount of metabolite 2 excreted in urine = 100 μmol − 37.5 μmol = 62.25 μmol

9.

$$\text{Ratio} = \frac{Cpss_{(m\,1)}}{Cpss} = \frac{f_{m1} CL_T}{CL_{T\,(m1)}} = \frac{0.8 \times 4.33 \text{ L/hr}}{8 \text{ L/hr}} = 0.433$$

10. No, this cannot be determined because we do not have any information about the half-life and the excretion rate constant of the parent drug and the metabolites.

9.7 EFFECT OF CHANGING THE PHARMACOKINETIC PARAMETERS ON THE STEADY-STATE DRUG AND METABOLITE CONCENTRATIONS DURING REPEATED DRUG ADMINISTRATIONS

The following discussion deals with the effect of changing only one pharmacokinetic parameter (all the other parameters are kept constant) on the metabolite/drug concentration ratio at steady state during multiple drug administrations.

9.7.1 Drug Dose

Administration of higher doses of the drug causes a proportional increase in the steady-state drug and metabolite concentrations. The steady-state metabolite/drug concentration ratio stays constant because f_m is kept constant.

9.7.2 Drug Total Body Clearance CL_T

Lower drug clearance results in a higher steady-state drug concentration without affecting the amount of metabolite formation and the metabolite steady-state concentration because f_m is kept constant. This leads to a lower metabolite/drug concentration ratio.

9.7.3 Drug Volume of Distribution Vd

The change in the Vd of the drug does not affect the steady-state concentration of the drug or the metabolite. So, the metabolite/drug concentration ratio at steady state does not change.

9.7.4 Fraction of Drug Dose Converted to Metabolite f_m

Larger f_m leads to a proportional increase in the metabolite formation rate and steady-state concentration when the drug dose is constant. Larger f_m leads to a higher steady-state metabolite/drug concentration ratio.

9.7.5 Metabolite Total Body Clearance $CL_{T(m)}$

Lower $CL_{T(m)}$ causes a proportional increase in the metabolite steady-state concentration without affecting the drug steady-state concentration, that is, a higher metabolite/drug concentration ratio.

9.7.6 Metabolite Volume of Distribution $Vd_{(m)}$

The change in the metabolite Vd does not affect the steady-state concentration of the drug or the metabolite. So, the metabolite/drug concentration ratio at steady state does not change.

9.8 METABOLITE KINETICS AFTER EXTRAVASCULAR ADMINISTRATION OF THE PARENT DRUG

When the parent drug is given as an IV bolus, the highest concentration of the drug is achieved immediately after its administration. So, the rate of metabolite formation, which is a function of the amount of the drug in the body and the metabolic rate constant for that particular pathway, will be at its maximum value initially. Then, the rate of metabolite formation will decrease as the amount of drug in the body decreases because of drug elimination.

However, when the parent drug is administered extravascularly (e.g., orally), the amount of the parent drug in the systemic circulation will be zero initially, then it increases because of drug absorption until it reaches the maximum concentration when the rate of drug absorption is equal to its rate of elimination. Beyond this

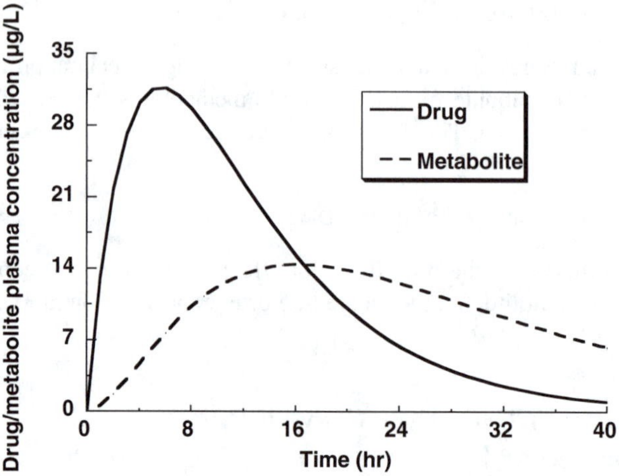

FIGURE 9.9 The drug and metabolite concentration–time profiles after oral administration of a single dose of the drug.

maximum concentration, the drug amount will decline because of drug elimination. Because the rate of metabolite formation is dependent on the amount of the drug in the body, the rate of metabolite formation will be low initially, then it starts to increase as the amount of the parent drug in the body increases until the maximum rate of metabolite formation is achieved when the amount of drug in the body is at its maximum value. After this point, the metabolite formation rate decreases. This makes the time to achieve the maximum metabolite concentration $t_{max(m)}$ usually larger than the time to achieve the maximum drug concentration t_{max}. The parent drug and the metabolite plasma concentration–time profiles after oral administration of the parent drug are illustrated in Figure 9.9.

The metabolite plasma concentration–time profile can be described by a triexponential expression. This expression describes three different processes: parent drug absorption, metabolite formation (or parent drug elimination to form the metabolite of interest), and metabolite elimination. The example presented here assumes that, during the absorption process, the parent drug does not undergo a significant first-pass effect. However, in many cases the parent drug can be metabolized during the absorption process. This will usually result in the appearance of the metabolite and the parent drug simultaneously in the systemic circulation. The resulting metabolite profile will be different from the profile described.

9.9 KINETICS OF SEQUENTIAL METABOLISM

Sequential metabolism means that when the parent drug is metabolized to form a metabolite, this formed metabolite is further metabolized to form a second metabolite. Many drugs are metabolized by sequential metabolism. Carbamazepine, which is an antiepileptic drug, is eliminated through different pathways; one pathway is

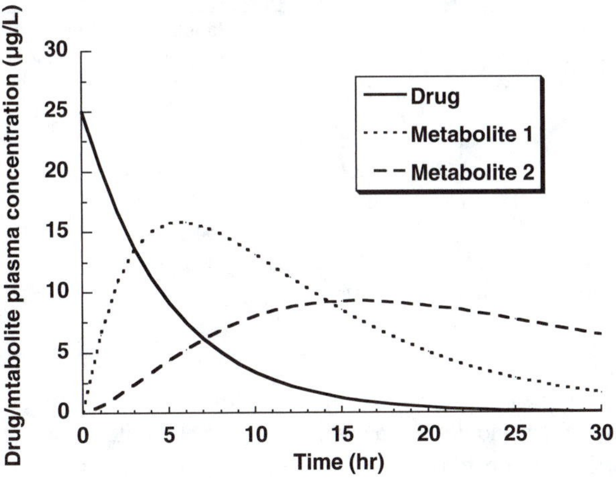

FIGURE 9.10 The drug and metabolite concentration–time profiles after IV administration of a single dose of a drug that is metabolized to metabolite 1, which is further metabolized to metabolite 2.

the formation of its major metabolite, carbamazepine epioxide. The epioxide metabolite is further metabolized to carbamazepine diol, which is then excreted in the urine.

After IV administration of the parent drug, the amount of the first metabolite in the body initially increases until it reaches a maximum concentration; then, it decreases because of metabolite elimination. The rate of the formation of the second metabolite, which is dependent on the amount of the first metabolite in the body, will be low initially and gradually increase until it reaches its maximum rate of formation. Beyond this point, the rate of formation of the second metabolite will decrease. This will result in the appearance of the maximum concentration of the second metabolite after the maximum concentration of the first metabolite. The drug and metabolites concentration-time profiles after IV administration of a drug that is sequentially metabolized to two metabolites is illustrated in Figure 9.10.

Assuming first-order elimination, the plasma metabolite profile of the second metabolite will be described by a triexponential expression. This expression describes three different processes: the formation of the first metabolite (or the parent drug elimination to form the first metabolite), the elimination of the first metabolite (or the elimination of the first metabolite to form the second metabolite), and the elimination of the second metabolite.

PRACTICE PROBLEMS

9.1. A drug is metabolized to three different metabolites through three parallel pathways. After administration of 1000 mg of the parent drug, plasma samples were obtained, and the concentrations of the parent drug and the metabolites were determined.

Time (hr)	Drug (mg/L)	Metabolite 1 (mg/L)	Metabolite 2 (mg/L)	Metabolite 3 (mg/L)
0	50	0	0	0
1	36.6	21.0	25.7	6.43
2	26.8	26.3	42.1	10.5
4	14.4	21.3	56.9	14.2
8	4.1	7.7	54.3	13.5
12	1.2	2.33	40.9	10.2
16	0.34	0.678	28.6	7.1
24	0.03	0.056	13.1	3.28

a. Plot the plasma concentration–time profiles for the parent drug and its metabolites and determine which of the metabolites follow a formation rate-limited profile and which follow an elimination rate-limited profile.

9.2. After administration of a drug to humans, it is eliminated by renal excretion and metabolism to two different metabolites that are completely excreted in urine according to the following scheme (Figure 9.11): After administration of 100 μmol of the parent drug to a normal volunteer, the total amounts of the parent drug, metabolite 1, and metabolite 2 recovered in the urine were 20, 30, and 50 μmol, respectively. The half-life of the parent drug is 4 hr, and its volume of distribution is 25 L.

a. Calculate the CL_T and the AUC of the parent drug after administration of the 100-μmol dose.
b. What is the renal clearance of the parent drug?
c. What is the fraction of the administered dose of the parent drug that is metabolized to metabolite 1?
d. If the observed AUC of metabolite 1 was 10 μmol-hr/L, what is the CL_T of metabolite 1?
e. What is the renal clearance of metabolite 1?
f. What is the formation clearance of metabolites 1 and 2?
g. If a dose of 300 μmol of the parent drug is administered to the same volunteer, then what are the expected AUCs of the parent drug and metabolite 1?

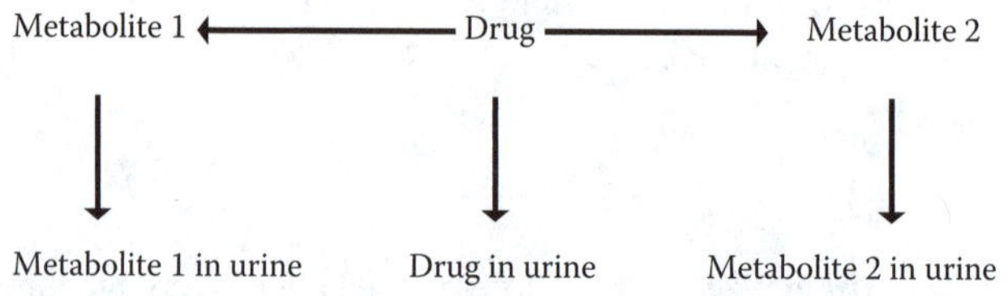

FIGURE 9.11 Schematic presentation of the different pathways involved in the elimination of the parent drug and its two metabolites.

h. If 100 μmol of metabolite 1 is administered to the same volunteer, then what are the total amounts of metabolites 1 and 2 that will be excreted in urine?
i. If a constant-rate IV infusion of the parent drug is administered to this volunteer, then what is the expected ratio of the metabolite concentration to that of the parent drug at steady state?
j. From the information provided, can you determine whether metabolites 1 and 2 follow a formation rate-limited or an elimination rate-limited profile?

9.3. After IV bolus administration of 1 μmol of a drug to a human volunteer, the following data were obtained:

Time (hr)	Parent Drug Concentration (μmol/L)	Metabolite Concentration (μmol/L)
0.5	13.0	0.56
1.5	10.8	1.15
3.0	9.5	2.5
5.0	7.5	4.7
7.0	5.6	6.0
9.0	4.5	6.4
12.5	2.8	4.3
17.5	1.5	2.3
23.5	0.74	1.1
30.0	0.32	0.48

On a separate occasion, 2 weeks later, the same volunteer received 1 mmol of the metabolites by IV bolus administration, and the following data were obtained:

Time (hr)	Metabolite Concentration (μmol/L)
1.0	21
3.5	9.9
6.0	4.5
8.5	2.0
11.0	0.94
16.0	0.2
20.0	0.059
25.0	0.013
32.0	0.0014

a. Calculate the following parameters:

- Fraction of parent drug converted to the metabolite
- Total body clearance of the metabolite
- Volume of distribution of the metabolite
- Formation clearance and formation rate constant of the metabolite

b. If the parent drug is to be given as a constant-rate infusion at 0.25 μmol/hr, then what will be the steady-state concentration of the metabolite?

c. What will be the concentration ratio of metabolite to parent drug at steady state during a constant-rate infusion of the drug?

9.4. An oral hypoglycemic drug is eliminated from the body by renal excretion or metabolism to a metabolite that is completely excreted in urine. After administration of 1000 mg of this drug to a normal volunteer, plasma samples were obtained, and the concentrations of the parent drug and its major metabolite were determined.

Time (hr)	Parent Drug Concentration (mg/L)	Metabolite Concentration (mg/L)
1	2.97	0.166
2	5.1	0.61
3	6.87	1.27
4	7.56	1.65
6	8.42	2.44
8	8.37	2.85
10	7.82	2.95
12	7.04	2.85
16	5.34	2.35
20	3.847	1.75
24	2.69	1.24

On a separate occasion, after IV bolus administration of 1000 mg of the metabolite to the same volunteer, the following concentrations were observed:

Time (hr)	Concentration (mg/L)
1	33.5
4	10.1
8	2.04
12	0.411
16	0.083

The bioavailability of this oral hypoglycemic drug is known to be 80% because of incomplete absorption from the gastrointestinal tract.

Because the difference in molecular weight between the parent drug and the metabolite is small, assume that the molecular weights are equal. The elimination rate constant of the parent drug is 0.2 hr^{-1}.

a. Calculate the CL_T and Vd of the metabolite.
b. What is the fraction of the parent drug (in the systemic circulation) that is converted to the metabolite?
c. What are the formation clearance and the formation rate constant of the metabolite?
d. What are the total amounts of the parent drug and its metabolite excreted in urine after administration of the 1000-mg dose orally?
e. If the parent drug is administered as 1000 mg every 12 hr, then what will be the average steady-state plasma concentrations of the parent drug and the metabolite?

9.5. After IV administration of an antihypertensive drug, 30% of the administered dose is excreted unchanged in urine, and 70% of the dose is metabolized to inactive metabolite that is completely eliminated in the urine. After administration of 50 μmol of this drug, its half-life was 1 hr, its volume of distribution was 20 L, and its AUC was 3.6 μmol-hr/L.

a. What is the renal clearance of the parent drug?
b. What is the metabolic clearance of the parent drug?
c. What is the formation clearance of the metabolite?
d. If the observed metabolite AUC was 5 μmole-hr/L, then what are the metabolite CL_T, metabolic clearance, and renal clearance?
e. If the metabolite volume of distribution is 30 L, determine whether this metabolite follows formation rate- or elimination rate-limited behavior.
f. If 120 μmol of the drug is administered, then what will be the expected parent drug and metabolite AUCs?
g. If the parent drug is administered by constant-rate IV infusion, then what will be the steady-state ratio of metabolite to parent drug concentration?

10 Disease State and Drug Pharmacokinetics

OBJECTIVES

After completing this chapter, you should be able to:

- Identify some causes of variability in drug pharmacokinetics in different individuals
- Determine the factors that affect the change in drug pharmacokinetics in patients with kidney failure during multiple drug administrations
- Analyze the effect of changing the kidney function and the liver function on the drug pharmacokinetics
- Recommend an appropriate dosing regimen in patients with kidney and liver dysfunction
- Evaluate the appropriateness of dosing regimens in patients with kidney and liver dysfunction

10.1 INTRODUCTION

Administration of the same dose of a drug may produce different drug responses in different patients. This difference in drug response can be attributed to differences in drug pharmacokinetics. This difference in the drug pharmacokinetics may result from differences in weight, age, disease, genetic factors, drug interactions, and other physiological and pathological conditions. So, individualization of drug therapy based on the patient's specific conditions is important to ensure that the drug produces the desired therapeutic response with minimal toxicity. The discussion in this chapter focuses on the individualization of the drug therapy in patients with dysfunction of the major eliminating organs. Specifically, strategies for calculating the dosing requirements in patients with kidney dysfunction and liver dysfunction are discussed.

10.2 PATIENTS WITH KIDNEY DYSFUNCTION

10.2.1 Factors Affecting the Change in Drug Pharmacokinetics in Patients with Kidney Dysfunction

10.2.1.1 Fraction of Dose Excreted Unchanged in Urine

Drugs that are excreted by the kidney to a larger extent (larger fraction of the drug dose excreted unchanged in urine) will be affected more by the decrease in kidney function. These drugs require larger reduction in doses to achieve therapeutic drug concentration in patients with renal dysfunction.

10.2.1.2 Degree of Kidney Dysfunction

The decrease in kidney function results in a proportional decrease in the rate of renal elimination of the drug. This decreases the renal clearance of the drug. Patients with lower kidney function require larger reduction of their doses to achieve therapeutic drug concentrations.

10.2.2 Dosage Adjustment in Patients with Renal Dysfunction

The Giusti and Hayton method and the Tozer approach for dosage adjustment in renal failure patients have the following assumptions:

- Kidney dysfunction does not affect the concentration–effect relationship; that is, the therapeutic range does not change because of the change in kidney function.
- The decrease in kidney function results in a proportional decrease in the rate of renal drug elimination.
- The decrease in kidney function does not affect the nonrenal drug elimination.
- The decrease in kidney function does not affect drug absorption or distribution.

Both methods require knowledge of the average drug dose in patients with normal kidney function, the kidney function, and the fraction of drug dose excreted unchanged in urine to calculate the dose required for patients with kidney dysfunction.

10.2.2.1 Determination of Kidney Function

The kidney function is expressed as the fraction of the normal kidney function. The creatinine clearance represents an accurate measure of the kidney function. The fraction remaining of kidney function is determined from the ratio of the creatinine clearance in the patient to the normal creatinine clearance.

$$\text{KF} = \frac{\text{Cr CL}_{\text{failure}}}{\text{Cr CL}_{\text{normal}}} \tag{10.1}$$

The creatinine clearance, which reflects the glomerular filtration rate, can be measured directly from 24-hr urine collection as discussed in Chapter 8. Also, mathematical expressions can be used to estimate the creatinine clearance from such patient information as age, weight, gender, and serum creatinine. These methods of CrCL estimation are empirical and are developed statistically to predict CrCL from patients' information. The CrCL estimation methods differ in the accuracy of the estimation in different patient populations. An example of these CrCL estimation methods is the Cockroft and Gault method, which can provide a reasonable estimate for the creatinine clearance in milliliters per minute from the age, weight, serum creatinine, and gender as in Equations 10.2 and 10.3. For males,

$$\text{Cr CL} = \frac{(140\text{-Age})\ (\text{Weight in kg})}{72\ (\text{Serum creatinine in mg/dl})} \tag{10.2}$$

and for females,

$$\text{Cr CL} = 0.85\left(\frac{(140\text{ - Age})\ (\text{Weight in kg})}{72\ (\text{Serum creatinine in mg/dl})}\right) \tag{10.3}$$

10.2.2.2 Determination of the Fraction of Dose Excreted Unchanged in Urine

The fraction of dose excreted unchanged in urine is determined from the ratio of the total amount of the drug excreted in urine and the intravenous (IV) dose:

$$\text{Fraction (f)} = \frac{A_{e\infty}}{\text{Dose}} \tag{10.4}$$

For the oral dose,

$$\text{Fraction (f)} = \frac{A_{e\infty}}{\text{F Dose}} \tag{10.5}$$

The fraction excreted unchanged in urine can be determined from the ratio of the renal excretion rate constant to the elimination rate constant or the ratio of the renal clearance to the total body clearance.

$$\text{Fraction (f)} = \frac{k_e}{k} = \frac{CL_R}{CL_T} \tag{10.6}$$

10.2.2.3 Determination of Dosage Requirements in Patients with Reduced Kidney Function

The dose for patients with kidney dysfunction can be calculated from the following expression:

$$\text{Dose}_{\text{failure}} = \text{Dose}_{\text{normal}}\ [\text{f (KF} - 1) + 1] \tag{10.7}$$

where f is the fraction of the drug dose normally excreted unchanged in the urine after an IV dose in patients with normal kidney function, and KF is the fraction remaining of the kidney function. Also, the half-life of the drug in patients with renal dysfunction can be determined from the following relationship:

$$t_{1/2\ \text{failure}} = \frac{t_{1/2\ \text{normal}}}{[\,f\,(KF - 1) + 1\,]} \tag{10.8}$$

Example

A patient admitted to the hospital because of acute myocardial infarction was started on oral antiarrhythmic medication. He was given the average recommended dose for patients with normal kidney function, which is 600 mg every 12 hr from an oral formulation known to be rapidly and completely absorbed. At steady state, the maximum and minimum plasma concentrations were 40 mg/ml and 10 mg/ml, respectively.

1. Calculate mathematically the half-life and the volume of distribution of this drug in this patient.
2. The patient suddenly developed acute renal failure, and the kidney function dropped to 30% of its normal value. If the renal clearance of this drug is 70% of the total body clearance, then recommend an appropriate dose for this patient after development of renal failure.
3. Calculate the maximum and minimum plasma concentration achieved at steady state from the regimen you recommended in part 2.

Answer

1.

$$Cp_{ss.\ max} - Cp_{ss.\ min} = \frac{\text{Dose}}{Vd}$$

$$40\ \text{mg/L} - 10\ \text{mg/L} = \frac{600\ \text{mg}}{Vd}$$

$$Vd = \frac{600\ \text{mg}}{30\ \text{mg/ L}} = 20\ \text{L}$$

$$Cp_{ss.\ min} = Cp_{ss.\ max}\ e^{-k\tau}$$

$$10\ \text{mg/L} = 40\ \text{mg/L}\ e^{-k\ 12\ \text{hr}}$$

$$\ln \frac{10\ \text{mg/L}}{40\ \text{mg/L}} = -k\ 12\ \text{hr}$$

$$-1.386 = -k\ 12\ \text{hr}$$

$$k = 0.1155\ \text{hr}^{-1} \qquad t_{1/2} = 6\ \text{hr}$$

2.

$$f = \frac{CL_R}{CL_T} = \frac{70}{100} = 0.7$$

$$KF = 0.3$$

$$\text{Dose}_{\text{failure}} = \text{Dose}_{\text{normal}}\ [\,f\,(KF - 1) + 1\,]$$

$$\text{Dose}_{\text{failure}} = 600\ \text{mg/12 hr}\ [\,0.7\,(0.3 - 1) + 1\,]$$

$$\text{Dose}_{\text{failure}} = 294\ \text{mg/12 hr}$$

3.

$$t_{1/2\ \text{failure}} = \frac{t_{1/2\ \text{normal}}}{[\,f\,(KF - 1) + 1\,]} = \frac{6\ \text{hr}}{[\,0.7\,(0.3 - 1) + 1\,]} = 12.24\ \text{hr}$$

$$k_{\text{failure}} = \frac{0.693}{12.24} = 0.0566\ \text{hr}^{-1}$$

$$Cp_{ss.\ \text{max}} = \frac{D}{Vd\,(1 - e^{-k\tau})}$$

$$Cp_{ss.\ \text{max}} = \frac{294\ \text{mg}}{20\ \text{L}\,(1 - e^{-0.0566\ \text{hr}^{-1}\ 12\ \text{hr}})} = 29.8\ \text{mg/L}$$

$$Cp_{ss.\ \text{min}} = Cp_{ss.\ \text{max}}\ e^{-k\tau}$$

$$Cp_{ss.\ \text{min}} = 29.8\ \text{mg/L}\ e^{-0.0566\ \text{hr}^{-1}\ 12\ \text{hr}} = 15.1\ \text{mg/L}$$

10.3 PATIENTS WITH LIVER DISEASES

Liver diseases can lead to hepatocyte damage, which results in reduction of the metabolic rate of the liver. Dosage reduction in patients with liver diseases may not be necessary unless there is significant reduction in the liver's metabolizing ability, such as in patients with liver cirrhosis. The reduction in the hepatic drug metabolism can lead to a slower rate of drug metabolism and reduction in the drug first-pass effect, leading to higher bioavailability. So, patients with advanced liver diseases may require dosage reduction for the drugs that are mainly eliminated by metabolism.

Dosage adjustment in patients with liver diseases is not as easy as in kidney diseases because there is no clinical laboratory test that can serve as a quantitative measure for the hepatic metabolic rate. Also, the different enzyme systems have different capacities for drug metabolism. So, for a limited-capacity enzyme system, the rate of drug metabolism may be significantly reduced with mild or moderate liver disease. On the other hand, significant reduction in the liver function may be necessary before the rate of metabolism is reduced in high-capacity enzyme systems. These two factors make the dosage adjustment in patients with liver disease a difficult task. There are several methods used for dosage calculations in patients with liver diseases, including the method dependent on the Child–Pugh score.

10.3.1 Child–Pugh Score

The liver's metabolizing ability is assessed in this method from the determination of the Child–Pugh score. This score is dependent on five different laboratory tests and clinical conditions: serum albumin, total bilirubin, prothrombin time, ascites, and encephalopathy. Each of these parameters can take a score from 1 (normal) to 3 (severely abnormal) as in Table 10.1. The total Child–Pugh score is calculated from the sum of the scores for all the parameters.

Patients with normal liver function can have a score of 5; patients with severe liver dysfunction can have a score of 15. Patients with a score of 8–9 require 25% reduction of their initial doses of drugs mainly eliminated from the body by hepatic metabolism (>60% metabolized); patients with a score of 10 or more require 50% reduction of their initial doses of drugs mainly eliminated from the body by hepatic metabolism. It is important to note that this is a recommendation for the starting doses of the drugs. After starting the drug therapy, the pharmacological and adverse effects of the drugs should be monitored, and further dosage adjustment should be made if necessary.

TABLE 10.1
Parameters Used in the Calculation of the Child–Pugh Score and the Breakdown of the Score for Each Parameter

	Score		
Parameters	**1**	**2**	**3**
Serum albumin (g/dL)	> 3.5	2.8–3.5	< 2.8
Total bilirubin (mg/dL)	< 2.0	2.0–3.0	> 3.0
Prothrombin time (seconds longer than control)	< 4	4–6	> 6
Ascites	Absent	Mild	Moderate
Encephalopathy	None	Moderate	Severe

Example

A 55-year-old female was admitted to the hospital after developing an episode of ventricular arrhythmia. The patient had a history of multiple medical problems, including liver cirrhosis, hypertension, and ischemic heart disease. Her laboratory values on admission were 1.1 mg/dL serum creatinine, 3.2 g/dL serum albumin, 4.5 mg/dL total bilirubin, and a prothrombin time 8 s longer than the control. Physical examination showed that the patient was alert without any signs of encephalopathy, and the patient had mild ascites. The physician wanted to start the patient on lidocaine and asked you to recommend an average starting dose of lidocaine.

Answer

Lidocaine is an antiarrhythmic drug that is completely metabolized. So, the patient's liver condition may affect the clearance of lidocaine. It is wise to calculate the Child–Pugh score for this patient to see if dosage reduction is necessary. For calculation of the Child–Pugh score based on Table 10.1:

Serum albumin	3.2 g/dL	Score = 2
Bilirubin	4.5 mg/dL	Score = 3
Prothromin time	8 s > Control	Score = 3
Ascites	Mild	Score = 2
Encephalopathy	Absent	Score = 1
	Total	Child–Pugh score = 11

Based on the Child–Pugh score, the starting dose of lidocaine for this patient should be 50% of the average recommended dose. Please note that the lidocaine dose can be adjusted after the start of therapy according to its therapeutic and adverse effects.

PRACTICE PROBLEMS

10.1. A patient admitted to the hospital because of acute myocardial infarction was started on oral antiarrhythmic medication. He was given 600 mg every 12 hr via an oral formulation known to be rapidly absorbed but only 80% bioavailable. At steady state, the maximum and minimum plasma concentrations were 30 μg/ml and 10.5 μg/ml, respectively.

a. Calculate mathematically the half-life and the volume of distribution of this drug in this patient.
b. The patient suddenly developed acute renal failure, and the kidney function dropped to 30% of its normal value. If the renal clearance of this drug is 75% of the total body clearance, then recommend an appropriate oral dose for this patient after development of renal failure.
c. Calculate the maximum and minimum plasma concentrations achieved at steady state from the regimen you recommended in problem 10.1b.

10.2. A 65-year-old man was taking 500 mg antihypertensive medication every 12 hr in the form of an oral tablet that is rapidly and completely absorbed. After administration of a single oral 500-mg dose, 375 mg is excreted unchanged in urine, and the drug half-life is 8 hr. The average plasma concentration of this antihypertensive drug in this patient while taking 500 mg every 12 hr was 20 mg/L.

a. Calculate the volume of distribution of this drug in this patient.
b. This patient developed acute renal failure, and his creatinine clearance decreased from the normal value of 120 ml/min to 30 ml/min. Calculate the new total body clearance for this drug in this patient after development of renal failure assuming that the deterioration in the kidney function does not affect the drug distribution characteristics.
c. Recommend a maintenance dose for this patient after he developed renal failure if the usual dose in patients with normal kidney function is 500 mg every 12 hr.
d. Calculate the maximum and minimum plasma concentrations achieved at steady state from the regimen you recommended in problem 10.2c.

10.3. A patient was admitted to the hospital because of severe pneumonia. An IV loading dose of an antibiotic followed by IV maintenance doses of 300 mg every 12 hr were prescribed. The creatinine clearance was 120 ml/min, which is considered normal for this patient. After 7 days of therapy (300 mg every 12 hr), the maximum and minimum plasma concentrations were 38 mg/l and 12.5 mg/L, respectively.

a. Calculate mathematically the half-life and the volume of distribution of this drug in this patient.
b. At steady state (while receiving 300 mg every 12 hr), 180 mg of the drug is excreted unchanged in urine during one dosing interval. What is the renal clearance of this drug?
c. After 15 days of antibiotic therapy, the kidney function of this patient deteriorated, and his creatinine clearance was 40 ml/min. What is the new half-life of the drug after this change in the patient's kidney function?
d. What will be the steady-state maximum and minimum plasma concentrations if this patient continues taking 300 mg every 12 hr intravenously despite the change in his kidney function?

10.4. After IV administration of procainamide (an antiarrhythmic drug), 60% of the administered dose is excreted unchanged in urine. The rest of the dose is metabolized in the liver. The average volume of distribution of procainamide is 140 L, the half-life is 3 hr in patients with normal kidney function, and the bioavailability is 100%.

a. Calculate the renal clearance of procainamide in patients with normal kidney function.
b. Calculate the half-life of procainamide in a patient with creatinine clearance of 30 ml/min (normal creatinine clearance is 120 ml/min).

c. Calculate the daily oral maintenance dose required in a patient with creatinine clearance of 30 ml/min (normal creatinine clearance is 120 ml/min). (The average daily oral maintenance dose in patients with normal kidney function is 3 g/day.)

d. If a patient with creatinine clearance of 30 ml/min (normal creatinine clearance is 120 ml/min) receives 750 mg every 6 hr, then calculate the maximum and minimum plasma concentrations at steady state in this patient.

10.5. A new antihypertensive drug is rapidly but incompletely absorbed. When 800 mg is given intravenously to normal volunteers, 600 mg can be recovered in the urine unchanged from time 0 to ∞, the AUC obtained from time 0 to ∞ is 400 mg-hr/L, and the elimination half-life is 8 hr. When 400 mg is given orally, the AUC from time 0 to ∞ is 125 mg-hr/L.

a. If a patient with normal kidney function is receiving 800 mg every 12 hr orally, what will be the average plasma concentration at steady state?

b. Calculate the maximum and the minimum plasma concentrations achieved at steady state for the regimen in problem 10.5a (800 mg every 12 hr orally) if the drug is rapidly absorbed after oral administration.

c. If the average maintenance dose for a patient with normal kidney function is 800 mg IV every 12 hr, what will be the maintenance dose for a patient whose creatinine clearance is only 10% of normal?

d. What will be the maximum and the minimum plasma concentrations at steady state for the IV regimen you recommended in problem 10.5c for the patient with 10% of normal kidney function assuming that the change in kidney function does not affect the volume of distribution?

11 Nonlinear Pharmacokinetics

OBJECTIVES

After completing this chapter, you should be able to:

- Describe the most common causes of nonlinear pharmacokinetic behavior and the common characteristics of nonlinear pharmacokinetics
- Define the Michaelis–Menten (M–M) pharmacokinetic parameters
- Describe the basic characteristics of M–M pharmacokinetics
- Analyze the effect of changing one or more of the pharmacokinetic parameters on the steady-state plasma concentration after single and multiple drug administrations
- Determine the nonlinear pharmacokinetic parameters using mathematical and graphical methods
- Recommend the dosing regimen required to achieve a therapeutic plasma concentration of drugs that follow nonlinear kinetics in patients

11.1 INTRODUCTION

Linear pharmacokinetics is observed when the pharmacokinetic parameters that describe the absorption, distribution, and elimination processes of the drug are constant and do not change with the change in dose or during chronic use of the drug. Nonlinear pharmacokinetics is observed when the absorption, distribution, or elimination processes can be saturated at a high drug concentration. At high drug concentrations, saturable processes follow zero-order kinetics, and nonlinear pharmacokinetics is observed.

11.1.1 Causes of Nonlinear Pharmacokinetics

11.1.1.1 Saturable Drug Absorption

Drugs that are absorbed by a saturable transport system in the gastrointestinal tract or undergo a saturable first-pass effect have dose-dependent bioavailability.

11.1.1.2 Saturable Protein Binding

Drugs that undergo saturable plasma protein binding or saturable tissue binding have concentration-dependent distribution. Also, this saturable protein binding can affect drug elimination because the rate of drug elimination is dependent on the free concentration for some drugs (drugs with a low extraction ratio).

11.1.1.3 Saturable Renal Elimination

Drugs that are actively secreted or actively reabsorbed in the renal tubules can have dose-dependent renal elimination after administration of large doses.

11.1.1.4 Saturable Drug Metabolism

Drugs that are metabolized by a saturable metabolic pathway can have dose-dependent pharmacokinetics after administration of large doses.

11.1.1.5 Others

Conditions such as enzyme induction, product inhibition, and drug-related pathological changes that affect drug excretion can result in nonlinear pharmacokinetics.

11.1.2 Evidence of Nonlinear Pharmacokinetics

The drug follows nonlinear pharmacokinetics when at least one of the following conditions is observed:

- The plasma concentration–time profile is not linear on a semilog scale.
- The area under the plasma concentration–time curve (AUC) is not proportional to the administered dose after administration of a single dose.
- The steady-state plasma concentration is not proportional to the administered dose during multiple drug administrations.
- The estimated pharmacokinetic parameters such as the half-life and total body clearance are different after administration of different doses.

11.2 MICHAELIS–MENTEN ENZYME KINETICS

Enzymes usually react with the substrate (drug) to form enzyme-substrate complexes; then, the product (metabolite) is formed. The enzyme can go back to react with another substrate to form another molecule of the product.

$$E + D \leftrightarrow ED \rightarrow E + M \tag{11.1}$$

where E is the enzyme, D is the drug, ED is the drug-enzyme complex, and M is the metabolite. According to the M–M kinetics, a quantitative relationship between the enzymatic reaction rate V and drug concentration Cp may be expressed as

$$V = \frac{V_{max}\ Cp}{K_m + Cp} \tag{11.2}$$

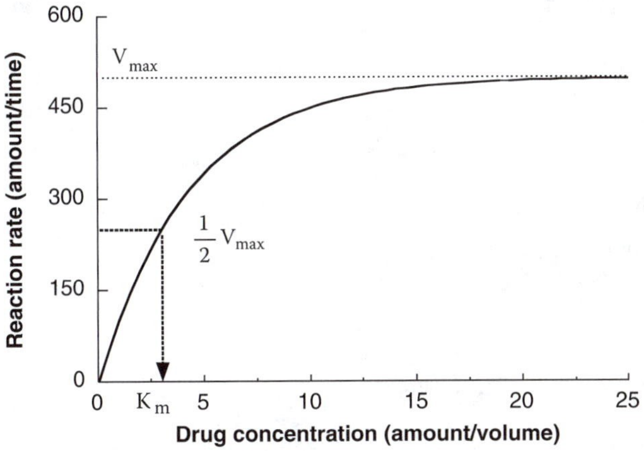

FIGURE 11.1 The relationship between the enzymatic reaction rate and the drug concentration. The V_{max} is the maximum reaction rate, and K_m is the drug concentration when the reaction rate is $V_{max}/2$.

where V_{max} is the maximum rate of the enzymatic reaction, and K_m is the M–M constant. Graphically, this relationship can be presented as in Figure 11.1. The rate of drug metabolism via a single metabolic pathway can be expressed as

$$\text{Rate of drug metabolism} = \frac{V_{max}\ Cp}{K_m + Cp} \tag{11.3}$$

where V_{max} is the maximum rate of drug metabolism, and K_m is the drug concentration when the rate of the drug metabolism is half the maximum rate ($V_{max}/2$). This hyperbolic relationship indicates that, as the drug concentration increases, the rate of drug metabolism increases until it reaches a plateau at a high drug concentration. At this plateau, the enzyme system is saturated, and the metabolic rate is at its maximum value. Theoretically, all metabolic pathways can be saturated at a high drug concentration. However, saturable drug metabolism is of great clinical significance when saturation occurs after administration of therapeutic doses.

The relationship between the enzymatic reaction rate and the drug concentration, which is presented in Figure 11.1, depends on the concentration of the drug. At low drug concentration (i.e., $K_m >> Cp$), Equation 11.3 is reduced to

$$\text{Rate} \cong \left(\frac{V_{max}}{K_m}\right) Cp \tag{11.4}$$

This means that the reaction rate becomes proportional to the drug concentration, and the metabolic process follows first-order kinetics.

However, at a high drug concentration (i.e., $K_m << Cp$), Equation 11.3 is reduced to

$$\text{Rate} \cong \left(\frac{V_{max}\ Cp}{Cp} \right) \cong V_{max} \qquad (11.5)$$

This means that the reaction rate becomes constant and independent of the drug concentration, and the metabolic process follows zero-order kinetics.

11.2.1 Pharmacokinetic Parameters

The V_{max} of a metabolic pathway is the maximum rate of drug metabolism through this particular metabolic pathway (units are amount/time, i.e., units of rate). Each metabolic pathway has its own maximum rate. V_{max} is dependent on the amount of enzymes involved in the metabolic process. Conditions like enzyme induction increase the available amount of the enzymes and can increase V_{max}. Enzyme induction increases the amount of the enzyme without affecting its affinity to react with drugs. This means that enzyme induction does not affect the K_m of the enzymatic process as in Figure 11.2.

The M–M constant K_m is a qualitative characteristic of how an enzyme interacts with the drug and is independent of the enzyme concentration. This constant is equal to the substrate concentration when the reaction rate is half its maximum value (units are mass/volume, i.e., concentration units). In the presence of a competitive inhibitor of the enzyme, the metabolic rate will be slower at any given drug concentration. However, as the drug concentration increases relative to the inhibitor concentration, the maximum metabolic rate will be achieved. This means that, in the presence of a competitive inhibitor, K_m will increase without affecting V_{max}, as illustrated in Figure 11.3.

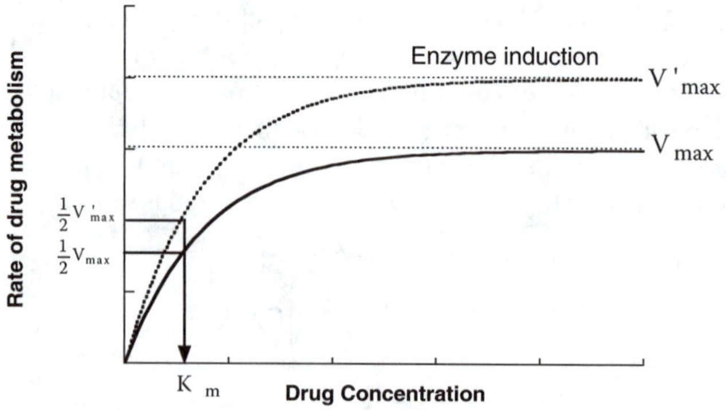

FIGURE 11.2 Enzyme induction causes increase in the V_{max} without affecting K_m.

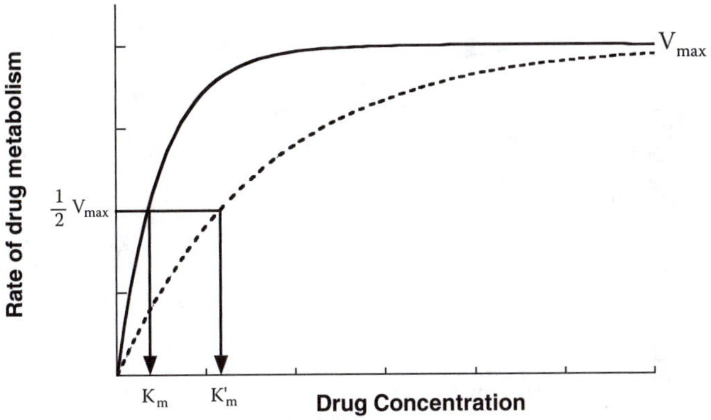

FIGURE 11.3 Competitive inhibition of the enzyme responsible for drug metabolism causes increase in K_m without affecting V_{max}.

11.2.2 Plasma Concentration–Time Profile after a Single Intravenous Dose of a Drug Eliminated by a Metabolic Pathway That Follows Michaelis–Menten Kinetics

11.2.2.1 After a Single Drug Administration

The model that describes the drug pharmacokinetic behavior after a single intravenous (IV) dose when the drug elimination is through a single metabolic pathway that follows M–M kinetics is presented in Figure 11.4. The plasma concentration–time profile after a single IV bolus dose of a drug that is eliminated by a single metabolic pathway that follows M–M kinetics is presented in Figure 11.5. The initial drug concentration is dependent on the dose and the volume of distribution. This means that administration of increasing doses produces initial drug concentrations that are proportional to the administered dose.

$$Cp_0 = \frac{\text{Dose}}{\text{Vd}} \tag{11.6}$$

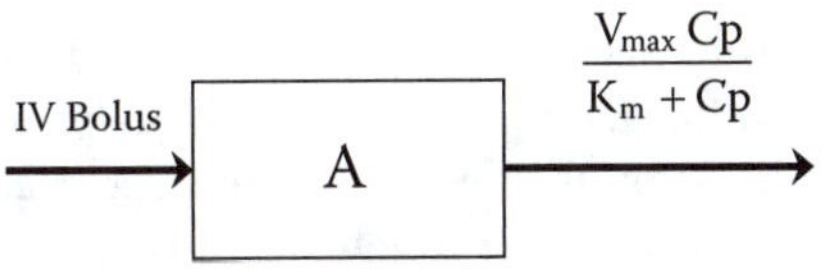

FIGURE 11.4 Schematic presentation of the pharmacokinetic model for a single IV bolus dose of a drug eliminated by a single pathway that follows M–M kinetics. A is the amount of the drug in the body.

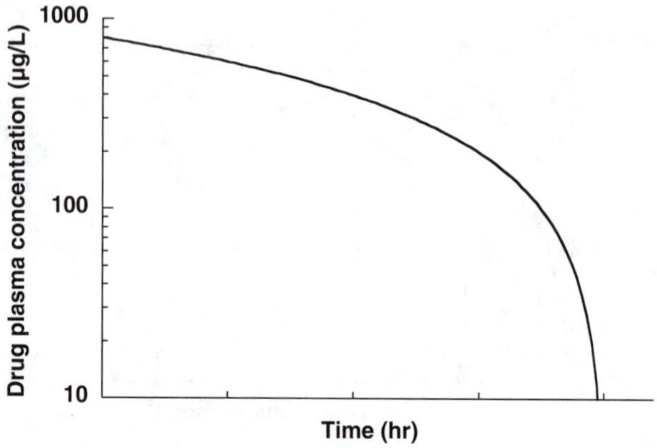

FIGURE 11.5 The plasma concentration–time profile after a single IV bolus dose of a drug eliminated by a single metabolic pathway that follows M–M kinetics.

The rate of decline in the amount of the drug in the body is equal to the rate of drug metabolism.

$$\frac{-dA}{dt} = \frac{V_{max}\ Cp}{K_m + Cp} \tag{11.7}$$

Integration of Equation 11.7 and division by the volume of distribution gives Equation 11.8:

$$Cp = Cp_0 + K_m \ln\left(\frac{Cp_0}{Cp}\right) - \frac{V_{max}\ t}{Vd} \tag{11.8}$$

Equation 11.8 is not an explicit expression for the plasma concentration-versus-time profile, which cannot be used to calculate the plasma concentration at specific times after drug administration because the term Cp is present in both sides of the equation and cannot be separated.

11.2.2.2 After Multiple Drug Administrations

The rate of drug administration is equal to the rate of drug elimination at steady state. When the drug is eliminated by a single metabolic pathway that follows M–M kinetics, the relationship between the dosing rate and steady-state drug plasma concentration can be described by the following equation:

$$\frac{F\,D}{\tau} = \frac{V_{max}\ Cp_{ss}}{K_m + Cp_{ss}} \tag{11.9}$$

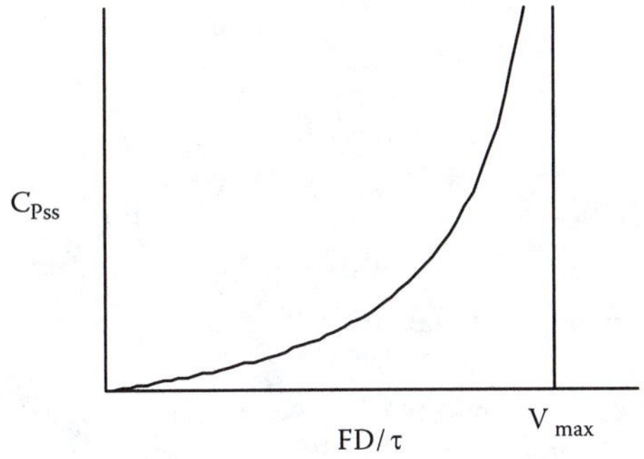

FIGURE 11.6 The relationship between the steady-state concentration and the dosing rate during multiple administrations of a drug when the drug elimination process follows M–M kinetics.

This relationship can be rearranged to obtain an expression for the steady-state drug plasma concentration:

$$Cp_{ss} = \frac{(FD/\tau)\ K_m}{V_{max} - (FD/\tau)} \qquad (11.10)$$

This expression means that administration of increasing doses of the drug results in more than proportional increase in the steady-state plasma drug concentration as presented in Figure 11.6. Note that in Equation 11.10 if the dosing rate D/τ exceeds V_{max}, the calculated steady-state concentration will be a negative value. The steady-state plasma concentration cannot be a negative value. From the definition of V_{max}, it is the maximum rate of drug elimination. So, if the dosing rate exceeds V_{max}, then steady state will never be achieved, and continuous accumulation of the drug in the body will occur.

11.3 DETERMINATION OF THE PHARMACOKINETIC PARAMETERS

11.3.1 Total Body Clearance

The total body clearance can be determined by dividing the drug excretion rate by the drug concentration:

$$CL_T = \frac{V_{max}}{K_m + Cp} \qquad (11.11)$$

The total body clearance is dependent on the drug concentration. As the drug concentration becomes higher, the total body clearance will be lower.

11.3.2 Half-Life

$$t_{1/2} = \frac{0.693\ Vd}{V_{max}} (K_m + Cp) \tag{11.12}$$

The half-life is dependent on the drug concentration. The half-life is longer when the drug concentration is higher.

The total body clearance and the half-life are different at different drug concentrations. So, these parameters have to be calculated at a specific drug concentration. After a single drug administration, the drug concentration will be changing, and the total body clearance and half-life will be changing. However, at steady state the plasma drug concentration will be fluctuating around an average steady-state concentration, and the total body clearance and half-life can be estimated at this average steady-state concentration.

11.4 EFFECT OF CHANGING THE PHARMACOKINETIC PARAMETERS ON PLASMA CONCENTRATION–TIME PROFILE

11.4.1 Dose

Administration of larger doses achieves higher initial drug plasma concentrations. Higher concentrations result in lower total body clearance and longer half-life. However, at any concentration the rate of decline of the drug concentration is similar because K_m and V_{max} are constant. Increasing the dose results in more than a proportional increase in the steady-state concentration during multiple drug administrations. It takes a longer time to achieve steady state following administration of larger doses.

11.4.2 V_{MAX}

A larger V_{max} results in higher drug total body clearance and shorter half-life, which lead to a faster rate of drug elimination and smaller area under the plasma concentration–time curve. Following multiple administrations of similar doses, the steady-state concentration will be lower when V_{max} is higher.

11.4.3 K_M

A larger K_m results in lower drug total body clearance and longer half-life, which lead to a slower rate of drug elimination and larger area under the plasma concentration–time curve. Following multiple administrations of similar doses, the steady-state concentration will be higher when K_m is higher.

11.5 ORAL ADMINISTRATION OF DRUGS ELIMINATED BY A MICHAELIS–MENTEN PROCESS

The rate of drug absorption significantly affects the plasma concentration–time profile after a single oral dose when drug elimination is nonlinear. After oral administration of the same dose of a drug, rapidly absorbed formulations will achieve higher drug concentrations (larger AUCs) compared to slowly absorbed formulations. This is because rapidly absorbed formulations achieve a higher maximum drug concentration. At a higher drug concentration, the total body clearance is lower, and the half-life is longer when drug elimination is nonlinear.

During multiple drug administration, the steady-state plasma drug concentration is dependent on the dose, V_{max}, and K_m. The rate of drug absorption does not affect the average steady-state plasma concentration. However, faster drug absorption may result in larger fluctuations in drug concentration at steady state.

The pharmacological effect of some drugs may be different after a single oral administration because of the difference in the rate of drug absorption. For example, alcohol is eliminated by a saturable metabolic process. Administration of the same amount of alcohol may produce different alcohol plasma concentration–time profiles depending on the rate of absorption. Alcohol intake on an empty stomach results in faster absorption, higher alcohol blood concentration, and more intense effects compared to intake on a full stomach, which may lead to slower absorption and lower alcohol blood concentration. Slower alcohol absorption also leads to a larger first-pass effect, which can result in lower alcohol blood concentration.

11.6 PHARMACOKINETIC PARAMETER DETERMINATION AND DOSAGE RECOMMENDATION

The method used to calculate the pharmacokinetic parameters has the following assumptions:

1. The drug is eliminated by a single metabolic pathway that follows M–M kinetics.
2. The drug is at steady state during repeated administration of a constant dose.
3. The method requires knowledge of two different steady-state concentrations during two different doses.

11.6.1 Mathematical Method

The relationship between the administered dose and the steady-state plasma concentration can be described by Equation 11.9:

$$\frac{F\,D}{\tau} = \frac{V_{max}\ Cp_{ss}}{K_m + Cp_{ss}}$$

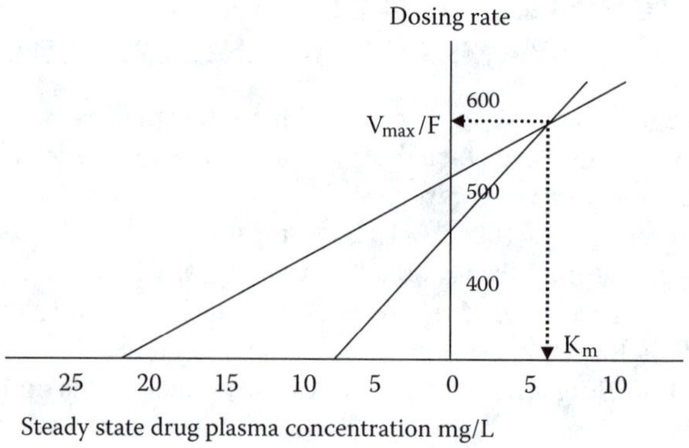

FIGURE 11.7 The direct linear plot.

When two different steady-state concentrations are achieved during administration of two different doses, two different equations can be constructed.

$$\frac{F D_1}{\tau} = \frac{V_{max}\ Cp_{ss\,1}}{K_m + Cp_{ss\,1}} \quad \text{and} \quad \frac{F D_2}{\tau} = \frac{V_{max}\ Cp_{ss\,2}}{K_m + Cp_{ss\,2}}$$

These two equations can be solved simultaneously to determine the pharmacokinetic parameters V_{max} and K_m.

11.6.2 Direct Linear Plot

The direct linear plot is a linear transformation method that is used to estimate the nonlinear pharmacokinetic parameters (V_{max} and K_m). This method requires the knowledge of two different dosing rates and the steady-state plasma concentration achieved with each dosing rate.

By plotting two lines between each of the dosing rates and their corresponding steady-state concentration and extrapolating the two lines, the two lines will intersect at a point. The X-coordinate of this point corresponds to the K_m, and the Y-coordinate of the point corresponds to the V_{max}/F as presented in Figure 11.7.

The direct linear plot can be used to predict the steady-state plasma concentration achieved after administration of a specific dose and to estimate the dose required to achieve a certain plasma concentration.

Example

A 32-year-old, 75-kg female has been taking 200 mg phenytoin daily. Because the average phenytoin plasma concentration was only 6 mg/L, her phenytoin dose was increased to 350 mg/day. The steady-state average phenytoin concentration was 21 mg/L. (Vd of phenytoin is 0.75 L/kg, and F = 1.)

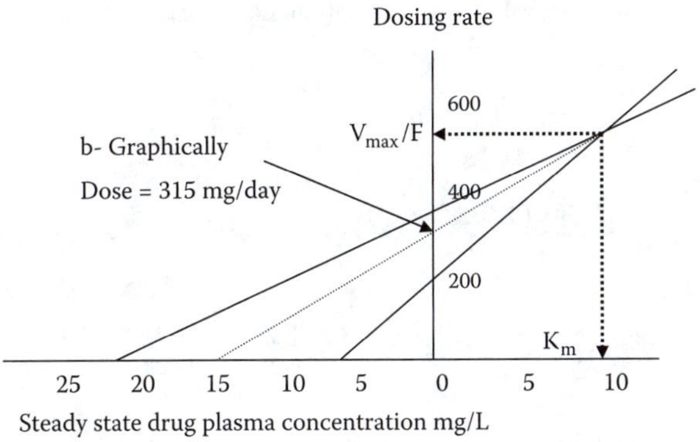

FIGURE 11.8 The V_{max}, K_m, and the dose that achieve certain steady-state concentration are determined from the direct linear plot.

1. Using the direct linear plot, calculate the phenytoin V_{max} and K_m in this patient.
2. Calculate the dose required to achieve an average steady-state phenytoin plasma concentration around 15 mg/L.
3. Calculate the phenytoin half-life at steady state while the patient was taking 350 mg/day.
4. Because of poor seizure control, phenobarbitone was added to the patient's medications. After several weeks, the phenytoin plasma concentration was 14 mg/L while taking 360 mg/day phenytoin. Comment on the decrease in phenytoin plasma concentration.

Answer

1. From the direct linear plot in Figure 11.8:

$$V_{max} = 500 \text{ mg/day}$$

$$K_m = 9 \text{ mg/L}$$

2. The dose required to achieve a steady-state concentration of 15 mg/L can be determined graphically and mathematically. Graphically, from Figure 11.8, the dose is approximately 315 mg/day. Mathematically,

$$\frac{F\,D}{\tau} = \frac{V_{max}\ Cp_{ss}}{K_m + Cp_{ss}}$$

$$\frac{F\,D}{\tau} = \frac{500 \text{ mg/day}\ \ 15 \text{ mg/L}}{9 \text{ mg/L} + 15 \text{ mg/L}} = 312.5 \text{ mg/day}$$

3. The steady state when the dose was 350 mg/day = 21 mg/L.

$$t_{1/2} = \frac{0.693\ Vd}{V_{max}}(K_m + Cp)$$

$$t_{1/2} = \frac{0.693\ (0.7\ L/kg \times 75\ kg)}{500\ mg/day}(9\ mg/L + 21\ mg/L) = 2.18\ days$$

4. Phenobarbitone is an enzyme inducer that can increase the rate of phenytoin metabolism (increase V_{max}) and decrease its steady-state concentration.

11.6.3 Linear Transformation Method

The linear transformation method is based on a linear transformation of the M–M equation. At steady state during multiple dose administrations, Equation 11.9 describes the relationship between the dosing rate and the plasma concentration at steady state:

$$\frac{F\,D}{\tau} = \frac{V_{max}\ Cp_{ss}}{K_m + Cp_{ss}}$$

The idea of the linear transformation method is to mathematically manipulate the M–M equation to put it in the form of a linear equation. Equation 11.9 can be written in the following form:

$$\frac{F\,D}{\tau}K_m + \frac{F\,D}{\tau}Cp_{ss} = V_{max}\ Cp_{ss} \tag{11.13}$$

Rearrangement and division by F Cp_{ss} gives

$$\frac{D}{\tau} = -K_m\frac{D/\tau}{Cp_{ss}} + \frac{V_{max}}{F} \tag{11.14}$$

This is the equation of a straight line. A plot of the dosing rate D/τ versus the dosing rate divided by the average steady-state level yields a straight line with a slope equal to $-K_m$, and the y-intercept equals V_{max}/F as in Figure 11.9. The slope and the intercept can be used to calculate a dosing rate required to produce a desired Cp_{ss} or conversely to calculate the expected Cp_{ss} from a given dosing rate.

11.7 MULTIPLE ELIMINATION PATHWAYS

Some drugs are eliminated by more than one elimination pathways, and one of these pathways is saturable. Administration of increasing doses will saturate the saturable pathway, and a larger fraction of the administered dose will be eliminated through the first-order pathways. In the presence of more than one saturable elimination pathway, these different pathways usually have different capacities. This makes the fraction of the administered dose that goes through each of the pathways different after administration of different doses.

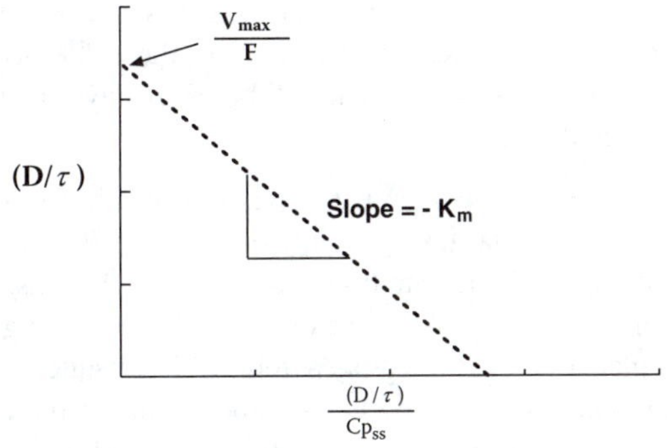

FIGURE 11.9 The linear transformation method.

PRACTICE PROBLEMS

11.1. A 78-kg, 28-year-old man is receiving phenytoin for the treatment of seizures. When this patient was taking a daily oral dose of 250 mg phenytoin, his steady-state plasma concentration was 7.2 mg/L. Because phenytoin plasma concentration was well below the therapeutic range, the patient's daily dose was increased to 450 mg phenytoin, which resulted in a steady-state plasma concentration of 30 mg/L. (Assume that the absolute bioavailability of oral phenytoin is 100%, and that the volume of distribution of phenytoin is 50 L.)

a. Graphically calculate the patient's V_{max} and K_m.
b. Calculate phenytoin half-life in this patient at steady state while he is taking 450 mg daily.
c. What is the steady-state concentration that should be achieved if the dose was 300 mg daily?
d. What is the daily phenytoin dose that should achieve a steady-state phenytoin plasma concentration of 20 mg/L in this patient?

11.2. A 65-kg male was started on 260 mg phenytoin daily at bedtime to control his seizures. After 3 months of phenytoin therapy, his serum phenytoin concentration was 5 mg/L. Because of the poor control of his seizures, his phenytoin dose was increased to 240 mg of phenytoin twice daily. At 1 month after starting this new dosage regimen, the serum phenytoin concentration was 24 mg/L. The volume of distribution of phenytoin is 0.7 L/kg and the bioavailability is 100%.

a. Calculate the V_{max} and K_m using a graphical method.
b. Because the therapeutic range of phenytoin is 10–20 mg/L, recommend a dosage regimen to maintain a steady-state serum phenytoin concentration around 15 mg/L.
c. What will be the half-life of phenytoin at steady state if a dose of 200 mg every 12 hr is given to this patient?

d. If the phenytoin dose was changed and the steady-state serum phenytoin concentration was exactly equal to the value of K_m you determined in problem 11.2a, what will be the phenytoin elimination rate during this dosage regimen?

11.3. A 65-kg, 21-year-old woman is receiving phenytoin for the treatment of seizures. When she was taking a daily oral dose of 300 mg phenytoin, her steady-state plasma concentration was 5.1 mg/L. Because the phenytoin plasma concentration was well below the therapeutic range, the patient's dose was increased to 500 mg phenytoin, which resulted in a steady-state plasma concentration of 20 mg/L. (Assume that the absolute bioavailability of oral phenytoin is 100% and the volume of distribution is 0.7 L/kg.)

a. Graphically calculate the patient's V_{max} and K_m.
b. Recommend a daily dose of phenytoin for this patient to achieve a phenytoin plasma concentration of 15 mg/L at steady state.
c. Calculate the half-life and the total body clearance when the plasma concentration is 15 mg/L.
d. What will be the steady-state concentration that should be achieved if the dose was 450 mg daily?

11.4. A 70-kg, 34-year-old man is receiving phenytoin for the treatment of seizures. When this patient was taking a daily oral dose of 350 mg phenytoin, his steady-state plasma concentration was 4.6 mg/L. Because the phenytoin plasma concentration was well below the therapeutic range, the patient's daily dose was increased to 600 mg phenytoin, which resulted in a steady-state plasma concentration of 18 mg/L. (Assume that the absolute bioavailability of oral phenytoin is 100% and the volume of distribution is 0.7 L/kg.)

a. Graphically calculate the patient's V_{max} and K_m.
b. Although the patient's phenytoin plasma concentration is in the therapeutic range, the seizures were not controlled. Phenobarbitone, another drug used in the treatment of seizures that is known to be an enzyme inducer, was added to the patient's drug therapy. At 4 months later, while still taking 600 mg phenytoin/day in addition to the phenobarbitone, the patient's phenytoin plasma concentration was 15 mg/L. Calculate the patient's new pharmacokinetic parameter responsible for this decrease in phenytoin plasma concentration (V_{max} and K_m).
c. Recommend a daily dose of phenytoin at this induction state for this patient to achieve a steady-state plasma concentration of 20 mg/L.

11.5. A 25-kg, 14-year-old female was admitted to the hospital because of frequent episodes of seizures. She was diagnosed as having epileptic seizures, and she was started on intravenous phenytoin. She received a loading dose of 5 mg/kg followed by 80 mg phenytoin intravenously. every 12 hr. At steady state, the average plasma phenytoin concentration was 8 mg/L. The phenytoin dose was increased to 100 mg phenytoin intravenously every 12 hr. At steady state, the plasma phenytoin concentration was 13.3 mg/L. Because the patient's condition was stable, the intravenous phenytoin was replaced with phenytoin oral suspension, which is known to have 100% bioavailability. The patient went home with a prescription for 225-mg phenytoin suspension at bedtime every day. (The volume of distribution of phenytoin is 0.8 L/kg.)

a. Graphically estimate phenytoin V_{max} and K_m in this patient.
b. What is the expected average steady-state phenytoin concentration in this patient while taking the 225-mg phenytoin suspension at night?
c. Calculate phenytoin CL_T and half-life in this patient while taking the phenytoin suspension (225 mg phenytoin at bedtime) at steady state.

12 Multicompartment Pharmacokinetic Models

OBJECTIVES

After completing this chapter, you should be able to:

- Describe the differences between the one-compartment and the two-compartment pharmacokinetic models
- Define all the parameters of the two-compartment pharmacokinetic model
- Describe the plasma concentration–time profile after a single intravenous (IV) and oral administration, during constant-rate IV infusion, and for multiple drug administrations of drugs that follow the two-compartment pharmacokinetic model.
- Utilize mathematical expressions to calculate the plasma concentration at any time after a single IV drug administration of drugs that follow the two-compartment pharmacokinetic model
- Determine the pharmacokinetic parameters of the two-compartment pharmacokinetic model from plasma concentrations obtained after a single IV administration
- Analyze the effect of changing one or more of the pharmacokinetic parameters on the plasma concentration–time profile and the drug distribution between the central and the peripheral compartments after administration of drugs that follow the two-compartment pharmacokinetic model

12.1 INTRODUCTION

In the previous discussion of the pharmacokinetics of drugs, it was assumed that once the drug enters the systemic circulation it is rapidly distributed to all parts of the body. This means that the body behaves as a single vessel or one compartment, and that the distribution process to the tissues is rapid. This does not mean that the concentration of the drug in all tissues is similar. In fact, the drug's concentration in the different tissues is different depending on the affinity of the drug to each tissue.

This principle can be illustrated if we assume that we have a beaker with porous coating material covering its inner wall. If we fill the beaker with water and then add a drop of dye to the beaker, the dye will dissolve and distribute in the water inside the beaker and to the coating material of the beaker wall. If the dye is rapidly distributed to the coating material (i.e., equilibrium between the drug in solution and the drug in the beaker coating material is achieved rapidly) and we take serial samples from the dye solution in the beaker, then the dye concentration will be

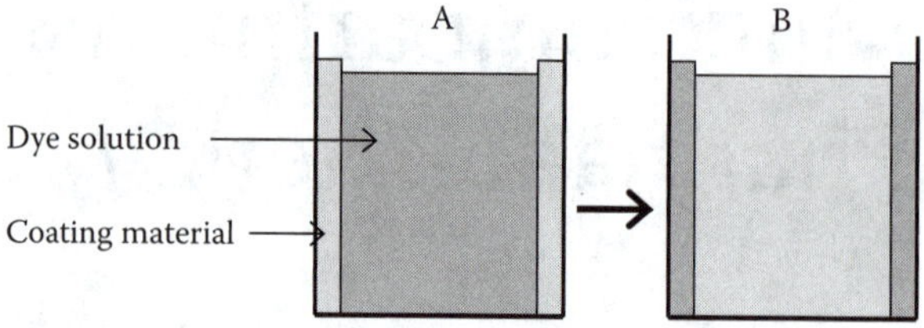

FIGURE 12.1 A diagrammatic presentation of the distribution of the dye from the solution in the beaker to the beaker coating material. The distribution process causes a decrease in the dye concentration in solution and an increase in the dye concentration in the coating material.

constant with time. This means that the beaker acts as a single compartment. However, the concentration of the dye in the solution is different from the concentration of the dye in the beaker coating material. This situation is similar to when the drug is distributed rapidly to all tissues after IV administration, and equilibrium is established between the plasma and the tissues quickly. The drugs that follow this behavior are designated as drugs that follow a one-compartment pharmacokinetic model. When these drugs are administered by a rapid IV bolus dose, the drug plasma concentration declines monoexponentially, and the plasma concentration–time profile can be presented by a straight line on the semilog scale.

For some drugs, the distribution of the drug from the systemic circulation to the different tissues is slow. The example of the beaker can be used to explain this situation. After adding the dye, initially the dye will dissolve and distribute in the water inside the beaker. Then, the dye will distribute slowly to the coating material of the beaker wall. The distribution of the dye from the solution to the beaker coating material results in decreasing the dye concentration in solution and increasing the dye concentration in the beaker coating material as illustrated in Figure 12.1.

If we take serial samples from the dye solution in the beaker, then we will notice that the concentration decreases gradually until it reaches a constant value as presented in Figure 12.2. The decrease in the dye concentration in the beaker will represent its distribution to the coating material. After the distribution is completed, equilibrium is achieved between the dye solution in the beaker and the dye in the coating material, and between the dye concentration in the solution and in the coating material stays constant. Drugs that are distributed slowly to different parts of the body and the equilibrium between the drug in plasma and the drug in different tissues is established slowly over a period of time will not follow the one-compartment pharmacokinetic model. These drugs follow a two-compartment pharmacokinetic model.

12.2 Two-Compartment Pharmacokinetic Model

After administration of a rapid IV dose of drugs that follow the two-compartment pharmacokinetic model, a plot of the plasma concentration–time profile is not a straight line on the semilog scale. This is because the plasma concentration–time profile will be described by a biexponential equation if the distribution process is a first-order process. The first exponent describes the distribution process, and the second exponent describes the elimination process.

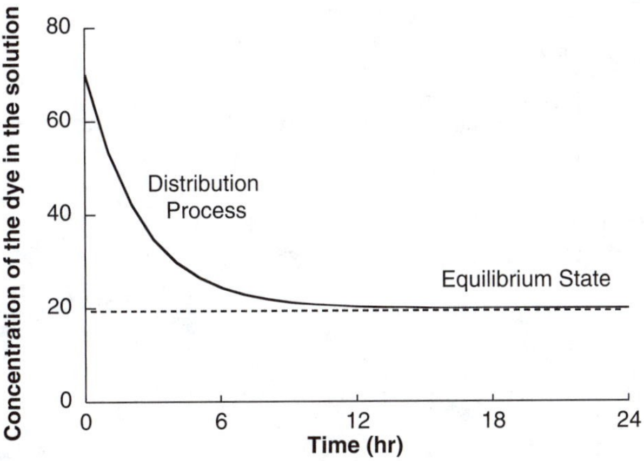

FIGURE 12.2 The dye concentration–time profile in the beaker with the decrease in the dye concentration representing the distribution of the dye from the solution to the coating material.

After IV administration of the drug, it is distributed rapidly in certain body spaces that represent the central compartment. Then, the drug is distributed by a first-order process from the central compartment to other body spaces and tissues that represent the peripheral compartment. Because the blood is usually part of the central compartment, the drug can be transported into the eliminating organs once the drug is in the central compartment. So, the distribution and elimination processes occur simultaneously after drug administration, and the drug concentration in the central compartment will decline depending on the rate of the two processes. After the distribution process is completed, the drug concentration in the central compartment will decline depending on the rate of the elimination process. A typical plasma concentration–time profile after IV bolus administration of drugs that follow the two-compartment pharmacokinetic model is presented in Figure 12.3.

This two-compartment pharmacokinetic model assumes that at time zero there is no drug in the tissue (peripheral) compartment. After an IV bolus dose, the drug is rapidly transferred to the peripheral compartment. The amount of drug in the central compartment declines rapidly because of the transfer of drug out of the central compartment to the peripheral compartment and because of drug elimination that occurs simultaneously. The drug in the central compartment is transferred to the peripheral compartment by a first-order process, and the drug that reaches the peripheral compartment can return back to the central compartment by a first-order process. Because initially the amount of the drug in the central compartment is larger than the amount of the drug in the peripheral compartment, the net transfer will be from the central compartment to the peripheral compartment. This means that initially the amount of drug in the peripheral compartment increases with time.

As the amount of drug in the peripheral compartment increases, the rate of drug transfer from the peripheral compartment to the central compartment approaches the rate of drug transfer from the central compartment to the peripheral compartment. When these two rates become equal, the amount of drug in the peripheral compartment

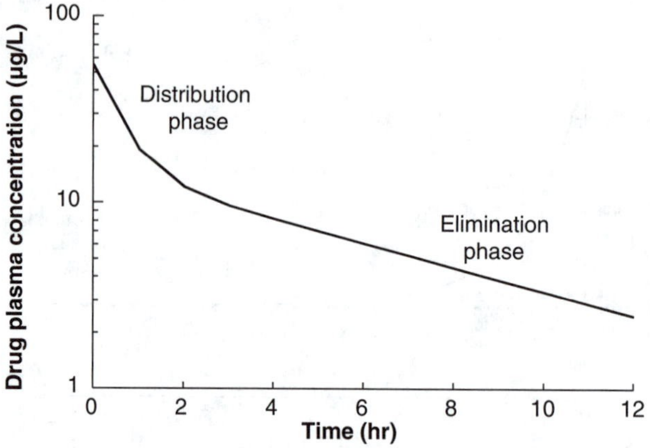

FIGURE 12.3 The plasma concentration–time profile for a drug that follows a two-compartment pharmacokinetic model after administration of a single IV bolus dose.

reaches a maximum value. Because the drug is continually eliminated from the central compartment, the amount of drug in the central compartment decreases, and the rate of drug transfer from the peripheral compartment to the central compartment becomes larger than the rate of transfer from the central compartment to the peripheral compartment to compensate for the drug elimination from the central compartment. The net drug transfer is from the peripheral compartment to the central compartment, and the amount of drug in the peripheral compartment starts to decline parallel to the amount of the drug in the central compartment. Figure 12.4 illustrates the drug concentration–time profile in the central and peripheral compartments after administration of a single IV bolus dose.

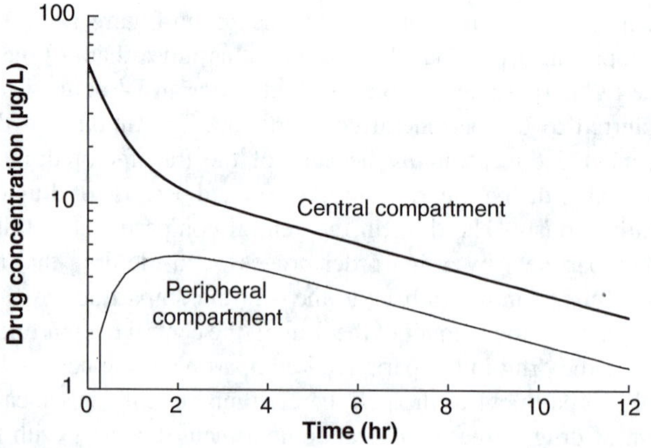

FIGURE 12.4 The drug concentration–time profile in the central and peripheral compartments after administration of a single IV bolus dose of a drug that follows a two-compartment pharmacokinetic model.

The concentration of drug in the central compartment is determined by dividing the amount of drug in the central compartment by the volume of the central compartment. Likewise, the concentration of drug in the peripheral compartment is determined by dividing the amount of the drug in the peripheral compartment by the volume of the peripheral compartment.

12.3 TWO-COMPARTMENT PHARMACOKINETIC MODEL PARAMETERS

The two-compartment pharmacokinetic model can be presented by the diagram in Figure 12.5. This model assumes that the drug transport between the central compartment and the peripheral compartment follows first-order kinetics, and that the drug is eliminated from the central compartment by a first-order process.

12.3.1 Definition of Pharmacokinetic Parameters

k_1 The first-order transfer rate constant from the central compartment to the peripheral compartment; has units of $time^{-1}$.

k_2 The first-order transfer rate constant from the peripheral compartment to the central compartment; has units of $time^{-1}$.

k_3 The first-order elimination rate constant from the central compartment; has units of $time^{-1}$.

X The amount of drug in the central compartment; has units of mass.

Y The amount of drug in the peripheral compartment; has units of mass.

A and B The hybrid coefficients; have units of concentration.

α The hybrid first-order rate constant for the distribution process; has units of $time^{-1}$.

β The hybrid first-order rate constant for the elimination process; has units of $time^{-1}$.

$\alpha_{t1/2}$ The half-life of the distribution process; has units of time.

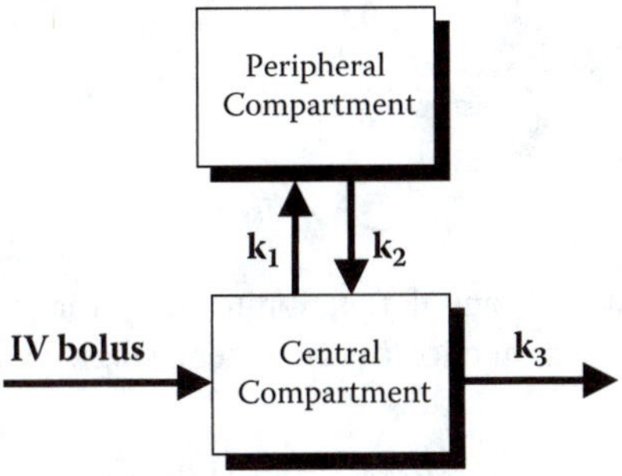

FIGURE 12.5 A diagram representing the two-compartment pharmacokinetic model with drug elimination from the central compartment.

$\beta_{t1/2}$ The half-life of the elimination process; has units of time.

V_c The volume of the central compartment; has units of volume. This term relates the dose of the drug administered intravenously and the initial drug plasma concentration (Cp_0) according to Equation 12.1.

$$Cp_0 = \frac{Dose}{V_c} \tag{12.1}$$

Vd_{ss} The volume of distribution of the drug at steady state; has units of volume. This term relates the amount of the drug in the body and the drug plasma concentration at steady state. The amount of the drug in the body at steady state is equal to $Vd_{ss}Cp_{ss}$.

Vd_β or Vd_{area} The volume of distribution during the elimination phase; has units of volume. This term relates the amount of the drug in the body and the drug plasma concentration during the elimination phase (β-phase). The amount of the drug in the body during the elimination phase is equal to $Vd_\beta Cp$.

12.3.2 Mathematical Equation That Describes the Plasma Concentration–Time Profile

The rate of change of the amount of drug in the central compartment X at any time after a single IV bolus dose is equal to the rate of drug transfer from the peripheral compartment to the central compartment minus the rate of drug transfer from the central compartment to the peripheral compartment minus the rate of drug elimination. Also, the rate of change of the amount of drug in the peripheral compartment Y is equal to the rate of drug transfer from the central compartment to the peripheral compartment minus the rate of drug transfer from the peripheral compartment to the central compartment.

The differential equations that describe these two rates are as follows:

$$\frac{dX}{dt} = k_2 Y - k_1 X - k_3 X \tag{12.2}$$

and

$$\frac{dY}{dt} = k_1 X - k_2 Y \tag{12.3}$$

Integrating the first differential equation to solve for the amount of drug in the central compartment X as a function of time after a single IV bolus dose D, we obtain

$$X = \frac{D(\alpha - k_2)}{(\alpha - \beta)} e^{-\alpha t} + \frac{D(k_2 - \beta)}{(\alpha - \beta)} e^{-\beta t} \tag{12.4}$$

Divide by the volume of the central compartment V_c to get the expression for the drug concentration at any time in the central compartment:

$$Cp = \frac{D\,(\alpha - k_2)}{V_c\,(\alpha - \beta)}\, e^{-\alpha t} + \frac{D\,(k_2 - \beta)}{V_c\,(\alpha - \beta)}\, e^{-\beta t} \tag{12.5}$$

which can be simplified to

$$Cp = A\ e^{-\alpha t} + B\ e^{-\beta t} \tag{12.6}$$

where

$$A = \frac{D\,(\alpha - k_2)}{V_c\,(\alpha - \beta)} \quad \text{and} \quad B = \frac{D\,(k_2 - \beta)}{V_c\,(\alpha - \beta)}$$

12.4 DETERMINATION OF TWO-COMPARTMENT PHARMACOKINETIC MODEL PARAMETERS

The parameters A, B, α, and β can be estimated from the drug plasma concentrations obtained after a single IV dose D of the drug by nonlinear regression analysis. Also, these parameters can be determined graphically from the plasma concentration-versus-time data. These four parameters can be used to calculate all the other parameters of the model. The pharmacokinetic parameters allow prediction of the drug steady-state plasma concentration during repeated drug administration and determination of the dose required to achieve a certain drug concentration at steady state.

12.4.1 Method of Residuals

The method of residuals is a graphical method that can be utilized to estimate the two-compartment model parameters after a single IV dose. The utilization of this graphical method to estimate the model parameters is illustrated in Figure 12.6. The basic principle of the method of residuals is to separate the two exponential terms of Equation 12.6, which describes the plasma concentration–time profile of drugs that follow the two-compartment pharmacokinetic model after a single IV dose.

The plasma concentration-time data are plotted on a semilog scale. The linear elimination phase (β-phase) is identified, and the line is back-extrapolated to the y-axis. This line is corresponding to the ($Be^{-\beta t}$) term in the biexponential equation. The y-intercept of the extrapolated line is equal to the coefficient B in the equation. The hybrid rate constant β is determined from the slope of the line representing the β-phase (Slope = $-\beta/2.303$), or the $\beta_{t1/2}$ is determined directly from the graph by calculating the time required for any concentration on the line to decrease by 50%. Then, β is calculated as:

$$\beta = \frac{0.693}{\beta_{t\,1/2}} \tag{12.7}$$

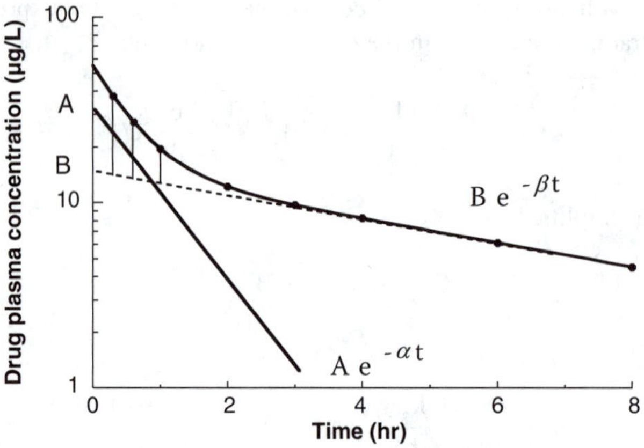

FIGURE 12.6 The method of residuals applied to separate the two exponential terms of the equation that describes the plasma concentration–time profile of drugs that follow the two-compartment pharmacokinetic model after a single IV dose.

The residuals are calculated from the difference between the original plasma concentration-time data and the corresponding value on the extrapolated elimination phase. These residuals are plotted versus their corresponding times. The residual-versus-time plot is linear on the semilog scale and corresponds to the ($Ae^{-\alpha t}$) term in the biexponential equation. The y-intercept of this line is equal to the coefficient A in the equation. The hybrid rate constant α is determined from the slope of the line (Slope = −α/2.303), or the $\alpha_{t\,1/2}$ is determined directly from the graph by calculating the time required for any point on the line representing the α-phase to decrease by 50%. Then, α is calculated as

$$\alpha = \frac{0.693}{\alpha_{t\,1/2}} \tag{12.8}$$

A is always the intercept of the faster process (the process with shorter $t_{1/2}$, which is usually the distribution process), and B is always the intercept of the slower process (the process with longer $t_{1/2}$, which is usually the elimination process).

12.4.2 Determination of Model Parameters

From the integration of Equation 12.2 to solve for the amount of drug in the central compartment, the following two relationships are determined:

$$k_1 + k_2 + k_3 = \alpha + \beta \tag{12.9}$$

and

$$k_2 \,.\, k_3 = \alpha \,.\, \beta \tag{12.10}$$

12.4.2.1 Volume of Central Compartment V_c

The drug is distributed initially in the central compartment. So, the volume of the central compartment can be determined from the dose and the initial drug concentration. If you substitute in Equation 12.6 for the time by zero, you obtain the initial drug concentration ($Cp_0 = A + B$).

$$V_c = \frac{\text{Dose}}{Cp_0} = \frac{\text{Dose}}{A + B} \tag{12.11}$$

12.4.2.2 Area under the Curve (AUC)

The area under the curve (AUC) can be determined by integrating the equation that describes the plasma concentration–time profile (Equation 12.6).

$$\text{AUC}\,\Big|_{t=0}^{t=\infty} = \frac{A}{\alpha} + \frac{B}{\beta} \tag{12.12}$$

12.4.2.3 Total Body Clearance CL_T

The total body clearance CL_T can be determined from the dose and the AUC.

$$CL_T = \frac{\text{Dose}}{\text{AUC}\,\Big|_{t=0}^{t=\infty}} \tag{12.13}$$

12.4.2.4 First-Order Elimination Rate Constant from Central Compartment k_3

The first-order elimination rate constant from the central compartment k_3 is determined from the CL_T and the volume of the central compartment.

$$CL_T = k_3\, V_c \tag{12.14}$$

$$k_3 = \frac{CL_T}{V_c} \tag{12.15}$$

12.4.2.5 First-Order Transfer Rate Constant from Peripheral Compartment to Central Compartment k_2

The first-order transfer rate constant from the peripheral compartment to the central compartment k_2 is obtained from Equation 12.10.

$$k_2 = \frac{\alpha\ \beta}{k_3} \tag{12.16}$$

12.4.2.6 First-Order Transfer Rate Constant from Central Compartment to Peripheral Compartment k_1

The first-order transfer rate constant from the peripheral compartment to the central compartment k_1 is obtained from Equation 12.9.

$$k_1 = (\alpha + \beta) - (k_2 + k_3) \tag{12.17}$$

12.4.2.7 Volume of Distribution at Steady State Vd_{ss}

$$Vd_{ss} = V_c\left(1 + \frac{k_1}{k_2}\right) \tag{12.18}$$

12.4.2.8 Volume of Distribution in Elimination Phase Vd_β

$$Vd_\beta = \frac{CL_T}{\beta} = \frac{V_c\ k_3}{\beta} \tag{12.19}$$

EXAMPLE

After a single IV bolus dose of 1000 mg of an antiarrhythmic drug, the following concentrations were obtained:

Time (hr)	Concentration (mg/L)
0.2	120
0.5	84
1.0	53
2.0	29
4.0	18
6.0	15
8.0	12.5
12.0	8.8

1. Using the method of residuals, calculate the following parameters: $\alpha_{t1/2}$, $\beta_{t1/2}$, k_1, k_2, k_3, V_c, Vd_β, Vd_{ss}, AUC, and CL_T.
2. What will be the amount of drug remaining in the body after 15 hr?

Answer

1. The method of residuals used to solve the problem and presented in Figure 12.7 can be performed by the following procedures:

   a. Plot the concentration versus time on a semilog scale.
   b. Identify the best line that represents the drug elimination process.

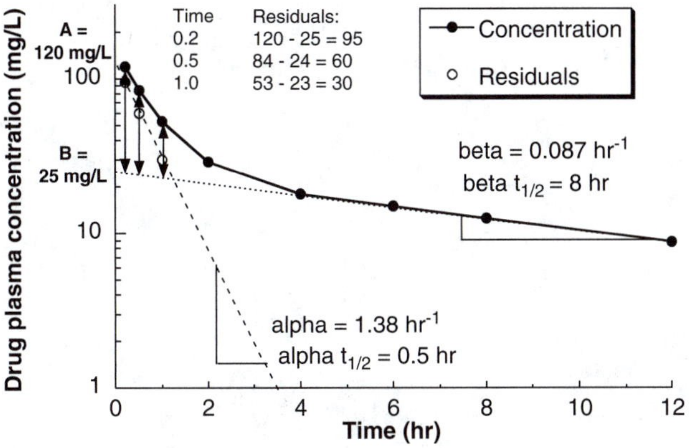

FIGURE 12.7 Application of the method of residuals to obtain the two-compartment model parameters.

c. The y-intercept is equal to B. The hybrid elimination rate constant β and β half-life can be determined from the line.
d. Calculate the residuals during the distribution phase.
e. Plot the residuals versus time and draw the best line that goes through the points.
f. The y-intercept is equal to A. The hybrid distribution rate constant α and α half-life can be determined from the line.

From Figure 12.7, the estimated values for A, B, α, and β are as follows:

A	120 mg/L
B	25 mg/L
$\alpha = 1.38\ \text{hr}^{-1}$	$\alpha t_{1/2} = 0.5$ hr
$\beta = 0.087\ \text{hr}^{-1}$	$\beta t_{1/2} = 8$ hr

For calculation of the other pharmacokinetic parameters,

$$V_c = \frac{\text{Dose}}{A+B} = \frac{1000}{120\text{ mg/L} + 25\text{ mg/L}} = 6.9\text{ L}$$

$$\text{AUC} = \frac{A}{\alpha} + \frac{B}{\beta} = \frac{120\text{ mg/L}}{1.38\text{ hr}^{-1}} + \frac{25\text{ mg/L}}{0.087\text{ hr}^{-1}} = 374.4\text{ mg-hr/L}$$

$$CL_T = \frac{\text{Dose}}{\text{AUC}} = \frac{1000\text{ mg}}{374.4\text{ mg-hr/L}} = 2.67\text{ L/hr}$$

$$k_3 = \frac{CL_T}{V_c} = \frac{2.67\text{ L/hr}}{6.9\text{ L}} = 0.387\text{ hr}^{-1}$$

$$k_2 = \frac{\alpha\,\beta}{k_3} = \frac{1.38\ \text{hr}^{-1} \times 0.087\ \text{hr}^{-1}}{0.387\ \text{hr}^{-1}} = 0.310\ \text{hr}^{-1}$$

$$k_1 = (\alpha + \beta) - (k_2 + k_3) = (1.38\ \text{hr}^{-1} + 0.087\ \text{hr}^{-1}) - (0.310\ \text{hr}^{-1} + 0.387\ \text{hr}^{-1}) = 0.77\ \text{hr}^{-1}$$

$$Vd_\beta = \frac{CL_T}{\beta} = \frac{2.67\ \text{l/hr}}{0.087\ \text{hr}^{-1}} = 30.7\ \text{L}$$

$$Vd_{ss} = V_c\ (1 + \frac{k_1}{k_2}) = 6.7\ \text{L}\ (1 + \frac{0.77\ \text{hr}^{-1}}{0.310\ \text{hr}^{-1}}) = 23.3\ \text{L}$$

2.

$$Cp = A\ e^{-\alpha t} + B\ e^{-\beta t}$$

$$Cp_{15\ \text{hr}} = 120\ \text{mg/L}\ e^{-1.38\ \text{hr}^{-1}\ 15\ \text{hr}} + 25\ \text{mg/L}\ e^{-0.087\ \text{hr}^{-1}\ 15\ \text{hr}} = 6.78\ \text{mg/L}$$

Amount of the drug in the body during the elimination phase = $Cp \times Vd_\beta$

$$\text{Amount}_{15\ \text{hr}} = Cp_{15\ \text{hr}} \times Vd_\beta = 6.78\ \text{mg/L} \times 30.7\ \text{L} = 208\ \text{mg}$$

12.5 EFFECT OF CHANGING THE PHARMACOKINETIC PARAMETERS ON DRUG CONCENTRATION–TIME PROFILE AFTER A SINGLE IV DOSE

12.5.1 Dose

Administration of higher doses results in a proportional increase in the plasma concentration. However, the plasma concentration–time profiles will be parallel to each other.

12.5.2 Volume of Distribution

The change in the volume of the central compartment will be accompanied by a proportional change in the volume of distribution at steady state and during the elimination phase. A larger volume of distribution results in a lower initial drug plasma concentration after administration of the same dose and similar AUC if the CL_T does not change. If the volume of distribution changes and the CL_T remains constant, then the elimination rate constant will be different.

12.5.3 Hybrid Distribution Rate Constant α

A larger distribution rate constant results in faster completion of the distribution process without affecting the rate of drug elimination. This is assuming that the three micro rate constants k_1, k_2, and k_3 change in a way that will change the rate of the distribution process without affecting the rate of the elimination process.

12.5.4 Hybrid Elimination Rate Constant β

A larger elimination rate constant results in faster drug elimination without affecting the rate of drug distribution. This is assuming that the three micro rate constants k_1, k_2, and k_3 change in a way that will change the rate of the elimination process without affecting the rate of the distribution process.

12.6 ORAL ADMINISTRATION OF DRUGS THAT FOLLOW THE TWO-COMPARTMENT PHARMACOKINETIC MODEL

After oral administration of drugs that follow a two-compartment pharmacokinetic model, the drugs are absorbed to the systemic circulation, which is part of the central compartment. Once in the central compartment, the drug can be eliminated from the body and distributed to the peripheral compartment. If the absorption of the drug is fast relative to the distribution and elimination processes, then the decline in the plasma concentration–time profile after the end of the absorption phase will be biexponential, representing the distribution and the elimination phases. However, if the drug absorption is slow, then the biexponential decline in the plasma concentration after the end of the absorption may not be clear. Figure 12.8 represents the plasma concentration–time profile after a single oral dose of a drug that follows a

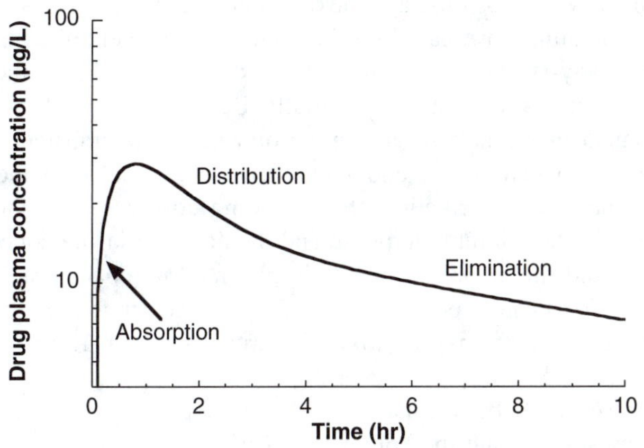

FIGURE 12.8 The plasma concentration–time profile for a drug that follows a two-compartment pharmacokinetic model after administration of a single oral dose.

two-compartment pharmacokinetic model. The decline of the drug concentration in the postabsorption phase is biexponential. The plasma concentration–time profile after oral administration of drugs that follow a two-compartment pharmacokinetic model can be described by a triexponential equation that represents the absorption, the distribution, and the elimination processes.

12.7 CONSTANT RATE IV ADMINISTRATION OF DRUGS THAT FOLLOW THE TWO-COMPARTMENT PHARMACOKINETIC MODEL

The plasma concentration–time profile of drugs that follow two-compartment pharmacokinetic model during constant rate IV infusion increases gradually until it reaches a steady state. At steady state, the rate of drug administration is equal to the rate of drug elimination. The steady-state plasma concentration is dependent on the rate of the IV infusion and the CL_T of the drug. This is similar to the drugs that follow a one-compartment pharmacokinetic model.

$$Cp_{ss} = \frac{\text{Infusion rate}}{CL_T} = \frac{K_0}{CL_T} \qquad (12.20)$$

The time to reach steady state during constant-rate IV infusion of drugs that follow a two-compartment pharmacokinetic model is dependent on the drug elimination half-life $\beta_{t1/2}$. It takes five to six elimination half-lives to reach the steady state. Termination of the IV infusion will result in a biexponential decline in the drug plasma concentration, a rapid distribution phase, and a slow elimination phase.

Administration of a loading dose may be necessary to achieve a faster approach to steady state, especially in emergency situations. In this case, simultaneous administration of an IV loading dose and the constant-rate IV infusion is necessary. Calculation of the loading dose based on the volume of the central compartment and the desired steady-state concentration ($Cp_{ss} \times V_c$) will achieve the desired concentration in the central compartment initially. Because of drug distribution to the peripheral compartment, the drug concentration will decline transiently (maybe to a subtherapeutic concentration) and then increase gradually to the desired steady-state concentration. Calculation of the loading dose based on the volume of distribution during the elimination phase and the desired plasma concentration ($Cp_{ss} \times Vd_\beta$) can avoid this transient decline in plasma drug concentration. However, this loading dose can produce a high drug concentration in the central compartment initially, which may be toxic for drugs with a narrow therapeutic range.

The loading dose should be calculated based on an average value for the volume of the central compartment and the volume of distribution during the elimination phase. Another approach may be to give a loading dose calculated based on the volume of the central compartment and then give smaller IV doses to compensate for the transient decline in drug concentration after the loading dose.

12.8 MULTIPLE DRUG ADMINISTRATIONS

Drugs that follow a two-compartment pharmacokinetic model accumulate during repeated administration until steady state is achieved. At steady state, the plasma concentration will be changing during each dosing interval; however, the maximum and minimum plasma concentrations will be similar if the drug is administered at equally spaced dosing intervals. The average steady-state concentration is directly proportional to the dosing rate and inversely proportional to the total body clearance.

$$Cp_{ss\ average} = \frac{F\ Dose}{CL_T\ \tau} \qquad (12.21)$$

where τ is the dosing interval, and F is the bioavailability. This relationship is similar for one- and two-compartment models. It takes five to six elimination half-lives $\beta_{t1/2}$ to reach the steady state during multiple administrations of drugs that follow a two-compartment pharmacokinetic model. Administration of a loading dose achieves a faster approach to the steady state.

12.9 RENAL EXCRETION OF DRUGS THAT FOLLOW THE TWO-COMPARTMENT PHARMACOKINETIC MODEL

For a drug that follows a two-compartment pharmacokinetic model, the amount of the drug in the central compartment declines biexponentially. So, the profile of renal excretion rate dA_e/dt versus time will also decline biexponentially.

$$\frac{d\,A_e}{d\,t} = A'e^{-\alpha t} + B'\ e^{-\beta t} \qquad (12.22)$$

The renal clearance can be determined from the renal excretion rate and the average plasma concentration during the urine collection interval. This is similar to drugs that follow a one-compartment pharmacokinetic model.

$$CL_R = \frac{\Delta A_e / \Delta t}{Cp_{t\text{-}mid}} \qquad (12.23)$$

The renal clearance can also be determined from the total amount of the drug excreted in urine and the drug AUC. This is similar to the drugs that follow a one-compartment pharmacokinetic model.

$$CL_R = \frac{A_{e\infty}}{AUC\,|_{t=0}^{t=\infty}} \qquad (12.24)$$

The fraction of the drug dose excreted in urine is determined from the ratio of the renal clearance to the total body clearance.

12.10 EFFECT OF CHANGING THE PHARMACOKINETIC PARAMETERS ON DRUG DISTRIBUTION BETWEEN CENTRAL AND PERIPHERAL COMPARTMENTS

Drugs that follow a one-compartment pharmacokinetic model are distributed rapidly to all parts of the body after IV administration. Although the drug concentration is different in different tissues, the body behaves as a kinetically homogeneous compartment (i.e., a 50% decrease in plasma concentration will be accompanied by a 50% decrease in concentration of all tissues). However, for drugs that follow a two-compartment pharmacokinetic model, the drug profile in the tissues that represent the central compartment is different from the drug profile in the tissues that represent the peripheral compartment.

12.10.1 Dose

The change in dose results in a proportional change in the amount of the drug in the central and peripheral compartments. However, the distribution ratio between the central and peripheral compartments does not change. Changing the dose does not affect the ratio of the amount of the drug in the peripheral compartment to the amount of the drug in the central compartment.

12.10.2 First-Order Transfer Rate Constant from Central to Peripheral Compartment k_1

The change in k_1 affects the drug distribution rate, elimination rate, and tissue distribution. A larger k_1 results in more drug distributing to the peripheral compartment, a faster distribution rate, and a slower elimination rate, assuming that the other parameters do not change. The ratio of the amount of the drug in the peripheral compartment to the amount of the drug in the central compartment at steady state increases because of the increase in the k_1/k_2 ratio.

12.10.3 First-Order Transfer Rate Constant from Peripheral to Central Compartment k_2

The change in k_2 affects the drug distribution rate, elimination rate, and tissue distribution. A larger k_2 results in less drug distributing to the peripheral compartment, a faster distribution rate, and a faster elimination rate, assuming that the other parameters do not change. The ratio of the amount of the drug in the peripheral compartment to the amount of the drug in the central compartment at steady state decreases because of the decrease in the k_1/k_2 ratio.

12.10.4 First-Order Elimination Rate Constant from Central Compartment k_3

The change in k_3 affects the drug distribution rate and the elimination rate. A larger k_3 results in a faster distribution rate and a faster elimination rate, assuming that the other parameters do not change. However, the drug distribution ratio between the central and the peripheral compartments does not change. The ratio of the amount of the drug in the peripheral compartment to the amount of the drug in the central compartment at steady state does not change because the ratio k_1/k_2 does not change.

12.11 THREE-COMPARTMENT PHARMACOKINETIC MODEL

With the development of accurate sampling strategies and sensitive analytical techniques, some drugs have been shown to follow a three-compartment pharmacokinetic model. After drug administration into the central compartment, the drug is distributed slowly to the tissues. However, the distribution of the drug to some tissues is much slower than its distribution to other tissues. This results in two distinct rates of distribution and a biexponential distribution phase followed by a terminal slower elimination phase. Figure 12.9 is an example of the plasma concentration–time profile for a drug that follows a three-compartment pharmacokinetic model

The diagram presented in Figure 12.10 is an example of a three-compartment pharmacokinetic model in which the elimination of the drug is from the central compartment, and the two peripheral compartments are connected to the central compartment. The equation that describes the plasma concentration–time profile after a single IV bolus dose is triexponential (includes three exponents). Equation 12.25

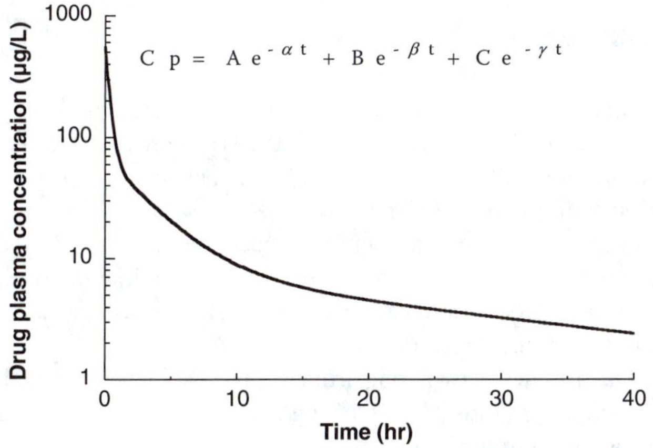

FIGURE 12.9 The plasma concentration–time profile for a drug that follows a three-compartment pharmacokinetic model after administration of a single IV bolus dose.

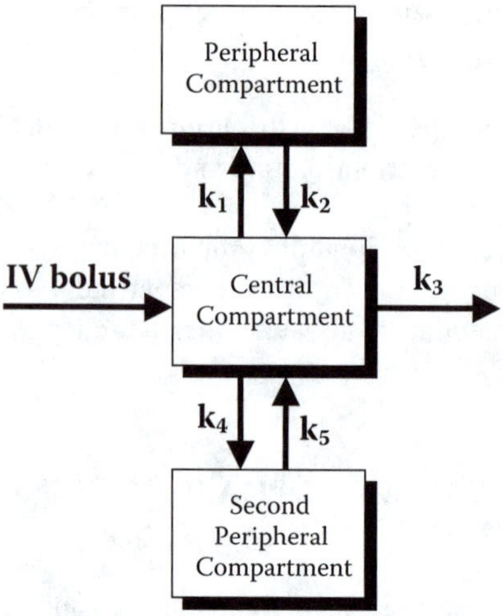

FIGURE 12.10 A diagram representing the three-compartment pharmacokinetic model with the two peripheral compartments connected to the central compartment and drug elimination from the central compartment.

represents the expression that describes the plasma concentration–time profile for a drug that follows a three-compartment pharmacokinetic model after administration of a single IV bolus dose.

$$Cp = A\ e^{-\alpha t} + B\ e^{-\beta t} + C\ e^{-\gamma t} \tag{12.25}$$

The pharmacokinetic parameters for three-compartment pharmacokinetic models can be obtained by nonlinear regression analysis, which requires the use of computers.

PRACTICE PROBLEMS

12.1. A drug that follows a two-compartment pharmacokinetic model is given to a patient by rapid IV injection. Would the drug concentration in each tissue be the same after the drug equilibrates between the plasma and all the tissues in the body? Explain.

12.2. A drug follows a two-compartment pharmacokinetic model. If a single IV bolus dose is given, then what is the cause of the initial rapid decline in the plasma concentration (α-phase)? What is the cause of the slower decline in the plasma concentration (β-phase)?

12.3. A drug that follows a two-compartment pharmacokinetic model was given as a single IV bolus dose of 5.6 mg/kg. The equation that describes the plasma concentration-time data is

$$Cp\ (mg/L) = 18\ e^{-2.8t} + 6\ e^{-0.11t}$$

a. Calculate the plasma concentration after 0.5, 3, and 12 hr of drug administration.
b. What will be the equation that describes the plasma concentration–time profile if the dose given was 11.2 mg/kg?

12.4. After administration of a single IV bolus dose of 75 mg of a drug to a healthy volunteer, the pharmacokinetics of this drug followed a two-compartment model. The following parameters were obtained:

A = 4.62 mg/L	B = 0.64 mg/L
α = 8.94 hr^{-1}	β = 0.19 hr^{-1}

a. Calculate the following parameters: $\alpha_{t1/2}$, $\beta_{t1/2}$, k_1, k_2, k_3, Vc, Vd_β, Vd_{ss}, AUC, and CL_T.
b. What will be the amount of drug remaining in the body after 8 hr?

12.5. A single dose of 500 mg of a drug was administered by a rapid IV injection into a 70-kg patient. Plasma samples were obtained over a 7-hr period and assayed for the drug. The results are as follows:

Time (hr)	Concentration (mg/L)
0.00	70.0
0.25	53.8
0.5	43.3
0.75	35.0
1.0	29.1
1.5	21.2
2.0	17.0
2.5	14.3
3.0	12.6
4.0	10.5
5.0	9.0
6.0	8.0
7.0	7.0

a. Calculate the following parameters: $\alpha_{t1/2}$, $\beta_{t1/2}$, k_1, k_2, k_3, Vc, Vd_β, Vd_{ss}, AUC, and CL_T.
b. What will be the plasma concentration 12 hr after drug administration?
c. What will be the initial plasma concentration if a dose of 1500 mg is administered as an IV bolus?
d. Which of the pharmacokinetic parameters above will change with the increase in the dose to 1500 mg?
e. Calculate the new values for these parameters.
f. What will be the IV infusion rate required to achieve a steady-state plasma concentration of 10 mg/L?

12.6. The plasma concentration time data following a 50-mg IV bolus dose of lidocaine is as follows:

Time (min)	Concentration (mg/L)
2.0	1.51
4.0	1.20
10	0.796
15	0.639
20	0.462
40	0.329
60	0.271
90	0.242
120	0.179
180	0.112
240	0.081

a. Using the method of residuals, calculate the following parameters: $\alpha_{t1/2}$, $\beta_{t1/2}$, k_1, k_2, k_3, Vc, Vd_β, Vd_{ss}, AUC, and CL_T.
b. Calculate the plasma concentration at the time of each sample from the equation that describes the plasma concentration–time profile and comment on the differences between the measured and the calculated concentrations.
c. What will be the amount of lidocaine remaining in the body after 240 min?
d. What will be the plasma concentration when 90% of the administered dosc is eliminated?

13 Drug Pharmacokinetics Following Administration by Intermittent Intravenous Infusion

OBJECTIVES

After completing this chapter, you should be able to:

- Describe the plasma concentration–time profile during multiple intermittent intravenous (IV) infusion.
- Analyze the effect of changing one or more of the pharmacokinetic parameters on the maximum and minimum steady-state drug concentration
- Determine the steady-state maximum and minimum drug concentrations during repeated intermittent IV infusions
- Predict aminoglycoside half-life based on the patient's kidney function
- Determine the patient's specific aminoglycoside pharmacokinetic parameters
- Recommend the appropriate aminoglycoside dosing regimen based on the patient's specific pharmacokinetic parameters
- Evaluate the appropriateness of certain aminoglycoside dosing regimens in patients

13.1 INTRODUCTION

Intermittent IV infusion means drug administration by constant-rate IV infusion over a short period of time. Following repeated administration of these short IV infusions, the drug will accumulate in the body until steady state is achieved. At steady state, the maximum and minimum plasma concentrations will be constant if the dose, infusion duration, and dosing interval are kept constant.

During intermittent IV infusion, the drug is administered over a period of t', and the dose is repeated every τ. The time between the maximum and the minimum drug concentrations is $\tau - t'$, as illustrated in Figure 13.1. The maximum plasma concentration achieved after the end of drug administration is lower than the maximum concentration achieved if the drug dose is administered by IV bolus dose. This is because a fraction of the administered dose is eliminated during the drug infusion period t'.

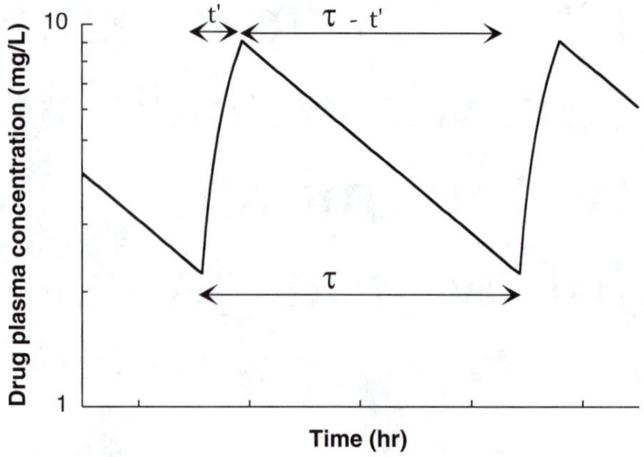

FIGURE 13.1 The drug plasma concentration–time profile during repeated intermittent IV administration. The dosing interval is the sum of the duration of the infusion t′ and the postinfusion time $\tau' - t'$.

If we neglect the time of the IV infusion in our pharmacokinetic study (i.e., if we assume that the drug is administered as an IV bolus dose), then we would miss the amount of drug eliminated from the body during drug administration (the time of infusion). For drugs with short half-lives, a significant amount of the drug is eliminated during the time of drug administration. This may result in significant errors in our calculation of the pharmacokinetic parameters. For this reason, studying the drug pharmacokinetics after administration of an intermittent IV infusion is necessary.

13.2 DRUG CONCENTRATION–TIME PROFILE DURING INTERMITTENT IV INFUSION

13.2.1 After First Dose

The rate of change of the amount of drug in the body during a constant-rate IV infusion is equal to the difference between the rate of drug administration and the rate of drug elimination (assuming first-order elimination and a one-compartment model):

$$\frac{dA}{dt} = K_0 - k\,A \tag{13.1}$$

where K_0 is the rate of the IV infusion, which is equal to (dose/infusion time); k is the first-order elimination rate constant; and A is the amount of drug in the body. Integrating Equation 13.1 gives the equation that describes the change in the amount of drug in the body during a constant-rate IV infusion.

$$A = \frac{K_0}{k}\,(1 - e^{-kt}) \tag{13.2}$$

Dividing by the volume of distribution gives the expression for the plasma concentration during the constant-rate IV infusion.

$$Cp = \frac{K_0}{k\ Vd}\ (1 - e^{-kt}) \tag{13.3}$$

Notice that if the drug infusion continues for a long time (t is large), then Equation 13.3 is reduced to the equation that describes the steady-state plasma concentration during a constant-rate IV infusion.

$$Cp_{ss} = \frac{K_0}{k\ Vd} \tag{13.4}$$

The plasma concentration at the end of an IV infusion administered over a period of t′ can be determined from the following equation:

$$Cp = \frac{K_0}{k\ Vd}\ (1 - e^{-kt'}) \tag{13.5}$$

If the drug IV infusion is terminated after time equal to t′, then the drug concentration declines monoexponentially as shown in Figure 13.2. The equation that describes the drug concentration during or after the drug infusion is

$$Cp = \left[\frac{K_0}{k\ Vd}\ (1 - e^{-kt'})\right] e^{-k(t - t')} \tag{13.6}$$

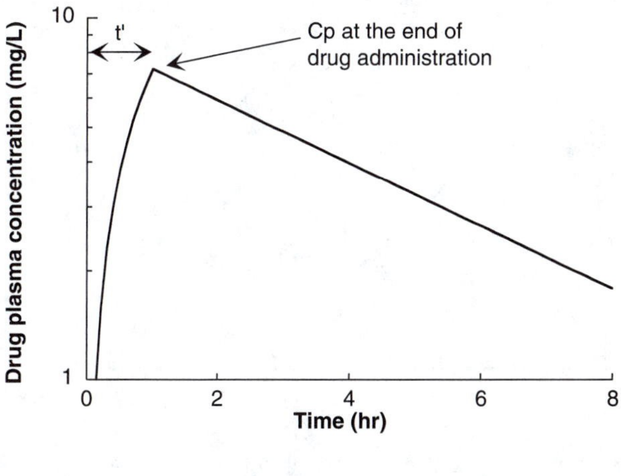

FIGURE 13.2 The plasma concentration–time profile during and after administration of the first dose as a short-time IV infusion of duration t′.

where t is the time from starting the drug administration, and t′ is the infusion time. Notice that this is the general equation that describes the drug concentration during and after a constant-rate IV infusion. During the IV infusion, t is equal to t′, and Equation 13.6 is reduced to Equation 13.5. After termination of the IV infusion, t becomes larger than t′.

13.2.2 After Repeated Administration before Reaching Steady State

During repeated intermittent IV infusions, when a second dose is administered the drug concentration during the second IV infusion is the sum of the drug concentration resulting from drug infusion plus the drug concentration remaining from the first dose. If we assume that the drug concentration just before the second IV infusion is equal to Cp_x, as illustrated in Figure 13.3, the drug concentration at the end of the second infusion (Duration = t′) can be obtained from the following equation:

$$Cp = \frac{K_0}{k\,Vd}\,(1 - e^{-k t'}) + Cp_x\, e^{-k t'} \tag{13.7}$$

If the second dose administered by IV infusion is terminated after time equal to t′, then the drug concentration declines monoexponentially as shown in Figure 13.3. The drug concentration after termination of the IV infusion can be described by the following equation:

$$Cp = \left[\frac{K_0}{k\,Vd}\,(1 - e^{-k t'}) + Cp_x\, e^{-k t'}\right] e^{-k(t - t')} \tag{13.8}$$

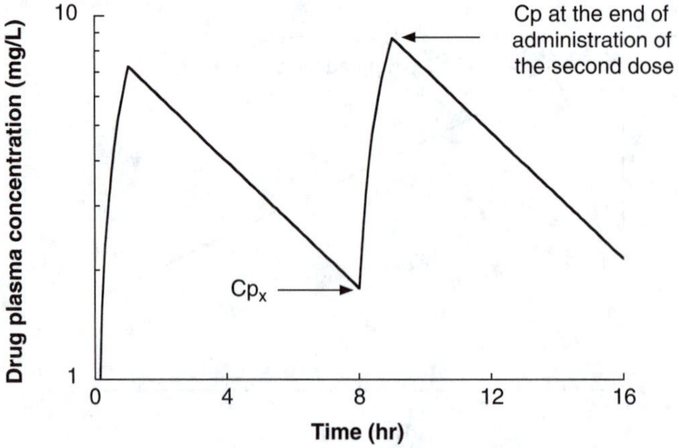

FIGURE 13.3 The plasma concentration–time profile during repeated administration of intermittent IV infusions before achieving steady state.

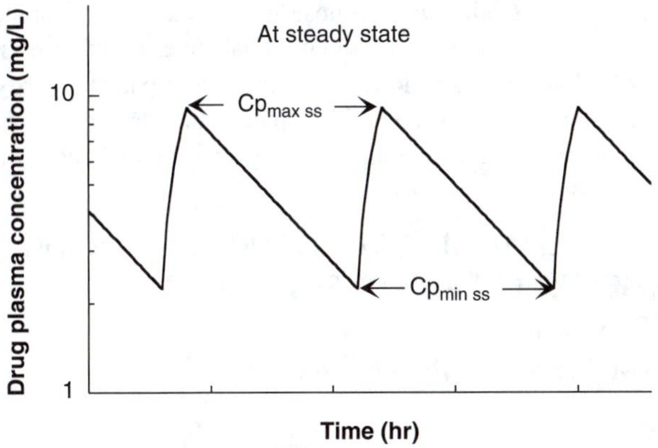

FIGURE 13.4 The plasma concentration–time profile during repeated administration of intermittent IV infusions at steady state.

Equation 13.8 is the general equation for drug administration as a short constant-rate IV infusion. During drug administration, t is equal to t′, and Equation 13.8 is reduced to Equation 13.7. Also, if the drug is administered for the first time, then Cp_x is equal to zero, and the equation is reduced to Equation 13.5 or 13.6.

13.2.3 At Steady State

Repeated drug administration by intermittent IV infusion will lead to drug accumulation in the body until steady state is achieved. At steady state, the drug concentration right after the end of drug administration is equal to $Cp_{max\ ss}$, and the drug concentration just before drug administration is equal to $Cp_{min\ ss}$, as shown in Figure 13.4. The drug concentration just after drug administration by a short IV infusion over a period of time equal to t′ at steady state is equal to

$$Cp_{max\ ss} = \frac{K_0}{k\ Vd}(1 - e^{-k t'}) + Cp_{min\ ss}\ e^{-k\ t'} \tag{13.9}$$

Because $Cp_{min\ ss}$ is equal to the concentration remaining from $Cp_{max\ ss}$ after the postinfusion period (τ – t′), $Cp_{min\ ss}$ can be expressed as

$$Cp_{min\ ss} = Cp_{max\ ss}\ e^{-k\ (\tau - t')} \tag{13.10}$$

By substitution for the value of $Cp_{min\ ss}$ in Equation 13.9 and solving for $Cp_{max\ ss}$, we get the following relationship:

$$Cp_{max\ ss} = \frac{K_0\ (1 - e^{-k t'})}{k\ Vd\ (1 - e^{-k \tau})} \tag{13.11}$$

Repeated drug administration by intermittent IV infusion will lead to drug accumulation in the body until steady state is achieved. The steady-state plasma concentration will be proportional to the administered dose if the total body clearance of the drug remains constant. It takes five to six elimination half-lives to achieve the steady state. Administration of a loading dose can lead to a faster approach to steady state without affecting the steady-state concentration. The steady-state drug concentration depends only on the drug administration rate and the drug total body clearance.

13.3 EFFECT OF CHANGING THE PHARMACOKINETIC PARAMETERS ON STEADY-STATE PLASMA CONCENTRATION DURING REPEATED INTERMITTENT IV INFUSION

13.3.1 Dose

The steady-state plasma concentration is directly proportional to the administered dose. Increasing the dose will result in a proportional increase in the steady-state maximum and minimum plasma concentrations if the total body clearance of the drug remains constant.

13.3.2 Infusion Time

Administration of the same dose of the drug over a longer duration will result in lower maximum drug plasma concentration and higher minimum drug plasma concentration at steady state. This is because a larger amount of the drug is eliminated during the longer infusion time.

13.3.3 Total Body Clearance

The steady-state drug concentration is inversely proportional to the total body clearance. Higher total body clearance leads to a faster rate of drug elimination (if Vd remains constant) and a lower steady-state plasma concentration. Patients with lower total body clearance will have a higher steady-state concentration if the dose and the volume of distribution remain constant.

13.3.4 Volume of Distribution

The steady-state concentration is dependent on the dose and the total body clearance. Differences in Vd do not affect the steady-state drug concentration if the dose and the total body clearance are constant.

13.4 APPLICATION OF PHARMACOKINETIC PRINCIPLES FOR INTERMITTENT IV INFUSION TO THERAPEUTIC USE OF AMINOGLYCOSIDE

The classical example of drugs administered by intermittent IV infusion and frequently monitored in patients is aminoglycoside antibiotics such as gentamicin, tobramycin, amikacin, and netilmicin. Aminoglycosides are antibacterial agents that have bactericidal activity against Gram-negative aerobic bacteria.

13.4.1 Pharmacokinetic Characteristics

13.4.1.1 Absorption

These drugs are not absorbed after oral administration. However, some aminoglycoside antibiotics, such as neomycin and streptomycin, are administered orally for their local gastrointestinal tract effect. After intramuscular administration, the maximum aminoglycoside plasma concentration is achieved after 30–60 min in patients with normal kidney function and after 2–5 hr in patients with reduced kidney function, depending on the severity of the kidney dysfunction.

13.4.1.2 Distribution

Aminoglycosides are distributed primarily in the extracellular fluid because of their poor lipid solubility. Their average volume of distribution is 0.2–0.25 L/kg.

13.4.1.3 Excretion

After parenteral drug administration, aminoglycosides are almost completely eliminated unchanged in urine.

13.4.2 Guidelines for Aminoglycoside Plasma Concentration

The most common adverse effects of aminoglycosides are nephrotoxicity, ototoxicity, and neuromuscular blockade. The goal of conventional aminoglycoside dosing adjustment strategies is to maintain the steady-state maximum and minimum plasma concentrations within a certain range to ensure optimal efficacy with minimal toxicity. Table 13.1 lists the guidelines for the desired maximum and minimum aminoglycoside plasma concentration at steady state using the conventional dosing approach.

TABLE 13.1
Guidelines for Steady-State Aminoglycoside Concentrations While Using Conventional Dosing Regimen

	Drug	
	Gentamicin, Tobramycin, Netilmicin (mg/L)	Amikacin (mg/L)
Maximum (peak) concentration		
Serious infections	6–8	20–25
Life-threatening infections	8–10	25–30
Minimum (trough) concentration		
Serious infections	0.5–1	1–4
Life-threatening infections	1–2	4–8

13.4.3 Extended-Interval Aminoglycoside Dosing Regimen

The total daily dose of aminoglycosides administered once a day has been utilized effectively to treat systemic infections. Administration of larger doses results in higher plasma aminoglycoside concentrations and should produce a more bactericidal effect. Also, the duration of the bactericidal effect of aminoglycosides is prolonged for a period of time after the plasma concentration of aminoglycoside falls below the minimum inhibitory concentration. These two factors provide the basis for the rationale of once-daily aminoglycoside dosing. The effectiveness of once-daily aminoglycoside dosing in all patients to treat all infections is yet to be determined. There are no known optimal maximum and minimum drug plasma concentrations when aminoglycosides are administered once daily. The guidelines in Table 13.1 do not apply to the once-daily dosing method. The following discussion covers the conventional aminoglycoside dosing adjustment method.

13.5 INDIVIDUALIZATION OF AMINOGLYCOSIDE THERAPY

Individualization of drug therapy in general follows three steps:

- Determination of the initial dosing regimen based on the population parameters
- Determination of the patient's specific pharmacokinetic parameters
- Determination of the dosing regimen based on the patient-specific parameters

13.5.1 Determination of Initial Dosing Regimen Based on Population Parameters

The patient's information is used to estimate the patient's pharmacokinetic parameters based on the reported parameters for different patient populations. Aminoglycosides are completely eliminated by the kidney. This makes their elimination half-lives highly correlated with the patient's kidney function. The patient's kidney function can be determined from the creatinine clearance. The creatinine clearance can be determined directly or can be estimated from the serum creatinine and some patients' specific information. The method of Cockroft and Gault, discussed in Chapter 10, can provide a reasonable estimate for the creatinine clearance in milliliters per minute from the age, weight, serum creatinine, and gender. The creatinine clearance is estimated for men from Equation 13.12 and for women from Equation 13.13.

$$\text{CrCL} = \frac{(140\text{-Age})\ (\text{Weight in kg})}{72\ (\text{Serum creatinine in mg/dL})} \tag{13.12}$$

$$\text{CrCL} = 0.85\left[\frac{(140\text{-Age})\ (\text{Weight in kg})}{72\ (\text{Serum creatinine in mg/dL})}\right] \tag{13.13}$$

By knowing the creatinine clearance of the patient, we can estimate the fraction remaining of the patient's kidney function (KF) by comparing the estimated creatinine clearance with the normal creatinine clearance, which is usually in the range of 120 ml/min.

$$\text{Fraction of KF} = \frac{\text{Patient Cr CL}}{120 \text{ ml/min}} \tag{13.14}$$

The aminoglycoside half-life can be estimated as follows:

$$\text{Estimated } t_{1/2} = \frac{\text{Normal } t_{1/2} \text{ (2.5 hr)}}{\text{Fraction of KF}} \tag{13.15}$$

The relationship used for the estimation of aminoglycoside half-life is valid only for drugs that are eliminated completely unchanged in urine. When the estimated creatinine clearance is more than 120 ml/min, the fraction remaining of the kidney function is considered equal to unity, and the half-life in this case can be estimated as the average half-life of aminoglycosides. The estimated aminoglycoside half-life and an average estimate for the volume of distribution (0.25 L/kg) are used to determine the initial dosing regimen for aminoglycosides.

13.5.2 Determination of Patient-Specific Pharmacokinetic Parameters

After the patient receives the initial drug treatment, the patient's specific parameters should be determined by designing an appropriate sampling schedule that allows parameter determination. The Sawchuk-Zaske method is one of the widely used methods for individualization of an aminoglycoside dosing regimen in a variety of different patient populations. This method assumes that aminoglycosides are administered by intermittent constant-rate IV infusions over a period of t′, and drug administration is repeated every one dosing interval τ. Also, the method assumes that aminoglycosides follow a one-compartment pharmacokinetic model. Although aminoglycosides follow a multicompartment pharmacokinetic model, the use of a one-compartment pharmacokinetic model can generally provide clinically acceptable estimates for aminoglycoside disposition.

13.5.2.1 If the Patient Is to Receive the First Aminoglycoside Dose

After administration of the first dose of the drug as a constant-rate IV infusion over a period of t′ and at a rate equal to K_0 (equal to dose/t), the drug plasma concentration at the end of the drug administration can be determined from Equation 13.3.

$$Cp = \frac{K_0}{k\,Vd}\left(1 - e^{-k t'}\right)$$

To estimate the pharmacokinetic parameters, three samples are obtained over a period of time equivalent approximately to the estimated aminoglycoside half-life. For example, for a patient with normal kidney function, samples should be drawn over a 2.5-hr period (at 0.5, 1.5, and 3 hr) after the end of drug administration.

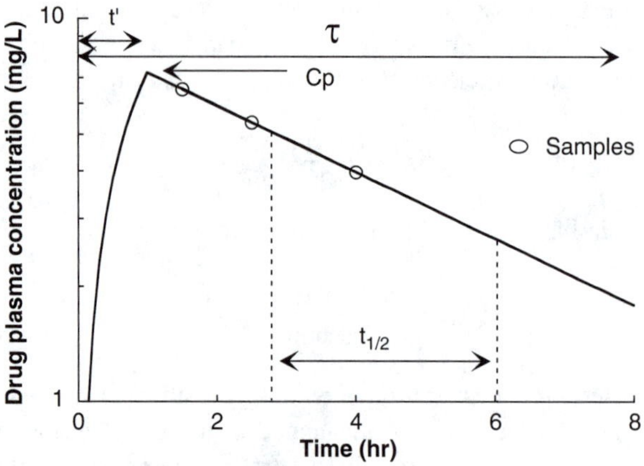

FIGURE 13.5 Graphical determination of the drug half-life and drug concentration at the end of drug administration from the drug plasma concentration–time profile during and after administration of the first dose of a short-time IV infusion of duration t′.

Patients with reduced kidney function may require obtaining the samples over a longer period of time according to their estimated aminoglycoside half-life. The samples are analyzed for aminoglycosides, and the measured drug concentrations are plotted on semilog graph paper as in Figure 13.5.

The best line that fits the three points is drawn and back-extrapolated to the time when the infusion was terminated to determine the drug concentration at the end of the drug administration Cp. Figure 13.5 represents the entire aminoglycoside plasma concentration–time profile during and after the end of drug administration. However, for the determination of the drug half-life and the drug concentration right at the end of drug administration, a plot of the drug concentration versus time after the end of drug administration may be sufficient. In this plot, the y-intercept will be equal to the drug plasma concentration at the end of drug administration, and the elimination rate constant or the half-life is determined from the plasma concentrations as in Figure 13.6.

The elimination rate constant can be calculated from the slope of the line (Slope = −k/2.303). Also, the half-life can be determined from the graph by calculating the time required for the drug concentration to decrease by 50%. By knowing either the elimination rate constant or the half-life, the other parameter can be calculated from the following relationship:

$$k = \frac{0.693}{t_{1/2}} \tag{13.16}$$

The drug elimination rate constant can also be determined mathematically by using any two plasma drug concentrations on the fitted line from Equation 13.17.

$$Cp_{t2} = Cp_{t1}\, e^{-kt} \tag{13.17}$$

where Cp_{t1} and Cp_{t2} are two different plasma concentrations, Cp_{t1} is the sample obtained first and Cp_{t2} is the sample obtained at later time; k is the first-order

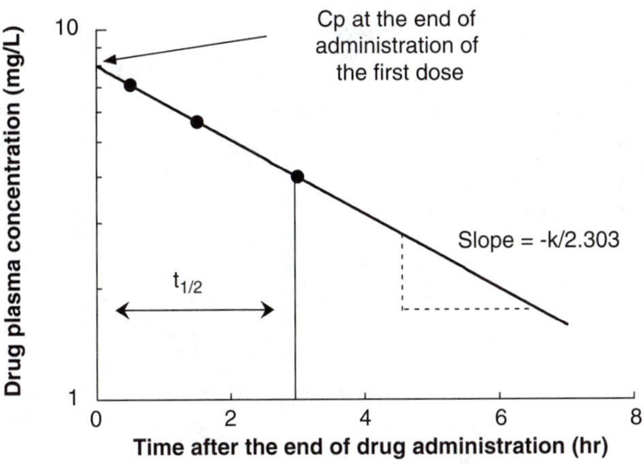

FIGURE 13.6 Graphical determination of the drug half-life and drug concentration at the end of drug administration from a plot of the drug concentrations versus time after the end of drug administration.

elimination rate constant; and t is the time difference between the two samples. After determination of the elimination rate constant, the half-life can be calculated. After determination of Cp graphically and the elimination rate constant, the volume of distribution of aminoglycosides can be determined by substitution in Equation 13.3.

13.5.2.2 If the Patient Received Aminoglycosides before but the Steady State Was Not Achieved

The plasma concentration after the end of administration of the second dose of the drug by a constant-rate IV infusion (or repeated administration before steady state is achieved) is the sum of the drug concentration resulting from the administered drug and the drug remaining from previous doses. In this case, the drug concentration at the end of drug administration can be expressed by Equation 13.7 as described previously.

$$Cp = \frac{K_0}{k\,Vd}\,(1 - e^{-k\,t'}) + Cp_x\,e^{-k\,t'}$$

To determine the drug elimination rate constant, the half-life, and the volume of distribution, one plasma sample should be obtained just before drug administration, and two or three samples are obtained after the end of drug administration as shown in Figure 13.7. The drug plasma concentration obtained just before drug administration is equal to Cp_x in Equation 13.7. The samples obtained after the end of drug administration should be obtained over a period of time equal approximately to the estimated aminoglycoside half-life in the patient. The elimination rate constant or the half-life can be determined as mentioned from the plasma concentrations obtained after the end of drug administration. The plasma concentration at the end of drug administration can be determined graphically by back-extrapolation to the time of termination of the infusion as mentioned. By substitution for Cp, Cp_x, and k in Equation 13.7, the volume of distribution can be determined.

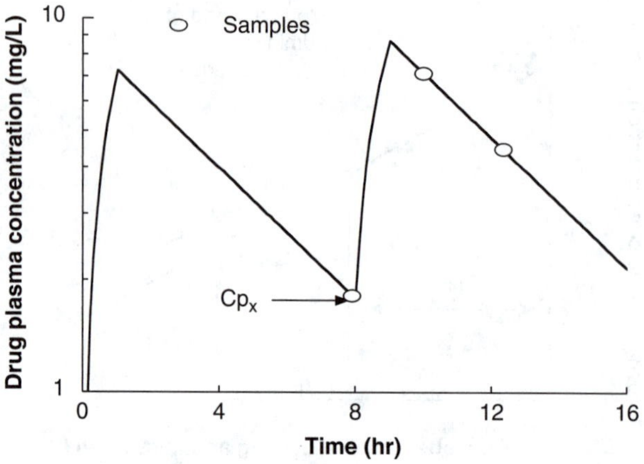

FIGURE 13.7 The plasma samples obtained for the determination of the pharmacokinetic parameters during repeated intermittent IV infusions before achieving steady state.

13.5.2.3 If the Patient Received Aminoglycosides and Steady State Has Been Achieved

Because the patient is at steady state, the $Cp_{max\ ss}$ and $Cp_{min\ ss}$ should be constant in consecutive dosing intervals. So, the drug concentration in the sample obtained just before the drug administration should be equal to the drug concentration at the end of the following dosing interval. So, two plasma samples are obtained, one sample just before drug administration and then 1 hr after the end of drug administration as shown in Figure 13.8.

The elimination rate constant can be calculated from the two different drug plasma concentrations obtained before and after drug administration. The two different

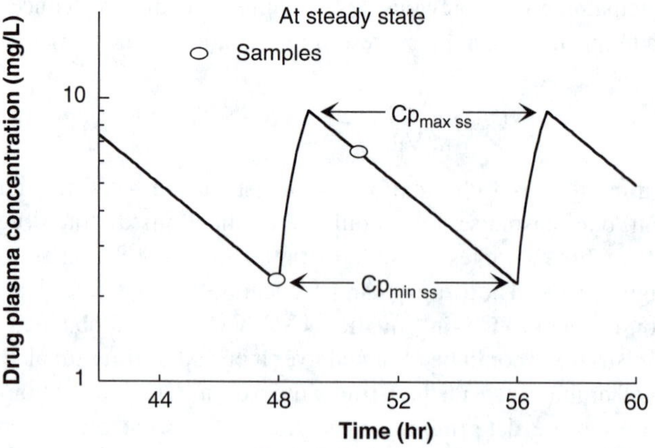

FIGURE 13.8 The plasma samples obtained for the determination of the pharmacokinetic parameters during repeated intermittent IV infusions at steady state.

concentrations are known, and the time difference between the two concentrations is known, so the elimination rate constant can be capsulated. Also, the drug concentration right after the end of drug administration can be determined graphically or mathematically. By substitution for the elimination rate constant and the $Cp_{max\ ss}$ in Equation 13.11, the volume of distribution can be determined:

$$Cp_{max\ ss} = \frac{K_0\ (1 - e^{-k t'})}{k\ Vd\ (1 - e^{-k \tau})}$$

13.5.3 Determination of the Dosing Regimen Based on the Patient's Specific Parameters

The estimated aminoglycoside elimination rate constant and volume of distribution are used to determine the dose D and the dosing interval τ that should achieve the desired $Cp_{max\ ss}$ (peak) and $Cp_{min\ ss}$ (trough).

13.5.3.1 Selection of Dosing Interval τ

After selecting the drug infusion time t′ and the desired $Cp_{max\ ss}$ and $Cp_{min\ ss}$, the dosing interval τ can be calculated from Equation 13.10. The calculated dosing interval τ should be approximated to the nearest practical dosing interval, that is, 4, 6, 8, 12, 18, 24, 48, or 72 hr.

13.5.3.2 Selection of Dose

The approximated value of the dosing interval τ, the predetermined infusion time t′, the desired $Cp_{max\ ss}$, and the calculated pharmacokinetic parameters are used to calculate the aminoglycoside dose from Equation 13.11. The calculated dose should be approximated to the nearest practical dose (approximate to the nearest 5 mg).

13.5.3.3 Selection of Loading Dose

When administration of a loading dose is necessary, the loading dose should be selected to achieve a plasma concentration equal to the desired maximum steady-state plasma concentration after the loading dose. The loading dose is calculated from Equation 13.5 after substation for t′, k, Vd, and the Cp.

The actual values of the $Cp_{max\ ss}$ (peak) and $Cp_{min\ ss}$ (trough) that should be achieved by using the approximated values of the dose and the dosing interval can be calculated from Equation 13.10 and Equation 13.11. The patient response and the dosage requirement should be monitored after initiation of drug therapy. Reassessment of aminoglycoside regimen is necessary when the patient's condition changes in a way that can alter aminoglycoside pharmacokinetics.

Example

A 43-year-old, 68-kg male was admitted to the hospital to treat a lung infection with gentamicin. He received his first dose of 140 mg administered by constant-rate IV infusion over a period of 1 hr. Three plasma samples were drawn after the end of drug administration, and the concentrations were as follows:

Time after end of administration	2 hr	4 hr	8 hr
Gentamicin concentration (mg/L)	8.4	5.85	2.84

1. Estimate the half-life and volume of distribution of gentamicin in this patient.
2. Recommend a dosing regimen (dose and dosing regimen) that should achieve maximum and minimum steady-state plasma gentamicin concentrations of 8 and 1 mg/L, respectively. Gentamicin is administered by constant-rate IV infusion over 1 hr.

Answer

The half-life and the plasma concentration achieved at the end of drug administration can be determined graphically as in Figure 13.9:

Half-life = 3.85 hr

Plasma concentration at the end of drug administration = 12 mg/L

$$Cp = \frac{K_0}{k\,Vd}\,(1 - e^{-kt'})$$

$$12\ \text{mg/L} = \frac{140\ \text{mg/hr}}{0.18\ \text{hr}^{-1}\ Vd}\,(1 - e^{-0.18\ \text{hr}^{-1}\ 1\ \text{hr}})$$

$$Vd = 10.68\ \text{L}$$

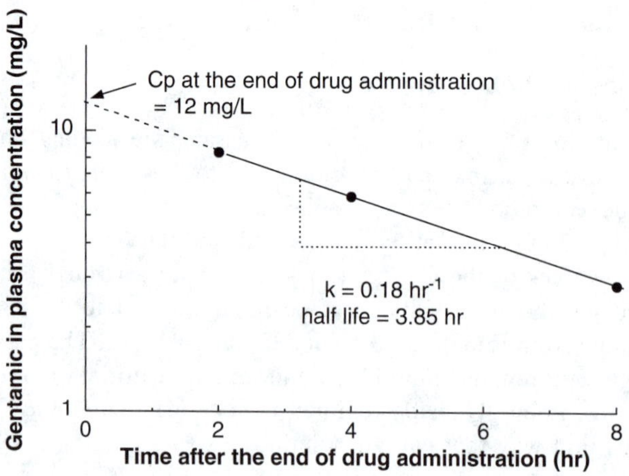

FIGURE 13.9 Graphical determination of the drug half-life and drug concentration at the end of drug administration from a plot of the drug concentrations versus time after the end of drug administration.

2. For the dosing regimen,

$$Cp_{\text{min ss}} = Cp_{\text{max ss}}\ e^{-k\,(\tau - t')}$$

$$1\ \text{mg/L} = 8\ \text{mg/L}\ e^{-0.18\ \text{hr}^{-1}\ (\tau - 1\ \text{hr})}$$

$$(\tau - t') = 11.55\ \text{hr}$$

$$\text{An appropriate dosing interval} = 12\ \text{hr}$$

$$Cp_{\text{max ss}} = \frac{K_0\ (1 - e^{-kt'})}{k\ Vd\ (1 - e^{-k\tau})}$$

$$8\ \text{mg/L} = \frac{K_0\ (1 - e^{-0.18\ \text{hr}^{-1}\ 1\ \text{hr}})}{0.18\ \text{hr}^{-1}\ \ 10.68\ \text{L}\ (1 - e^{-0.18\ \text{hr}^{-1}\ 12\ \text{hr}})}$$

$$K_0 = 82.6\ \text{mg administered over 1 hr}$$

The recommendation is 85 mg gentamicin administered as a constant-rate IV infusion over 1 hr and repeated every 12 hr.

Example

A 38-year-old, 68 kg male was admitted to the hospital because of acute pneumonia, and he is to receive tobramycin. His serum creatinine was 1.6 mg/dL on admission to the hospital.

1. Estimate the half-life of tobramycin in this patient based on his kidney function.
2. A loading dose of 2 mg/kg tobramycin given as a constant-rate infusion for 1 hr followed by 150 mg tobramycin every 8 hr given as a constant-rate infusion for 1 hr were prescribed. The patient received his first dose of tobramycin, and before administration of the second dose you are asked to determine the pharmacokinetic parameters of tobramycin in this patient. Recommend a sampling schedule around the second dose that can allow the determination of tobramycin pharmacokinetic parameters in this patient (please give the exact number and time of sampling).
3. Despite the pharmacokinetic consultation, the patient continued to receive 150 mg tobramycin every 8 hr given as a constant-rate infusion for 1 hr. At steady state, the maximum and the minimum plasma concentrations of tobramycin (measured immediately after the end of drug administration and just before drug administration at steady state) were 11.3 and 3.85 mg/L, respectively. Calculate the half-life and the volume of distribution of tobramycin in this patient.
4. Recommend a dosing regimen (a dose and dosing interval) that will achieve steady-state maximum and minimum plasma concentrations of 6 and 1 mg/L, respectively.

Answer

1.

$$CrCL = \frac{(140\text{-Age})\ (\text{Weight in kg})}{72\ (\text{Serum creatinine in mg/dL})}$$

$$CrCL = \frac{(140\text{-}38\ \text{yr})\ (68\ \text{kg})}{72\ (1.6\ \text{mg/dL})} = 60\ \text{ml/min}$$

$$\text{Fraction of KF} = \frac{\text{Patient Cr CL}}{120\ \text{ml/min}} = \frac{60\ \text{ml/min}}{120\ \text{ml/min}} = 0.5$$

$$\text{Estimated tobramicin } t_{1/2} = \frac{\text{Normal } t_{1/2}\ (2.5\ \text{hr})}{\text{Fraction of KF}} = \frac{2.5\ \text{hr}}{0.5} = 5\ \text{hr}$$

2. The blood samples will be obtained around the second sample (before reaching steady state). So, one sample should be obtained before administration of the second dose, and two or three samples should be obtained after the end of drug administration over a period of time equal approximately to the estimated tobramycin half-life (5 hr).

First sample	Just before drug administration
Second sample	0.5 hr after the end of drug administration
Third sample	2 hr after the end of drug administration
Fourth sample	5 hr after the end of drug administration

3.

$$Cp_{\text{min ss}} = Cp_{\text{max ss}}\ e^{-k\,(\tau - t')}$$

$$3.85\ \text{mg/L} = 11.3\ \text{mg/L}\ e^{-k\,(8\ \text{hr} - 1\ \text{hr})}$$

$$k = 0.154\ \text{hr}^{-1} \qquad t_{1/2} = 4.5\ \text{hr}$$

$$Cp_{\text{max ss}} = \frac{K_0\ (1 - e^{-kt'})}{k\ Vd\ (1 - e^{-k\tau'})}$$

$$11.3\ \text{mg/L} = \frac{150\ \text{mg/hr}\ (1 - e^{-0.154\ \text{hr}^{-1}\ 1\ \text{hr}})}{0.154\ \text{hr}^{-1}\ Vd\ (1 - e^{-0.154\ \text{hr}^{-1}\ 8\ \text{hr}})}$$

$$Vd = 17.4\ \text{L}$$

4. For the dosing regimen,

$$Cp_{\text{min ss}} = Cp_{\text{max ss}}\ e^{-k\,(\tau - t')}$$

$$1\ \text{mg/L} = 6\ \text{mg/L}\ e^{-0.154\ \text{hr}^{-1}\ (\tau\ -\ 1\ \text{hr})}$$

$$(\tau - t') = 11.6\ \text{hr}$$

$$\text{An appropriate dosing interval} = 12\ \text{hr}$$

$$Cp_{\text{max ss}} = \frac{K_0\ (1 - e^{-k\,t'})}{k\ Vd\ (1 - e^{-k\,\tau})}$$

$$6\ \text{mg/L} = \frac{K_0\ (1 - e^{-0.154\ \text{hr}^{-1}\ 1\ \text{hr}})}{0.154\ \text{hr}^{-1}\ \ 17.4\ \text{L}\ (1 - e^{-0.154\ \text{hr}^{-1}\ 12\ \text{hr}})}$$

$$K_0 = 95\ \text{ mg administered over 1 hr}$$

The recommendation is for 95 mg tobramycin administered as a constant-rate IV infusion over 1 hr and repeated every 12 hr.

PRACTICE PROBLEMS

13.1. A 60-kg patient received a 1-hr infusion of gentamicin, and the pharmacokinetic study showed that the half-life was 2.7 hr and the volume of distribution was 0.21 L/kg. The desired maximum and minimum steady-state concentrations for this patient are 6 and 1 mg/L, respectively.

a. Calculate the dosing regimen to achieve steady-state concentrations around these desired concentrations.
b. Calculate the actual steady-state maximum and minimum plasma concentrations for the regimen you recommended.

13.2. A patient is receiving 75 mg gentamicin every 4 hr as an infusion for 1 hr duration. The maximum and minimum plasma gentamicin concentrations achieved at steady state are 6 and 2.35 mg/L, respectively.

a. Calculate gentamicin half-life in this patient.
b. Calculate gentamicin volume of distribution in this patient.
c. Recommend a dosing regimen to achieve steady-state maximum and minimum plasma gentamicin concentrations around 8 and 1 mg/L, respectively.
d. Calculate the actual steady-state maximum and minimum plasma concentrations that should be achieved with the regimen you recommended in problem 13.2c.

13.3. A patient is receiving 50 mg tobramycin every 6 hr of as intermittent IV infusions for 1 hr duration. At steady state, three plasma samples were obtained, and tobramycin concentrations were as follows:

Time	Before the Dose	0.5 hr After the Infusion	2 hr After the Infusion
Concentration (mg/L)	1.26	3.56	2.52

a. Calculate tobramycin half-life in this patient.
b. Calculate tobramycin volume of distribution in this patient.
c. Recommend a dosing regimen to achieve steady-state maximum and minimum plasma tobramycin concentrations around 10 and 1.5 mg/L, respectively.
d. Calculate the actual steady-state maximum and minimum plasma concentrations that should be achieved with the regimen you recommended in problem 13.3c.

13.4. A 60-yr-old, 60-kg male was admitted to the hospital because of acute pneumonia. Gentamicin 75 mg every 12 hr given as a short infusion for 1 hr was prescribed. Because his serum creatinine was 2.5 mg/dL, the pharmacokinetic service was consulted to adjust the gentamicin dosing regimen.

a. Estimate the creatinine clearance in this patient.
b. What is the percentage renal function remaining in this patient?
c. What is the estimated half-life of gentamicin in this patient?

Four plasma samples were drawn around the second dose, just before giving the second dose and 1, 4, and 10 hr after the second dose. Samples were analyzed for gentamicin, and the results were as follows:

Time	Just Before	1 hr Post	4 hr Post	10 hr Post
Concentration (mg/L)	2.1	6.5	5.11	3.13

d. Calculate the half-life and the volume of distribution of gentamicin in this patient.
e. What was the maximum plasma concentration after the first dose?
f. What would be the steady-state maximum and the minimum plasma concentrations if 75 mg gentamicin every 12 hr were continued?
g. Comment on the difference between the maximum plasma concentration after the first dose and the maximum plasma concentration at steady state (during the regimen of 75 mg every 12 hr regimen).
h. Recommend a dosing regimen (dose and dosing interval) to achieve steady-state maximum and minimum plasma concentrations of 7 and 1 mg/L, respectively.

13.5. A patient is receiving tobramycin as 100 mg every 8 hr as a short infusion over 0.5 hr. His serum creatinine was 1 mg/dL. At steady state, two plasma samples were obtained, 0.5 hr before the administration of the dose and 1 hr after the end of the infusion; the tobramycin plasma concentrations were 2.18 and 8.73 mg/L in the two samples, respectively.

a. Calculate the half-life and volume of distribution of tobramycin in this patient.
b. Recommend a dosing regimen to achieve steady-state maximum and minimum plasma concentrations of 9 and 1 mg/L, respectively.
c. Calculate the actual maximum and minimum plasma concentrations achieved at steady state with the regimen you recommended in problem 13.5b.
d. The patient came back to the hospital 6 months later, and his serum creatinine was 2 mg/dL. What is the estimated new half-life of tobramycin in this patient?

13.6. An 84-year-old, 50-kg male is admitted to the hospital, and he is to receive gentamicin. His serum creatinine was 1.2 mg/dL. Dosing of 65 mg gentamicin every 12 hr given as short infusion for 1 hr was prescribed.

a. Estimate the half-life of gentamicin in this patient.
b. Recommend a sampling schedule around the second dose that will allow the determination of the pharmacokinetic parameters in this patient. Samples were obtained and a dose of 75 mg every 24 hr as short infusion (1 hr duration) was recommended. At steady state, two samples were obtained, 1 and 8 hr after the end of the dose; the gentamicin plasma concentrations were 9.25 and 5.4 mg/L, respectively.
c. Calculate the half-life and volume of distribution of gentamicin in this patient.
d. Recommend a dosing regimen to achieve steady-state maximum and minimum plasma concentrations of 9 and 1 mg/L, respectively.
e. Calculate the actual maximum and minimum plasma concentrations achieved at steady state with the regimen you recommended in problem 13.6d.

14 Noncompartmental Approach to Pharmacokinetic Data Analysis

OBJECTIVES

After completing this chapter, you should be able to:

- Describe the advantages of the noncompartmental approach in pharmacokinetic data analysis
- Define the mean residence time
- Calculate the area under the curve (AUC), the area under the first-moment curve (AUMC), and the mean residence time (MRT) from the plasma concentration-time data
- Analyze the drug absorption characteristics after extravascular administration using the noncompartmental approach
- Determine the pharmacokinetic parameters using the noncompartmental approach and describe how they are related to their estimates from the compartmental approach

14.1 INTRODUCTION

In all the previous discussions, we used the compartmental approach in analyzing the pharmacokinetic behavior of the drug in the body. It was assumed that the drug behavior in the body can be described by one-compartment or multicompartment pharmacokinetic models. When the drug is rapidly distributed to all parts of the body, the body behaves as one compartment, and the drug profile in the body can be described by a one-compartment pharmacokinetic model. On the other hand, when the distribution of the drug in a group of tissues or organs is faster than its distribution to other tissues or organs, the body behaves as two different compartments, and the drug profile in the body can be described by a two-compartment pharmacokinetic model. The body can also behave as multiple compartments when the drug is distributed to different groups of tissues at different rates.

The compartmental model characteristics, including the number of compartments, the arrangements of the compartments, and the compartment from which drug elimination takes place, are determined from the plasma concentration–time profile obtained after drug administration. The pharmacokinetic model is selected to describe the obtained drug concentration–time profile. For example, if the drug concentration–time profile after a single intravenous (IV) bolus administration is linear on the semilog scale, this means that the drug behavior in the body can be described by a one-compartment pharmacokinetic model. The drug behavior in the body can be described by a two-compartment pharmacokinetic model when the plasma concentration–time profile after a single IV bolus dose is curvilinear on the semilog scale.

The compartmental approach in data analysis sometimes is faced with some difficulties, such as when the drug concentration–time profile after IV administration is described by a two-compartment pharmacokinetic model, but after the oral administration of the same drug, the profile is similar to that of the one-compartment model because the rates of the absorption and distribution processes are not distinctively different. Also, the compartmental analysis is usually performed utilizing computer software, which requires special skills and knowledge of pharmacokinetics and statistics to ensure proper model specification and accuracy of the obtained results. Furthermore, the use of complex pharmacokinetic models (multicompartment models) usually describes the drug profile in the body better than the simpler models, which makes it important to test statistically if going to complex pharmacokinetic models significantly improves the description of the drug concentration–time profile in the body. To avoid these difficulties, a different approach, known as the *noncompartmental approach*, can be used for data analysis when the pharmacokinetic question under investigation can be examined without the need to assume a certain compartmental model.

14.2 NONCOMPARTMENTAL APPROACH IN DATA ANALYSIS

The noncompartmental approach in pharmacokinetic data analysis is based on the statistical moment theory, which has been utilized in chemical engineering. This theory views the drug molecules in the body as randomly distributed, and each molecule has a certain probability to be eliminated at a certain time t. So, according to this theory, the time course for the drug concentration in plasma can be regarded as a probability density function. This probability density function multiplied by time raised to a certain power (0, 1, or 2) and integrated over time yields the area under the moment curve. For example, the area under the zero-moment curve can be determined from Equation 14.1, which is equal to the AUC. Also, the area under the first-moment curve (AUMC) can be determined according to Equation 14.2. Only the areas under the zero and first moments are utilized in pharmacokinetics because higher moments are subjected to large computational errors.

$$\text{Area under the zero-moment curve} = \int_{t=0}^{t=\infty} t^0\,\text{Cp dt} = \int_{t=0}^{t=\infty} \text{Cp dt} = \text{AUC} \tag{14.1}$$

$$\text{Area under the first-moment curve} = \int_{t=0}^{t=\infty} t^1\,\text{Cp dt} = \int_{t=0}^{t=\infty} \text{t Cp dt} = \text{AUMC} \tag{14.2}$$

The principle of moment analysis has been utilized to estimate pharmacokinetic parameters such as the MRT, drug clearance, and the volume of distribution at steady state.

14.3 MEAN RESIDENCE TIME

The drug molecules are distributed throughout the body after IV administration. Some drug molecules are eliminated from the body faster than other molecules, which stay longer despite the fact that all the molecules are similar. The difference in the residence time for each molecule in the body occurs by chance according to statistical moment theory. The MRT is defined as the average time for the residence of all the drug molecules in the body. In other words, the MRT can be calculated from the total residence time for all drug molecules (by adding the residence time for all molecules) divided by the number of the drug molecules as in Equation 14.3:

$$\text{MRT} = \frac{\text{Total residence time for all drug molecules}}{\text{Number of drug molecules}} \tag{14.3}$$

Equation 14.3 help explain the meaning of the MRT; however, practically it cannot be used in the calculation. The MRT can be calculated from the area under the zero- and first-moment curves according to Equation 14.4.

$$\text{MRT} = \frac{\text{AUMC}}{\text{AUC}} \tag{14.4}$$

where AUMC is the area under the first moment–time curve, and AUC is the area under the zero moment-time curve or the area under the plasma concentration–time curve. The MRT has units of time.

14.3.1 Calculation of AUC and AUMC

14.3.1.1 Area Under the Plasma Concentration–Time Curve

The AUC can be calculated utilizing the trapezoidal rule as described in Chapter 5 The plasma concentration–time profile is divided into trapezoids, and the area of each trapezoid is calculated according to Equation 14.5.

$$\text{Area of a trapezoid} = \left(\frac{C_n + C_{n+1}}{2}\right) . (t_{n+1} - t_n) \tag{14.5}$$

The $AUC_{0\text{-}t}$ is calculated by adding the area of all the trapezoids. The $AUC_{t-\infty}$ is calculated as in Equation 14.6.

$$AUC_{t-\infty} = \frac{Cp_{last}}{\lambda} \tag{14.6}$$

where Cp_{last} is the last-measured drug plasma concentration, and λ is the rate constant for the terminal decline in the drug plasma concentration. The total $AUC_{0-\infty}$ is calculated as in Equation 14.7.

$$AUC_{0-\infty} = AUC_{0-t} + AUC_{t-\infty} \tag{14.7}$$

14.3.1.2 Area Under the First Moment–Time Curve

The AUMC can also be calculated utilizing the trapezoidal rule after dividing the curve into trapezoids. The area of each trapezoid is calculated according to Equation 14.8:

$$\text{Area of a trapezoid} = \left(\frac{t_n\, C_n + t_{n+1}\, C_{n+1}}{2}\right) . (t_{n+1} - t_n) \tag{14.8}$$

The $AUMC_{0\text{-}t}$ is calculated by adding the area of all the trapezoids. The $AUMC_{0-\infty}$ is calculated as in Equation 14.9:

$$AUMC_{t-\infty} = \frac{t_{last}\, Cp_{last}}{\lambda} + \frac{Cp_{last}}{\lambda^2} \tag{14.9}$$

where Cp_{last} is the last-measured drug plasma concentration, t_{last} is the time of the last-measured drug plasma concentration, and λ is the rate constant for the terminal decline in the drug plasma concentration. The total $AUMC_{0\text{-}\infty}$ is calculated as in Equation 14.10:

$$AUMC_{0-\infty} = AUMC_{0-t} + AUMC_{t-\infty} \tag{14.10}$$

Example

After a single IV bolus administration of 50 mg of a drug, the following plasma concentrations were obtained:

Time (hr)	Concentrations (μg/L)
0	250
1	225
3	185
6	135
9	105
12	77
18	40
24	22

The terminal rate constant for the decline in the drug concentration is 0.1 hr^{-1}.

1. Calculate the MRT.

Answer

1. The MRT is calculated from the AUC and AUMC. For calculation of the AUC by the trapezoidal rule,

$$\text{Area of trapezoid 1} = \left(\frac{250+225}{2}\right).(1-0) = 237.5\ \mu\text{g-hr/L}$$

$$\text{Area of trapezoid 2} = \left(\frac{225+185}{2}\right).(3-1) = 410\ \mu\text{g-hr/L}$$

$$\text{Area of trapezoid 3} = \left(\frac{185+135}{2}\right).(6-3) = 480\ \mu\text{g-hr/L}$$

$$\text{Area of trapezoid 4} = \left(\frac{135+105}{2}\right).(9-6) = 360\ \mu\text{g-hr/L}$$

$$\text{Area of trapezoid 5} = \left(\frac{105+77}{2}\right).(12-9) = 273\ \mu\text{g-hr/L}$$

$$\text{Area of trapezoid 6} = \left(\frac{77+40}{2}\right).(18-12) = 351\ \mu\text{g-hr/L}$$

$$\text{Area of trapezoid 7} = \left(\frac{40+22}{2}\right).(24-18) = 186\ \mu\text{g-hr/L}$$

$$AUC_{t-\infty} = \frac{22}{0.1} = 220\ \mu g\text{-}hr/L$$

$$AUC_{0-\infty} = 237.5 + 410 + 480 + 360 + 273 + 351 + 186 + 220 = 2517.5\ \mu g\text{-}hr/L$$

For calculation of the AUMC, it is easier to add a column to the available data that includes the product of the time and the plasma concentration as follows:

Time (hr)	Concentration (μg/L)	Time × Concentration (μg-hr/L)
0	250	0
1	225	225
3	185	555
6	135	810
9	105	945
12	77	924
18	40	720
24	22	528

$$\text{Area of trapezoid } 1 = \left(\frac{0 + 225}{2}\right).(1 - 0) = 112.5\ \mu g\text{-}hr^2/L$$

$$\text{Area of trapezoid } 2 = \left(\frac{225 + 555}{2}\right).(3 - 1) = 780\ \mu g\text{-}hr^2/L$$

$$\text{Area of trapezoid } 3 = \left(\frac{555 + 810}{2}\right).(6 - 3) = 2047.5\ \mu g\text{-}hr^2/L$$

$$\text{Area of trapezoid } 4 = \left(\frac{810 + 945}{2}\right).(9 - 6) = 2632.5\ \mu g\text{-}hr^2/L$$

$$\text{Area of trapezoid } 5 = \left(\frac{945 + 924}{2}\right).(12 - 9) = 2803.5\ \mu g\text{-}hr^2/L$$

$$\text{Area of trapezoid } 6 = \left(\frac{924 + 720}{2}\right).(18 - 12) = 4932\ \mu g\text{-}hr^2/L$$

$$\text{Area of trapezoid } 7 = \left(\frac{720 + 528}{2}\right).(24 - 18) = 3744\ \mu g\text{-}hr^2/L$$

$$AUMC_{t-\infty} = \frac{t_{last}\ Cp_{last}}{\lambda} + \frac{Cp_{last}}{\lambda^2} = \frac{528}{0.1} + \frac{22}{(0.1)^2} = 7480\ \mu g\text{-}hr^2/L$$

$$AUC_{0-\infty} = 112.5 + 780 + 2047.5 + 2632.5 + 2803.5 + 4932 + 3744 + 7480$$
$$= 24532\ \mu g\text{-}hr^2/L$$

$$MRT = \frac{AUMC}{AUC} = \frac{24532\ \mu g\text{-}hr^2/L}{2517.5\ \mu g\text{-}hr/L} = 9.74\ hr$$

Note that the MRT was calculated without the need for any assumption of any compartmental model. The only information needed is the rate constant for the terminal elimination phase.

14.3.2 Mean Residence Time after Different Routes of Administration

14.3.2.1 Mean Residence Time after Extravascular Administration

The MRT for a specific drug in a given patient should be constant after a single IV bolus administration when the drug follows linear pharmacokinetics. However, after oral (or any extravascular) administration, for example, the drug spends additional time at the site of administration. In this case, the observed MRT_{oral} will be equal to the sum of the MRT in the body (similar to the MRT observed after a single IV dose) and the mean absorption time (MAT), which is the average time a drug molecule spends at the site of absorption.

$$MRT_{oral} = MRT_{IV} + MAT \tag{14.11}$$

This means that the noncompartmental data analysis can be used to compare the rate of drug absorption from different products for the same active drug. This is because, if the products contain the same active drug, then the MRT_{IV} in the body should be similar in a given patient. The difference in the observed MRT_{oral} for the different oral products results from the difference in the MAT. Longer MRT_{oral} indicates slower absorption. The MRT is calculated after oral administration from the plasma concentration-time data after calculating the AUC and AUMC as described.

This approach allows comparison of the rate of absorption of different drug products without the need to assume a specific compartmental model or knowledge of the order of drug absorption. If the objective of the study is to compare the rate of absorption of two different oral products for the same active drug, the MRT is calculated for the two products, and the difference will be the difference in the MAT for the two products. However, if the objective of the study is to calculate the MAT, in this case the drug has to be administered by IV and by oral administration on two different occasions, and the MAT is calculated from the difference in the MRT_{oral} and MRT_{IV} as in Equation 14.11.

Example

In an experiment to investigate drug absorption from two different oral products of the same active drug, a normal volunteer received a single IV bolus dose of 100 mg, a single oral 100-mg dose of formulation A, and a single oral 100-mg dose of formulation B on three different occasions. The following data were obtained:

Formulation	**AUC (μg-hr/L)**	**AUMC (μg-hr²/L)**
IV bolus (100 mg)	352	1232
Formulation A (100 mg)	264	1056
Formulation B (100 mg)	299	1495

How would you interpret these data?

Answer

The available information can be used to compare the rate and the extent of drug absorption from the two oral formulations. For the rate of absorption,

$$\text{MRT}_{\text{IV}} = \frac{\text{AUMC}_{\text{IV}}}{\text{AUC}_{\text{IV}}} = \frac{1232\ \mu\text{g-hr}^2/\text{L}}{352\ \mu\text{g-hr/L}} = 3.5\ \text{hr}$$

$$\text{MRT}_{\text{Formulation A}} = \frac{\text{AUMC}_{\text{Formulation A}}}{\text{AUC}_{\text{Formulation A}}} = \frac{1056\ \mu\text{g-hr}^2/\text{L}}{264\ \mu\text{g-hr/L}} = 4.0\ \text{hr}$$

$$\text{MRT}_{\text{Formulation B}} = \frac{\text{AUMC}_{\text{Formulation B}}}{\text{AUC}_{\text{Formulation B}}} = \frac{1495\ \mu\text{g-hr}^2/\text{L}}{299\ \mu\text{g-hr/L}} = 5.0\ \text{hr}$$

The MAT can be calculated for the two oral formulations to compare their rate of absorption:

$$\text{MAT}_{\text{Formulation A}} = \text{MRT}_{\text{Formulation A}} - \text{MRT}_{\text{IV}} = 4.0\ \text{hr} - 3.5\ \text{hr} = 0.5\ \text{hr}$$

$$\text{MAT}_{\text{Formulation B}} = \text{MRT}_{\text{Formulation B}} - \text{MRT}_{\text{IV}} = 5.0\ \text{hr} - 3.5\ \text{hr} = 1.5\ \text{hr}$$

This means that formulation A is absorbed faster than formulation B.

For the extent of absorption (bioavailability),

$$\text{F}_{\text{Formulation A}} = \frac{\text{AUC}_{\text{Formulation A}}}{\text{AUC}_{\text{IV}}} = \frac{264\ \mu\text{g-hr/L}}{352\ \mu\text{g-hr/L}} = 0.75$$

$$\text{F}_{\text{Formulation B}} = \frac{\text{AUC}_{\text{Formulation B}}}{\text{AUC}_{\text{IV}}} = \frac{299\ \mu\text{g-hr/L}}{352\ \mu\text{g-hr/L}} = 0.85$$

The absolute bioavailability of the drug from formulation A is 75%, and the absolute bioavailability of the drug from formulation B is 85%.

14.3.2.2 The Mean Residence Time after Constant-Rate IV Infusion

When the drug is administered by continuous constant-rate IV infusion for a duration of time equal to T, the MRT is usually longer than the MRT after IV bolus administration because the drug stays in the syringe for a period of time. So, the MRT after continuous constant-rate IV infusion can be determined as in Equation 14.12:

$$MRT_{IV\ infusion} = MRT_{IV} + \frac{T}{2} \quad (14.12)$$

where T is the IV infusion duration.

14.4 OTHER PHARMACOKINETIC PARAMETERS THAT CAN BE DETERMINED USING THE NONCOMPARTMENTAL APPROACH

The noncompartmental approach can also be used to calculate other pharmacokinetic parameters, such as the bioavailability, drug clearance, and the volume of distribution at steady state. Estimation of the bioavailability and the clearance has been discussed without stating that the methods were independent of any compartmental assumptions. The absolute bioavailability is determined from the ratio of the AUC after oral and IV administration as in Equation 14.13, and the relative bioavailability of two oral products is determined from the ratio of the AUC for the two different oral products as in Equation 14.14.

$$F_{Absolute} = \frac{AUC_{oral}}{AUC_{IV}} \quad (14.13)$$

$$F_{Relative} = \frac{AUC_{Product\ A}}{AUC_{Product\ B}} \quad (14.14)$$

The drug clearance can be determined after IV administration from the dose and the AUC as in Equation 14.15 and after oral administration as in Equation 14.16:

$$CL_T = \frac{Dose_{IV}}{AUC_{IV}} \quad (14.15)$$

$$\frac{CL_T}{F} = \frac{Dose_{oral}}{AUC_{oral}} \quad (14.16)$$

The volume of distribution at steady state or the Vd_{ss} represents the proportionality constant that relates the amount of the drug in the body at steady state during continuous IV infusion and the resulting steady-state drug blood concentration. Also, the Vd_{ss} relates the average amount of the drug in the body at steady state during multiple drug administrations and the resulting average steady-state drug blood concentration. At steady state, the drug is in a state of equilibrium in all parts of the body regardless of the number of compartments. Estimation of Vd_{ss} does not require drug administration to reach steady state because, according to the statistical moment theory, Vd_{ss} is the product of the clearance and MRT. So, after a single IV bolus administration, Vd_{ss} can be estimated as follows:

$$Vd_{ss} = CL_T \times MRT \tag{14.17}$$

$$Vd_{ss} = \frac{Dose_{IV}}{AUC} \times \frac{AUMC}{AUC} = \frac{Dose_{IV}\ AUMC}{AUC^2} \tag{14.18}$$

The volume of distribution at steady state can also be determined similarly after continuous constant-rate IV infusion as follows:

$$Vd_{ss} = CL_T \times MRT_{infusion} = CL_T\left(MRT - \frac{T}{2}\right) \tag{14.19}$$

which can be rearranged to

$$Vd_{ss} = \frac{\text{Infused dose} \times AUMC}{(AUC)^2} - \frac{\text{Infused dose} \times T}{2\ AUC} \tag{14.20}$$

where T is the duration of the IV infusion, and the infused dose is the total amount of drug administered during the IV infusion and can be calculated from the product of the infusion rate and the infusion duration. The volume of distribution at steady state after oral drug administration cannot be determined this way unless we make some assumptions regarding the bioavailability and the mean absorption time.

14.5 DETERMINATION OF MEAN RESIDENCE TIME FOR COMPARTMENTAL MODELS

The previous discussion dealt with the determination of the MRT using a noncompartmental approach. However, when the pharmacokinetic model is known, it is possible to use the equations that describe the models to calculate the MRT. The following is the MRT for selected compartmental models:

- A single IV bolus dose when the drug follows a one-compartment pharmacokinetic model:

$$MRT_{IV} = \frac{1}{k} \tag{14.21}$$

where k is the first-order elimination rate constant.

- A single oral dose when the drug follows a one-compartment pharmacokinetic model:

$$MRT_{oral} = \frac{1}{k} + \frac{1}{k_a} \tag{14.22}$$

and

$$MAT = \frac{1}{k_a} \tag{14.23}$$

where k is the first-order elimination rate constant, and k_a is the first-order absorption rate constant.

- Drug administration by constant-rate IV infusion when the drug follows a one-compartment pharmacokinetic model:

$$MRT_{infusion} = \frac{1}{k} + \frac{T}{2} \tag{14.24}$$

where k is the first-order elimination rate constant, and T is the duration of the IV infusion.

PRACTICE PROBLEMS

14.1. After administration of a single 1-mg intravenous bolus dose, the following plasma concentrations were obtained:

Time (hr)	Concentration (μg/L)
0	50
1	39
3	24
6	12
9	6.8
12	4.1
18	1.8
24	0.94

a. Calculate the MRT, clearance, and Vd_{ss} for this drug if the terminal rate for decline of the plasma dug concentration is 0.1 hr^{-1}.

14.2. In a study to compare the absorption characteristics of three different oral formulations for the same active drug, a group of volunteers received a single 25-mg dose as IV solution and the three oral formulations on four different occasions. The following data were obtained:

Formulation	AUC (μg-hr/L)	AUMC (μg-hr²/L)
IV solution	6250	40625
Formulation A	3750	31875
Formulation B	2500	17500
Formulation C	4375	39375

a. Arrange formulations A, B, and C according to the extent of drug absorption.
b. Arrange formulations A, B, and C according to the rate of drug absorption.

14.3. A volunteer received a single 20-mg dose of IV solution, capsule, and tablet for the same active drug on three different occasions. The following plasma concentrations were obtained:

Time (hr)	IV Solution Concentration (μg/L)	Oral Capsule Concentration (μg/L)	Oral Tablet Concentration (μg/L)
0	400	0	0
0.5	371	32	56
1	344	58	97
2	296	92	149
3	255	111	172
4	220	119	178
6	162	116	162
8	120	101	133
10	89	83	105
12	66	66	80
18	27	30	34
24	11	13	14

a. Calculate the MRT for this drug after IV administration.
b. Calculate the MRT after the two oral formulations.
c. Calculate the MAT for the two oral formulations.
d. Calculate the clearance and the Vd_{ss} for this drug.

15 Physiological Approach to Hepatic Clearance

OBJECTIVES

After completing this chapter, you should be able to:

- Describe the physiological meaning of the total body clearance in terms of organ blood flow, intrinsic clearance, and extraction ratio
- Describe the effect of changing the hepatic intrinsic clearance and blood flow on the efficiency of the liver to eliminate the drug (extraction ratio)
- Analyze the effect of changing the intrinsic clearance on the plasma concentration–time profile after intravenous (IV) and oral administration
- Analyze the effect of changing the liver blood flow on the plasma concentration–time profile after IV and oral administration

15.1 INTRODUCTION

The physiological approach to organ clearance is a simple approach that uses the organ's ability for drug elimination, organ blood flow, and protein binding to describe the rate of organ drug elimination and the drug profile in the body. This approach allows prediction of the change in drug disposition that occurs because of changes in organ blood flow, enzymatic activity, and drug protein binding. For example, the hepatic clearance of a drug is dependent on the liver's intrinsic ability to metabolize the drug and the rate of delivery of the drug to the liver (which is determined by liver blood flow). Enzyme induction and enzyme inhibition can alter the liver's ability to metabolize the drug and can lead to changes in hepatic clearance. Also, diseases such as congestive heart failure and drugs such as β-blockers can decrease the cardiac output and decrease the liver blood flow, which may change the hepatic clearance of the drug.

15.2 ORGAN CLEARANCE

Organ clearance is defined as the volume of the blood that is completely cleared from the drug per unit time by that particular organ. This is a measure of the efficiency of the organ in eliminating the drug from the blood reaching the organ. Based on this definition, the clearance can be estimated from the organ blood flow and the difference in the arterial and venous drug concentration across the organ.

$$CL_{organ} = \frac{\text{The rate of drug entering the organ} - \text{The rate of drug leaving the organ}}{\text{Concentration of drug entering the organ}}$$

The rate of drug entering the organ is equal to the product of drug concentration in the arterial side and the organ blood flow; the rate of drug leaving the organ is equal to the product of drug concentration in the venous side and the organ blood flow. The difference in the rate of drug entering the organ and the rate of drug leaving the organ is the rate of drug elimination by the organ. Based on this definition, the hepatic clearance CL_H can be expressed as

$$CL_H = \frac{Q\,Cp_a - Q\,Cp_v}{Cp_a} \tag{15.1}$$

where Q is the liver blood flow, Cp_a is the drug concentration in the arterial side of the liver (portal and arterial), and Cp_v is the drug concentration in the venous side of the liver.

$$CL_H = Q\left[\frac{Cp_a - Cp_v}{Cp_a}\right] \tag{15.2}$$

$$CL_H = Q\,E \tag{15.3}$$

where E is the extraction ratio.

15.3 HEPATIC EXTRACTION RATIO

The hepatic extraction ratio is the fraction of the drug amount presented to the liver that is eliminated during a single pass through the liver. When all drug presented to the liver is eliminated (i.e., the drug concentration in the blood leaving the liver Cp_v is equal to zero), then the hepatic extraction ratio becomes equal to unity. On the other hand, when no drug is eliminated in the liver (i.e., the drug concentration in the blood entering the liver is equal to the drug concentration in the blood leaving the liver, $Cp_v = Cp_a$), then the extraction ratio is equal to zero.

The extraction ratio can take values from 0 to 1, which can also be expressed as percentages from 0 to 100%. Drugs are classified as low extraction ratio drugs if their hepatic extraction ratio is less than 0.3 (e.g., diazepam, warfarin, salicylic acid, phenytoin, and procainamide) or as high extraction ratio drugs if their hepatic extraction ratio is larger than 0.7 (e.g., lidocaine, propranolol, morphine, verapamil, and propoxyphen). Drugs with a hepatic extraction ratio between 0.3 and 0.7 are classified as intermediate extraction ratio drugs. Drugs with similar hepatic extraction ratios usually share some common characteristics of how the change in the physiological parameters affects the overall elimination of the drug.

It is important to note that the hepatic extraction ratio is a measure of the elimination efficiency during a single pass of the drug through the liver. This is different from the fraction of the administered dose, which is metabolized. There are examples of drugs that are completely metabolized but have a low hepatic extraction ratio and drugs that have a high hepatic extraction ratio and are not completely metabolized.

The hepatic extraction ratio is a function of the intrinsic ability of the liver to eliminate the drug CL_{int} and the hepatic blood flow:

$$E = \frac{CL_{int}}{Q + CL_{int}} \tag{15.4}$$

15.4 INTRINSIC CLEARANCE (CL_{int})

The *intrinsic clearance* is the maximum ability of the organ to eliminate the drug in the absence of any flow limitation. The hepatic intrinsic clearance reflects the inherent ability of the hepatic enzyme systems to eliminate drugs. So, the intrinsic clearance is the maximum capacity of the liver to eliminate the drug; the hepatic clearance is the actual observed clearance of the drug. The hepatic clearance is determined by the liver blood flow and the intrinsic clearance of the liver.

$$CL_H = Q\,E = Q\left[\frac{CL_{int}}{Q + CL_{int}}\right] \tag{15.5}$$

By rearrangement, an empirical definition of this parameter can be obtained:

$$CL_{int} = \frac{Q\,E}{1 - E} \tag{15.6}$$

This relationship indicates that the intrinsic clearance for high extraction ratio drugs is much higher than the hepatic clearance, and for low extraction ratio drugs the value of the intrinsic clearance is close to that of the hepatic clearance.

15.5 SYSTEMIC BIOAVAILABILITY

When the orally administered drug is absorbed completely to the portal circulation, the only cause for incomplete bioavailability is hepatic metabolism during the first pass through the liver. In this case, the drug bioavailability is dependent on the hepatic extraction ratio.

$$F = 1 - E \tag{15.7}$$

This means that the bioavailability of drugs with a high hepatic extraction ratio is much less than the bioavailability of drugs with a low hepatic extraction ratio when the drugs are absorbed completely to the portal circulation. Factors that can alter the hepatic extraction ratio, such as the change in hepatic blood flow or intrinsic clearance, can affect the bioavailability of orally administered drugs. It is important to note that if the drug is not absorbed completely from the gastrointestinal tract to the portal circulation, Equation 15.7 cannot be applied, and the bioavailability will be determined from the fraction of dose absorbed and the fraction of dose that escapes hepatic metabolism.

15.6 EFFECT OF CHANGE IN INTRINSIC CLEARANCE AND HEPATIC BLOOD FLOW ON HEPATIC CLEARANCE, SYSTEMIC AVAILABILITY, AND DRUG CONCENTRATION–TIME PROFILE

The hepatic clearance of any drug is dependent on the drug intrinsic clearance and hepatic blood flow as presented in Equation 15.5. For a drug with small CL_{int} compared to the hepatic blood flow (i.e., $Q >> CL_{int}$), Equation 15.5 can be reduced to

$$CL_H = Q \frac{CL_{int}}{Q} = CL_{int} \tag{15.8}$$

Equation 15.8 indicates that the hepatic clearance for drugs with low intrinsic clearance relative to the hepatic blood flow (low extraction ratio drugs) is dependent on the drug intrinsic clearance, and any change in enzyme activity by induction or inhibition will affect the hepatic clearance and the rate of drug elimination. Changes in the hepatic blood flow will not have a significant effect on the hepatic clearance and the rate of elimination of low extraction ratio drugs.

On the other hand, when CL_{int} is large compared to the hepatic blood flow (i.e., $CL_{int} >> Q$), then Equation 15.5 will be reduced to

$$CL_H = Q \tag{15.9}$$

Equation 15.9 indicates that the hepatic clearance for the drugs with high intrinsic clearance relative to the hepatic blood flow (high extraction ratio drugs) is about equal to the hepatic blood flow, and any change in the hepatic blood flow will affect the hepatic clearance and the rate of drug elimination. Changes in the drug intrinsic clearance will not have a significant effect on the hepatic clearance and the rate of elimination of high extraction ratio drugs.

15.6.1 Low Extraction Ratio Drugs

Assume that we have a low extraction ratio drug that is completely metabolized, indicating that the hepatic clearance is equal to the total body clearance. After oral administration, the drug is completely absorbed to the portal circulation, which means that the hepatic metabolism during the first pass through the liver is the cause of its incomplete bioavailability. The drug extraction ratio E is equal to 0.05, and the hepatic blood flow Q is 1.5 L/min. The intrinsic clearance of this drug can be calculated from Equation 15.6.

$$CL_{int} = \frac{Q\,E}{1-E} = \frac{1.5\text{ L/min } 0.05}{1-0.05} = 0.079\text{ L/min}$$

The hepatic clearance can be calculated from Equation 15.3.

$$CL_H = Q\,E = 1.5\ \text{L/min} \times 0.05 = 0.075\ \text{L/min}$$

The bioavailability of the drug can be calculated from Equation 15.7.

$$F = 1 - E = 1 - 0.05 = 0.95$$

- If the drug's intrinsic clearance increases to double its original value because of enzyme induction and the hepatic blood flow stays the same, then the new intrinsic clearance after induction will be

$$CL_{int} = 0.079\ \text{L/min} \times 2 = 0.158\ \text{L/min}$$

For the extraction ratio after induction,

$$E = \frac{CL_{int}}{Q + CL_{int}} = \frac{0.158\ \text{L/min}}{1.5\ \text{L/min} + 0.158\ \text{L/min}} = 0.095$$

For the hepatic clearance after induction,

$$CL_H = Q\,E = 1.5\ \text{L/min} \times 0.095 = 0.143\ \text{L/min}$$

For the bioavailability after induction,

$$F = 1 - E = 1 - 0.095 = 0.905$$

Based on these calculations, enzyme induction resulted in the increase in the extraction ratio from 0.05 to 0.095 (about 90%), which resulted in a significant increase in the hepatic clearance from 0.075 to 0.143 L/min (about 90%) and a small decrease in bioavailability from 0.95 to 0.905 (about 5%). So, enzyme induction significantly increased the clearance of low extraction ratio drugs after IV and oral administration without significantly affecting the drug bioavailability, as illustrated in Figures 15.1A and 15.1B.

- If the hepatic blood flow decreases by 50% (new $Q = 0.75$ L/min) without affecting the intrinsic clearance, then the new extraction ratio after the reduction in the hepatic blood flow will be

$$E = \frac{CL_{int}}{Q + CL_{int}} = \frac{0.079\ \text{L/min}}{0.75\ \text{L/min} + 0.079\ \text{L/min}} = 0.095$$

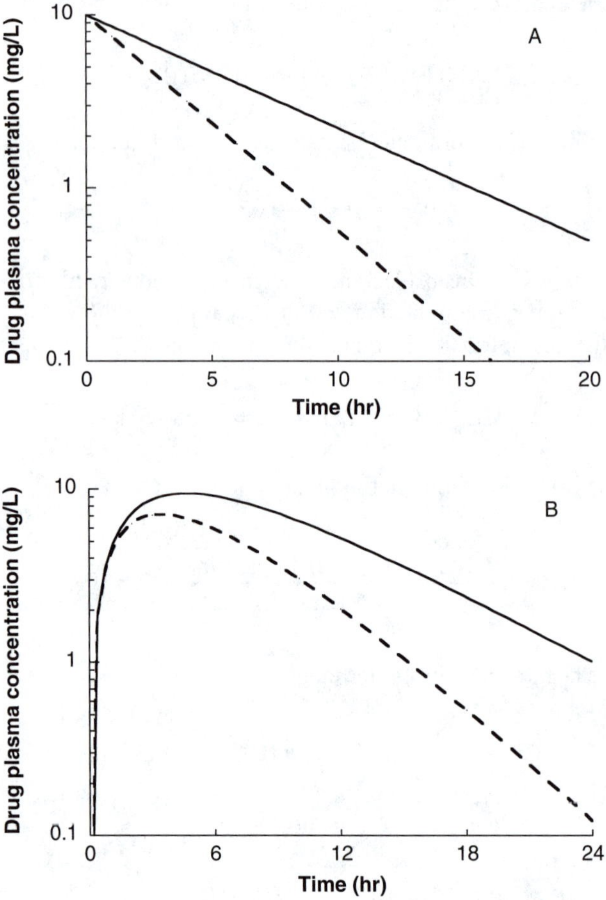

FIGURE 15.1 The plasma concentration–time profile for a low extraction ratio drug after administration of (A) a single IV bolus dose and (B) a single oral dose before (——) and after (------) enzyme induction.

Pharmacokinetic Parameters	Before Induction	After Induction
Q	1.5 L/min	1.5 L/min
E	0.05	0.095
CL_{int}	0.079 L/min	0.158 L/min
CL_H	0.075 L/min	0.143 L/min
F	0.95	0.905

For the hepatic clearance after the decrease in hepatic blood flow,

$$CL_H = Q\,E = 0.75\ \text{L/min} \times 0.095 = 0.0712\ \text{L/min}$$

For the bioavailability after the decrease in hepatic blood flow,

$$F = 1 - E = 1 - 0.095 = 0.905$$

Based on these calculations, the decrease in hepatic blood flow resulted in an increase in the extraction ratio from 0.05 to 0.095 (about 90%), a small decrease in the hepatic clearance from 0.075 to 0.0712 L/min (about 5%), and a small decrease in bioavailability from 0.95 to 0.905 (about 5%). So, the change in hepatic blood flow does not significantly affect the clearance and bioavailability of low extraction ratio drugs, which should not affect the plasma concentration–time profile of the drug after IV and oral administration, as illustrated in Figures 15.2A and 15.2B.

15.6.2 High Extraction Ratio Drugs

Assume that we have a high extraction ratio drug that is completely metabolized, indicating that the hepatic clearance is equal to the total body clearance. After oral administration, the drug is completely absorbed to the portal circulation, which means that the hepatic metabolism during the first pass through the liver is the cause of its incomplete bioavailability. The drug extraction ratio E is equal to 0.95, and the hepatic blood flow Q is 1.5 L/min. The intrinsic clearance of this drug can be calculated from Equation 15.6.

$$CL_{int} = \frac{Q\ E}{1 - E} = \frac{1.5\ \text{L/min}\ 0.95}{1 - 0.95} = 28.5\ \text{L/min}$$

The hepatic clearance can be calculated from Equation 15.3.

$$CL_H = Q\,E = 1.5\ \text{L/min} \times 0.95 = 1.425\ \text{L/min}$$

The bioavailability of the drug can be calculated from Equation 15.7.

$$F = 1 - E = 1 - 0.95 = 0.05$$

- If the drug's intrinsic clearance increases to double its original value because of enzyme induction and the hepatic blood flow stays the same, then the new intrinsic clearance will be

$$CL_{int} = 28.5\ \text{L/min} \times 2 = 57.0\ \text{L/min}$$

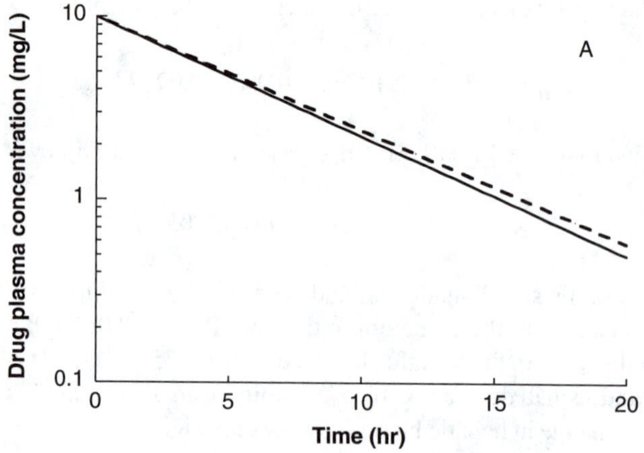

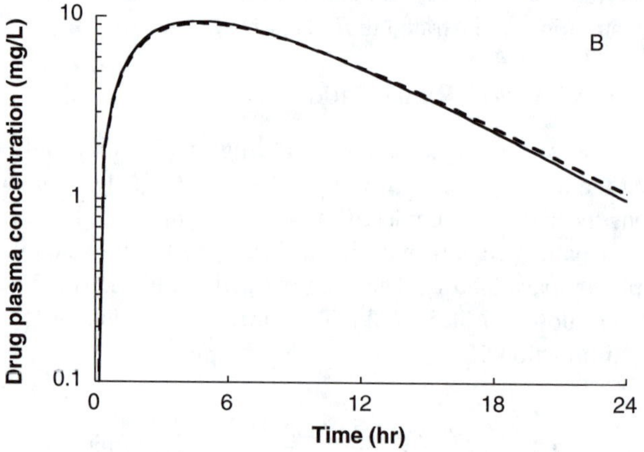

FIGURE 15.2 The plasma concentration–time profile for a low extraction ratio drug after administration of (A) a single IV bolus dose and (B) a single oral dose when the hepatic blood flow is 1.5 L/min (——) and after the reduction of the hepatic blood flow to 0.75 L/min (------).

Pharmacokinetic Parameters	Normal Hepatic Blood Flow	Low Hepatic Blood Flow
Q	1.5 L/min	0.75 L/min
E	0.05	0.095
CL_{int}	0.079 L/min	0.079 L/min
CL_H	0.075 L/min	0.0712 L/min
F	0.95	0.905

For the extraction ratio after induction,

$$E = \frac{CL_{int}}{Q + CL_{int}} = \frac{57\ \text{L/min}}{1.5\ \text{L/min} + 57\ \text{L/min}} = 0.974$$

For the hepatic clearance after induction,

$$CL_H = Q\,E = 1.5\ \text{L/min} \times 0.974 = 1.461\ \text{L/min}$$

For the bioavailability after induction,

$$F = 1 - E = 1 - 0.974 = 0.026$$

Based on these calculations, enzyme induction resulted in the increase in the extraction ratio from 0.95 to 0.974 (about 2.5%), which resulted in a small increase in the hepatic clearance from 1.425 to 1.461 L/min (about 2.5%) and a significant decrease in bioavailability from 0.05 to 0.026 (about 50%). So, enzyme induction does not significantly affect the clearance of high extraction ratio drugs, which will not affect the rate of decline of the plasma concentration–time profile after a single IV and oral drug administration. However, enzyme induction decreases the bioavailability of high extraction ratio drugs, which results in a significant decrease in the drug's AUC, as illustrated in Figures 15.3A and 15.3B.

- If the hepatic blood flow decreases by 50% (new $Q = 0.75$ L/min) without affecting the intrinsic clearance, then the extraction ratio after the reduction in the hepatic blood flow will be

$$E = \frac{CL_{int}}{Q + CL_{int}} = \frac{28.5\ \text{L/min}}{0.75\ \text{L/min} + 28.5\ \text{L/min}} = 0.974$$

For the hepatic clearance after the decrease in hepatic blood flow,

$$CL_H = Q\,E = 0.75\ \text{L/min} \times 0.974 = 0.7305\ \text{L/min}$$

For the bioavailability after the decrease in hepatic blood flow,

$$F = 1 - E = 1 - 0.974 = 0.026$$

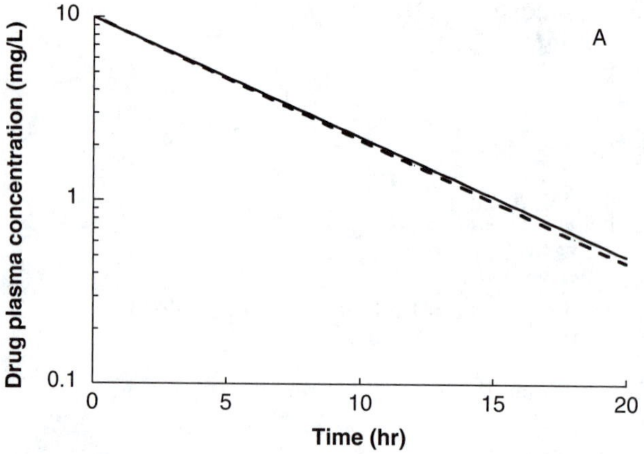

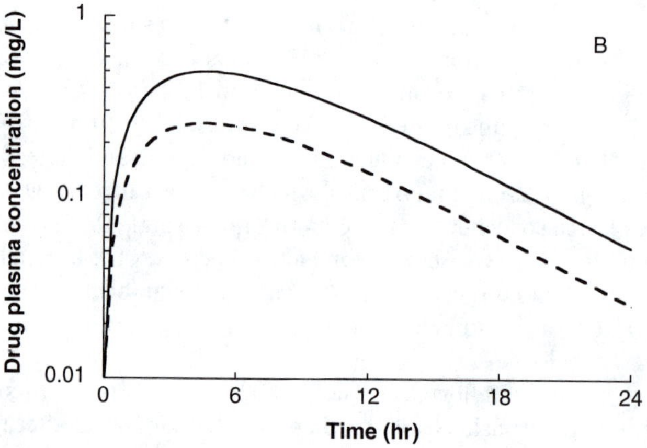

FIGURE 15.3 The plasma concentration–time profile for a high extraction ratio drug after administration of (A) a single IV bolus dose and (B) a single oral dose before (——) and after (------) enzyme induction.

Pharmacokinetic Parameters	Before Induction	After Induction
Q	1.5 L/min	1.5 L/min
E	0.95	0.974
CL_{int}	28.5 L/min	57.0 L/min
CL_H	1.425 L/min	1.461 L/min
F	0.05	0.026

> Based on these calculations, the decrease in hepatic blood flow resulted in the increase in the extraction ratio from 0.95 to 0.974 (about 2.5%), which resulted in a significant decrease in the hepatic clearance from 1.425 to 0.7305 L/min (about 50%) and a significant decrease in bioavailability from 0.05 to 0.026 (about 50%). So, the decrease in the hepatic blood flow significantly decreases the clearance of high extraction ratio drugs after IV and after oral administration, which is reflected by a slower rate of decline in the drug concentration–time profile. After oral administration, the decrease in the clearance of the high extraction ratio drugs caused by the decrease in hepatic blood flow should increase the drug's AUC. However, the decrease in the hepatic blood flow also causes a reduction in the bioavailability of the high extraction ratio drugs, which should decrease the AUC. So, the increase in the AUC caused by the reduction in drug clearance is compensated with the decrease in AUC caused by the reduction in drug bioavailability, and the drug's AUC does not change significantly, as illustrated in Figures 15.4A and 15.4B.

The effect of altered hepatic blood flow and changes in intrinsic clearance on the pharmacokinetics of drugs depends on whether the drug can be classified as a low or high extraction ratio drug. The systemic clearance of low extraction ratio drugs is affected mainly by changes in the intrinsic clearance and is not affected by changes in the hepatic blood flow; the systemic clearance of high extraction ratio drugs is affected mainly by the alteration in hepatic blood flow and is not affected by the change in intrinsic clearance. After oral administration, the bioavailability of low extraction ratio drugs is high, and changes in the extraction ratio caused by changes in intrinsic clearance or hepatic blood flow do not cause a significant change in the bioavailability. On the other hand, changes in the intrinsic clearance and the hepatic blood flow cause small changes in the extraction ratio and the bioavailability of high extraction ratio drugs after oral administration. However, because the bioavailability of high extraction ratio drugs is usually low, this small change in bioavailability causes a significant change in the bioavailable amount of the drug. For intermediate extraction ratio drugs, the systemic clearance and the half-life are partially dependent on liver blood flow to an extent that is only estimated by knowing the extraction ratio.

Example

An experimental antiarrhythmic drug (MAH96) is completely metabolized by the liver to inactive metabolites. In clinical trials, this drug was found to have a hepatic extraction ratio of 0.89 in a congestive heart failure patient who has hepatic blood flow of 1.22 L/min. This drug is 96% bound to plasma protein. Although the oral bioavailability of this drug is less than 100%, when it is administered orally the dose is absorbed completely from the gastrointestinal tract and reaches the portal circulation.

1. Calculate the total body clearance of this drug in this patient.
2. Calculate the intrinsic clearance of this drug in this patient.
3. What is the area under the plasma concentration–time curve produced after administration of a single 300-mg oral dose?

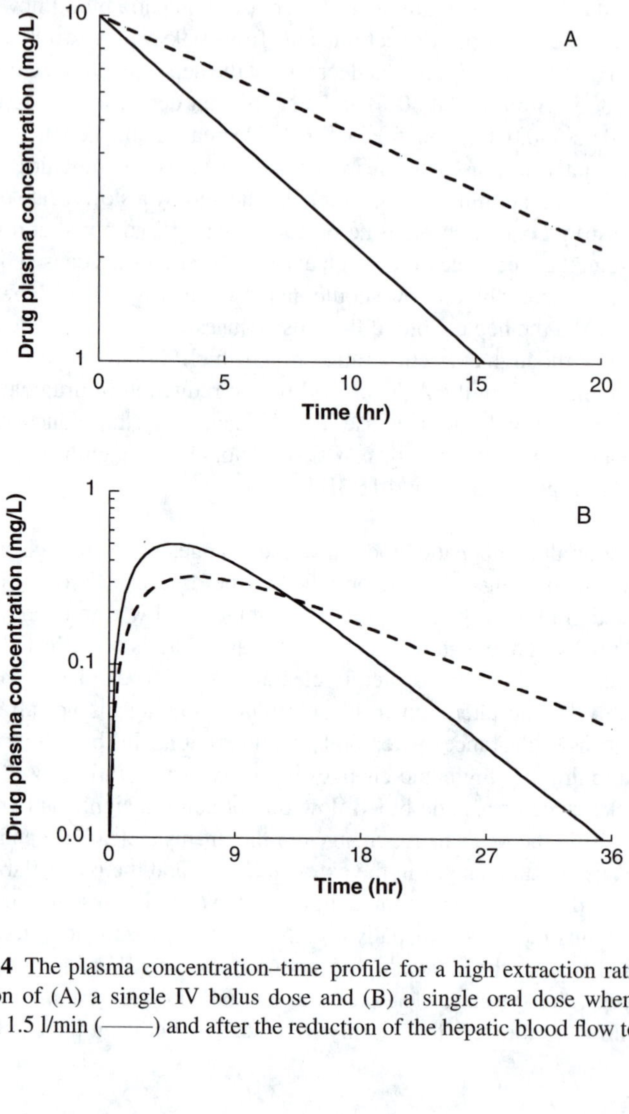

FIGURE 15.4 The plasma concentration–time profile for a high extraction ratio drug after administration of (A) a single IV bolus dose and (B) a single oral dose when the hepatic blood flow is 1.5 l/min (——) and after the reduction of the hepatic blood flow to 0.75 L/min (------).

Pharmacokinetic Parameters	Normal Hepatic Blood Flow	Low Hepatic Blood Flow
Q	1.5 L/min	0.75 L/min
E	0.95	0.974
CL_{int}	28.5 L/min	28.5 L/min
CL_H	1.425 L/min	0.7305 L/min
F	0.05	0.026

4. In addition to the antiarrhythmic drug, the patient started taking an inotropic drug, which increases the cardiac output with no effect on any other organs. Because of this increase in cardiac output, the liver blood flow increased to 1.62 L/min. How does the increase in the hepatic blood flow affect the value of each of the following parameters?

Hepatic intrinsic clearance	Increase	Decrease	No change
Hepatic extraction ratio	Increase	Decrease	No change
Total body clearance	Increase	Decrease	No change
Oral bioavailability	Increase	Decrease	No change

Answer

1. Because the drug is completely metabolized, CL_H is equal to CL_T:

$$CL_T = CL_H = Q\,E = 1.22\ \text{L/min} \times 0.89 = 1.086\ \text{L/min}$$

2.

$$CL_{int} = \frac{Q\,E}{1-E} = \frac{1.22\ \text{L/min} \times 0.89}{1-0.89} = 9.87\ \text{L/min}$$

3.

$$AUC = \frac{F\ \text{Dose}}{CL_T} = \frac{(1-E)\ \text{Dose}}{CL_T} = \frac{0.11 \times 300\ \text{mg}}{1.086\ \text{L/min}} = 30.4\ \text{mg-min/L}$$

4. Hepatic intrinsic clearance is dependent on the intrinsic ability of the liver to metabolize the drug and is independent of the hepatic blood flow. So, the hepatic intrinsic clearance will not change because of the increase in hepatic blood flow. For the hepatic extraction ratio,

$$E = \frac{CL_{int}}{Q + CL_{int}} = \frac{9.87\ \text{L/min}}{1.62\ \text{L/min} + 9.87\ \text{L/min}} = 0.859$$

The increase in hepatic blood flow decreases the extraction ratio.
For the total body clearance,

$$CL_T = CL_H = Q\,E = 1.62\ \text{L/min} \times 0.859 = 1.392\ \text{L/min}$$

The total body clearance, which is equal to the hepatic clearance for this drug, increases with the increase in the hepatic blood flow.

For the oral bioavailability,

$$\text{Bioavailability (F)} = 1 - E = 1 - 0.859 = 0.141$$

The oral bioavailability increases because the hepatic extraction ratio decreases in response to the increase in hepatic blood flow.

15.7 PROTEIN BINDING AND HEPATIC EXTRACTION

The preceding discussion has been concerned with the total drug concentration in the blood. However, it is known that almost all drugs are bound to blood constituents to some extent. So, it is important to consider the effect of protein binding on drug clearance and half-life. It is usually assumed that only the free (unbound) drug is available for elimination. However, many examples exist in which the hepatic extraction is sufficiently high that the drug can be stripped from its binding sites during passage through the liver. Two different extraction processes are usually observed, one restricted or limited to the free drug and one that is nonrestricted in which both free and bound drug can be removed by the liver. When the protein binding is taken into account, the following relationship can be obtained:

$$CL_H = Q\,E = Q\left[\frac{f_u\,CL'_{int}}{Q + f_u\,CL'_{int}}\right] \tag{15.10}$$

where f_u is the free unbound fraction of the drug in the blood, and CL'_{int} is the intrinsic clearance of the unbound free drug.

The effect of protein binding on the hepatic clearance of drugs is different depending on the drug characteristics. The clearance of high extraction ratio drugs is considered to be flow dependent, so changes in the protein binding of these drugs do not affect their hepatic clearance. This is because during drug passage through the liver, both free and bound drug molecules are extracted by the liver for elimination.

The hepatic clearance of drugs that have low extraction ratios and are not bound to a large extent (<75% protein bound) does not change significantly by the change in their protein binding. On the other hand, the hepatic clearance of drugs that have low extraction ratios and are highly bound to plasma protein is very sensitive to even a small change in protein binding. This is because a small displacement in the protein binding of these drugs will cause a large increase in the free drug concentration and will increase the liver's ability to eliminate the drug (because of the increase in f_u).

PRACTICE PROBLEMS

15.1. Why does a drug with a high extraction ratio (e.g., propranolol) demonstrate a greater difference between individuals after oral administration than after IV administration?

15.2. Why does a drug with a low hepatic extraction ratio (e.g., theophylline) demonstrate greater differences between individuals after hepatic enzyme induction than a drug with a high extraction ratio?

15.3. A drug has an intrinsic clearance of 40 ml/min in a normal adult patient whose hepatic blood flow is 1.5 L/min.

a. Calculate the hepatic clearance of this drug
b. If the patient develops congestive heart failure that reduces hepatic blood flow to 1.0 L/min without affecting the intrinsic clearance, then calculate the hepatic clearance of the drug in this patient.
c. If the patient was receiving medication such as phenobarbital that increased the intrinsic clearance to 90 ml/min but did not alter the hepatic blood flow (1.5 L/min), then calculate the hepatic clearance of the drug in this patient.

15.4. A drug has an intrinsic clearance of 12 L/min in a normal adult patient whose hepatic blood flow is 1.5 L/min.

a. Calculate the hepatic clearance of this drug.
b. If this patient develops congestive heart failure that reduces his hepatic blood flow to 1.0 L/min without affecting the intrinsic clearance, then calculate the hepatic clearance of the drug in this patient.
c. Calculate the extraction ratio for the liver in this patient before and after congestive heart failure develops.
d. From the information in this problem, estimate the drug bioavailability assuming that when the drug is given orally all the drug is absorbed to the portal vein.

15.5. Use the pharmacokinetic properties for the hypothetical group of drugs (A–H) listed in Table 15.1 to determine the expected changes in the total body clearance, the biological half-life, and the systemic bioavailability for each of the drugs in the following conditions:

a. Administration of an enzyme inducer that increases the activity of the metabolizing enzymes
b. Administration of an enzyme inhibitor that decreases the activity of the metabolizing enzymes
c. Administration of a highly protein bound drug that can displace the above drugs from their binding protein and increases their free fraction
d. Decrease in the hepatic blood flow because of congestive heart failure

TABLE 15.1
Pharmacokinetic Properties for a Group of Hypothetical Drugs (A–H)

Drug	A	B	C	D	E	F	G	H
Percentage of the dose metabolized (%)	98	10	94	50	10	90	50	95
Protein binding (%)	94	60	94	93	96	60	60	50
Extraction ratio	0.1	0.1	0.92	0.11	0.1	0.1	0.11	0.93

16 Pharmacokinetic–Pharmacodynamic Relationship

OBJECTIVES

After completing this chapter, you should be able to:

- Describe the different pharmacodynamic models that can relate the drug concentration at the site of action and the direct pharmacological effect
- Describe how the pharmacokinetic models can be linked to the pharmacodynamic models to predict the time course of the drug pharmacological effect
- Utilize the pharmacokinetic/pharmacodynamic principles to determine the duration of drug effect when the drug effect is dependent on the plasma drug concentration

16.1 INTRODUCTION

The main goal of clinical pharmacokinetics is the quantitative prediction of drug effect on humans. *Pharmacokinetics* is the study of the kinetics of drug absorption, distribution, and elimination. It defines the relationship between the dose and the time course of drug concentration in the body. However, *pharmacodynamics* is used to describe the drug effect once the drug has reached its site of action. This term is used to describe the relationship between drug concentration at the site of action, which is usually related to the drug concentration in the blood, and drug effects. This can be summarized as follows: pharmacokinetics is what the body does to the drug, and pharmacodynamics is what the drug does to the body. The relationship between pharmacokinetics and pharmacodynamics is illustrated in Figure 16.1.

The term *model* has been used in pharmacokinetics and pharmacodynamics to describe the observed drug concentration or effects. Several models have been developed in pharmacokinetics, such as the one-compartment model and the multi-compartment model. Also, physiological models have been used to describe the drug pharmacokinetic behavior. In this chapter, we discuss the different pharmacodynamic models and how these models can be related to the pharmacokinetic characteristics of the drug.

The pharmacodynamic models describe the relationship between drug concentration at the site of action and the observed drug effect. In these models, we assume that we know the drug concentration at the site of effect. In almost all cases, it is

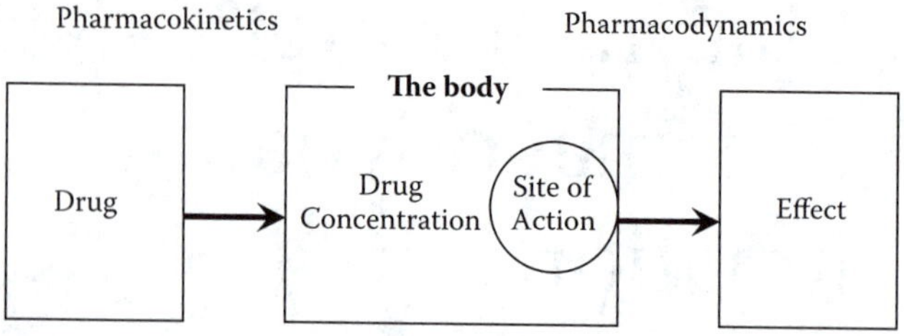

FIGURE 16.1 Schematic presentation of the relationship between pharmacokinetics and pharmacodynamics.

not possible to measure drug concentrations at the site of action. However, these concentrations can be estimated from the pharmacokinetic model. So, the pharmacokinetic parameters of the pharmacokinetic model are estimated from the drug concentration–time data. Then, these parameters are used in conjunction with the drug effect–time data to predict the appropriate pharmacodynamic model and to estimate the parameters of this model. If the pharmacokinetic model and the pharmacodynamic model are known, then the plasma concentration-time data and the drug effect–time data can be used simultaneously to estimate the pharmacokinetic and the pharmacodynamic parameters of the models.

16.2 PHARMACODYNAMIC MODELS

The time course of the drug effect, including the onset, intensity, and duration of effect, is dependent on the drug concentration–time profile at the site of action when there is a direct relationship between the drug concentration and the resulting drug effect. In general, the onset of the drug effect is observed once the drug reaches the site of action in adequate concentration, and the higher the drug concentration at the site of action, the higher the intensity of the drug effect will be. Also, the duration of effect is determined from the length of time the drug concentration is maintained above a certain concentration at the site of action.

For some drugs, there is no direct relationship between the drug concentration at the site of action and the observed drug effect. The drug may initiate or block a series of biological steps, which can lead to the appearance of the drug's pharmacological effect. So, the pharmacological effect may be observed after the drug is completely eliminated from the body. Examples of drugs that have this indirect pharmacological effect include anticancer drugs and oral anticoagulants. Indirect pharmacodynamic models have been developed to describe the drug concentration–effect relationship for these drugs. However, in this chapter only the pharmacodynamic models that describe the drug concentration–effect relationship for drugs that have a direct relationship between the drug concentration and the effect are discussed.

The pharmacodynamic models describe the relationship between the drug concentration at the site of action and the drug effect. When rapid equilibrium exists between the drug concentration in the blood and the drug concentration at the site of action, the drug concentration in the blood can be used in the modeling process.

The pharmacodynamic model that describes the drug concentration–effect relationship for a certain drug is determined experimentally by measuring the drug effect resulting from different drug concentrations. Characterization of the drug concentration–effect relationship will be better when the drug effect is measured over a wide range of concentrations. Then, the concentration-effect data are fitted to the different equations for the different pharmacodynamic models to determine which model can describe the concentration–effect relationship. The following are the different general models that can describe the relationship between the drug concentration at the effect site and the observed drug effect: fixed effect, linear, log-linear, E_{max}, and sigmoid E_{max}.

16.2.1 Fixed-Effect Model

The fixed-effect model is the simplest pharmacodynamic model that relates the drug concentration to a fixed effect that is either present or not, for example, as for cure or no cure, asleep or awake. Also, it may refer drug concentration to a certain degree of effect, such as for a 20% decease in blood glucose or 10% decrease in diastolic blood pressure. In this model, there is only one parameter, which is the drug concentration at which the effect appears.

16.2.2 Linear Model

The linear model assumes a linear relationship between the drug concentration at the site of action and the observed effect over a certain range of drug concentrations.

$$E = S\,C \tag{16.1}$$

where E is the intensity of effect, C is the drug concentration at the site of action, and S is the slope parameter that determines the rate of change of the intensity of effect with the change in drug concentration. The slope of this linear relationship reflects the potency of the drug.

The linear model expressed by Equation 16.1 and presented in Figure 16.2 assumes that the drug does not have an effect in the absence of the drug (Drug concentration = 0). If the measured effect has some value in the absence of the drug (e.g., blood pressure), then the model can be expressed as

$$E = E_0 + S\,C \tag{16.2}$$

where E_0 is the effect in the absence of the drug or the baseline effect. In this case, the concentration–effect relationship can be presented as in Figure 16.3. An example of this model is the measurement of blood pressure as a function of drug concentration of antihypertensive drugs.

If a linear relationship exists between the drug concentration and the observed effect, then linear regression can be performed to estimate the model parameters: the slope S and baseline effect E_0. This linear relationship between the effect and the drug concentration may exist only over a certain range of drug concentrations,

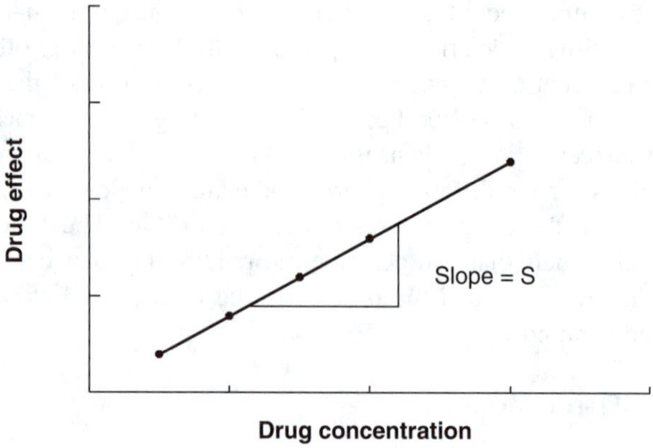

FIGURE 16.2 The drug concentration–effect relationship for a drug that follows the linear pharmacodynamic model.

and this linear relationship does not hold outside this range. In this case, it has to be specified that the model should be used only over this range of concentrations, and extrapolation outside this range is not appropriate.

16.2.3 Log-Linear Model

The log-linear model assumes a linear relationship between the effect and the logarithm of the drug concentration at the site of action over a certain range of drug concentrations.

$$E = S \text{ Log } C + I \tag{16.3}$$

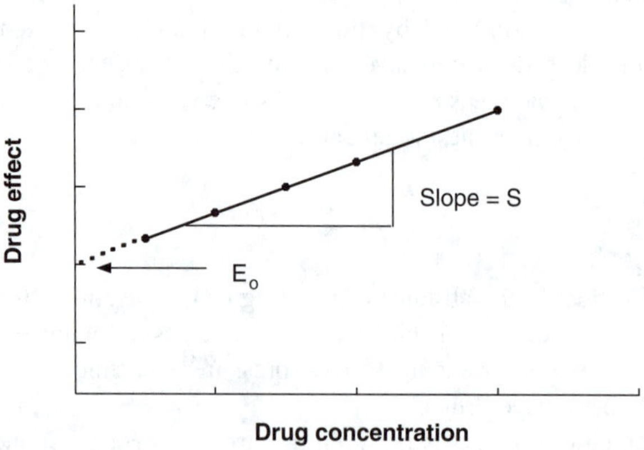

FIGURE 16.3 The drug concentration–effect relationship for a drug that follows the linear pharmacodynamic model in the presence of a baseline effect.

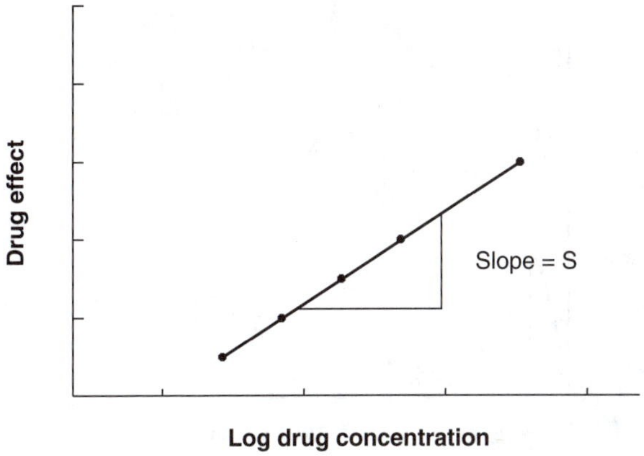

FIGURE 16.4 The drug concentration–effect relationship for a drug that follows the log-linear pharmacodynamic model.

where E is the drug effect, S is the slope of the line, C is the drug concentration at the effect site, and I is a constant. The slope of the line also reflects the potency of the drug as in the linear pharmacodynamic model. It is important to remember that the log-linear relationship between the drug concentration and effect exists over a certain range of drug concentrations as presented in Figure 16.4. This relationship may not hold outside this range of concentrations, and extrapolation outside this range is not appropriate.

This model has some disadvantages. It does not allow the prediction of the effect in the absence of the drug (Drug concentration = 0) and the inability to predict the maximum effect. The log-linear model has been applied extensively to the description of in vitro pharmacodynamic studies. The estimation of the slopes of this log-linear relationship can be used to compare the relative potencies of different drugs and the combined effects of drugs. When the concentration–effect relationship can be described by the log-linear model, linear regression can be performed between the effect and log drug concentration to determine the slope that is a measure of the potency of the drug.

16.2.4 E_{max} Model

The E_{max} model assumes that the effect of the drug increases as the drug concentration increases until it reaches a plateau (maximum effect) at a very high drug concentration as presented in Figure 16.5. The concentration–effect relationship can be described mathematically by a hyperbolic function:

$$E = \frac{E_{max}\, C}{EC_{50} + C} \tag{16.4}$$

where E_{max} is the maximum effect resulting from the drug, which actually represents the intrinsic activity of the drug; EC_{50} is the drug concentration when the effect is

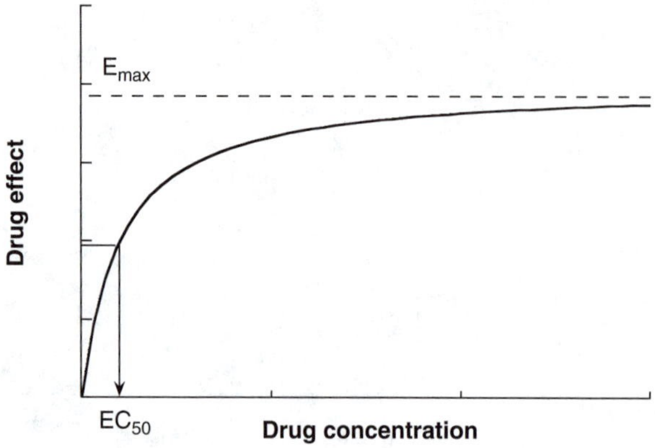

FIGURE 16.5 The drug concentration–effect relationship for a drug that follows the E_{max} pharmacodynamic model.

50% of the maximum effect, which is a measure of the drug potency; and C is the drug concentration at the site of action.

This model can be used to describe the concentration–effect relationship when there is a measured effect observed in the absence of the drug. In this case, Equation 16.4 can be modified to account for a constant E_0, which represents the baseline effect measurement in the absence of drug as in Equation 16.5.

$$E = E_0 + \frac{E_{max}\ C}{EC_{50} + C} \tag{16.5}$$

The model can also be used to describe the concentration–effect relationship when the drug causes a reduction in the value of the measured effect, such as lowering the blood pressure by antihypertensive drugs as in Equation 16.6.

$$E = E_o - \frac{E_{max}\ C}{EC_{50} + C} \tag{16.6}$$

In this case, the maximum effect E_{max} (maximum reduction in blood pressure) can be calculated from the difference between the baseline blood pressure (blood pressure before using the drug) and the lowest blood pressure observed while using increasing doses of the drug. When the drug concentration–effect relationship follows the E_{max} model, the observed effects at different drug concentrations are fitted to the model equation with nonlinear regression to estimate the model parameters, E_{max}, and EC_{50}.

16.2.5 Sigmoid E_{max} Model

When the concentration–effect relationship does not follow the typical hyperbolic function, the sigmoid E_{max} model can be used to describe the concentration–effect relationship. If the drug concentration-effect curve is S-shaped or if the response approaches E_{max} more slowly than expected above EC_{50}, then deviation from a simple hyperbola can be described by

$$E = \frac{E_{max}\ C^n}{EC_{50}{}^n + C^n} \quad (16.7)$$

where n is the parameter affecting the shape of the curve. If n is greater than 1, then the curve will be S-shaped, and if it is less than 1, then the initial portion of the curve has a slope greater than the simple hyperbola, and beyond EC_{50} the slope is less than the simple hyperbola as shown in Figure 16.6.

The sigmoid E_{max} model is applied when the interaction between one drug molecule and the receptor affects the interaction of the second molecule of the drug and the receptor; for example, if the interaction of one drug molecule makes the receptor more sensitive for accepting the second molecule ($n > 1$). On the other hand, the drug receptor interaction may decrease the sensitivity of the receptor to accept the next molecule ($n < 1$). The sigmoid E_{max} model should not be used if the maximum effect is not clearly defined. When the drug concentration–effect relationship follows the sigmoid E_{max} model, the observed effects at different drug concentrations are fitted to the model equation with nonlinear regression to estimate the model parameters, E_{max}, EC_{50}, and n.

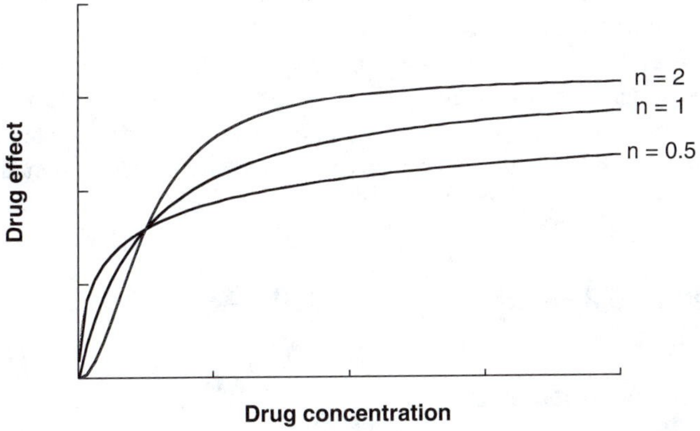

FIGURE 16.6 The drug concentration–effect relationship for a drug that follows the sigmoid E_{max} pharmacodynamic model.

16.3 LINK BETWEEN PHARMACOKINETIC AND PHARMACODYNAMIC MODELS

In the discussion, the different pharmacodynamic models that relate the drug concentration at the site of action to the drug effect were described. It is usually not possible to measure the drug concentration at the site of action. However, the pharmacokinetic model is used to estimate the drug concentration–time course at the site of action. Then, these estimated drug concentrations are used to choose the appropriate pharmacodynamic model that describes the drug concentration–effect relationship, and the pharmacodynamic parameters can be estimated.

The estimation of the drug concentration–time course at the site of action requires some knowledge about the pharmacokinetic characteristics of the drug. Also, some knowledge about the nature of the drug concentration–effect relationship may be required to determine the site of drug effect within the pharmacokinetic model. When rapid equilibrium exists between the drug in plasma and the site of action, and during steady state the drug plasma concentration can be used to reflect the drug concentration– time profile at the site of action.

For drugs that follow a multicompartment pharmacokinetic model, the drug concentration–time profile in the central compartment can be used to describe the drug concentration–time profile at the site of action if the drug in the central compartment is in equilibrium with the drug at the site of action. On the other hand, the tissue or the peripheral compartment in multicompartment pharmacokinetic models may represent the site of action or may be in equilibrium with the site of action. In these cases, the drug concentration in the peripheral compartment that can be estimated from the pharmacokinetic model can be used to describe the drug concentration–time profile at the site of action. More sophisticated models have been developed to describe the time course of the drug concentration in a hypothetical effect compartment that is connected to the pharmacokinetic model.

After determination of the time course of the drug concentration at the effect site, the drug concentration–effect relationship can be used to estimate the parameters of the pharmacodynamic model. When the models that describe the drug concentration–effect relationship and the pharmacokinetic behavior are known, the drug plasma concentration-time data and the drug concentration–effect data can be used simultaneously to fit both the pharmacokinetic and the pharmacodynamic models and to estimate the parameters of both models.

16.4 APPLICATION OF PHARMACODYNAMIC MODELS

16.4.1 Duration of Drug Effect

The pharmacodynamic models can be used to predict the effect of the drug at any time after drug administration. When there is a specific drug concentration required to produce the effect, the duration of effect will be the length of time the drug concentration remains above this particular concentration. The relationship between the elimination rate of a drug and the rate of loss of drug effect is different depending on the range of drug concentrations. If a drug follows the E_{max} pharmacodynamic model and the drug concentration is many times greater than EC_{50}, then the effect will be close to the maximum effect, and drug concentration in plasma may change severalfold with little change in the effect. However, when the drug concentration is much smaller than the EC_{50}, then the effect will change with the change in drug concentration.

16.4.2 Dosing Regimen

The combination of a pharmacokinetic model with a pharmacodynamic model such as the E_{max} model can help to explain the influence of dosing regimen on the overall drug effect. Some drug regimens can produce wide fluctuations in drug concentrations during the dosing interval without causing fluctuations in drug effect. In other instances, these fluctuations may cause fluctuations in drug effect within the dosing interval and may cause diminished effect during the latter part of the dosing interval. In general, the influence of dosing regimen can be expected to be of greatest significance when the average concentration is in the neighborhood of the EC_{50} and the dosing interval is longer than the drug elimination half-life.

In summary, pharmacokinetics is the study of the kinetics of drug absorption, distribution, and elimination, which will determine the time course of the drug profile in the body. Pharmacodynamics describes the relationship between the drug concentration at the site of action and the observed pharmacological effect. The pharmacokinetic properties of the drug determine the time course of the drug at the site of action. The pharmacodynamic models describe how the change in the drug profile at the site of action will be reflected on the observed drug effect. Linking the pharmacokinetics and pharmacodynamics of the drug can allow prediction of the time course of the drug effect.

PRACTICE PROBLEMS

16.1. A drug has a biological half-life of 6 hr, volume of distribution of 0.45 L/kg, and minimum effective concentration of 10 mg/L (i.e., the pharmacological effect is observed as long as the plasma concentration is above 10 mg/L).

a. What will be the expected duration of effect if a dose of 8 mg/kg of this drug is administered intravenously to a patient who did not receive this drug before?

b. What will be the expected duration of effect if a dose of 16 mg/kg is administered intravenously to a patient who did not receive this drug before?

16.2. A β-blocker has a biological half-life of 3.0 hr. Following an IV dose of 20 mg, the drug duration of response was 1.5 hr.

a. What is the expected duration of response following a single IV dose of 40 mg?

b. What is the minimum effective dose of this drug?

16.3. In a clinical study, it was found that a new antiarrhythmic can prevent arrhythmias for a period of 1.8 hr after a single IV dose of 14.3 mg/kg, whereas a dose of 21.5 mg/kg is effective for a period of 3.8 hr.

a. Calculate the minimum amount of the drug needed to prevent arrhythmias.

b. Calculate the half-life of this drug.

17 Therapeutic Drug Monitoring

OBJECTIVES

After completing this chapter, you should be able to:

- Describe the importance of therapeutic drug monitoring (TDM) in optimization of drug therapy
- Identify the causes of pharmacokinetic variability in different individuals
- Determine the criteria that make a drug suitable for TDM
- Describe the different steps involved in designing an appropriate dosing regimen utilizing TDM

17.1 INTRODUCTION

Therapeutic drug monitoring (TDM) is the use of drug blood concentration measurement as a tool for individualization of drug therapy and dosage adjustment. Many drugs exert their desired pharmacological effect with minimal adverse effects in most patients when their blood concentrations are within a certain range. For these drugs, it is necessary to maintain their blood concentrations within this range all the time. In any particular patient, the blood drug concentration achieved at steady state during multiple drug administration is dependent on the dosing rate of the drug and the drug total body clearance, which is different from one patient to another. This makes it possible to use the drug blood concentration as a guide for the determination of the dosage requirement in any particular patient. TDM is a concept that has been accepted as a result of the development in the area of biopharmaceutics and pharmacokinetics and the establishment of the drug blood concentration-therapeutic effect and the drug blood concentration-adverse effects relationship for many drugs. Also, application of this concept became possible after the development of analytical procedures and techniques for rapid determination of the drug blood concentration with reasonable accuracy. Furthermore, this concept became attractive because several studies have proven the cost-effectiveness of applying this service.

17.2 GENERAL PRINCIPLES OF INITIATION AND MANAGEMENT OF DRUG THERAPY

Drugs are usually administered to achieve a certain therapeutic goal with minimal undesired effects. Usually, the drug and the drug dosing regimen are chosen to achieve this goal. Patients are usually monitored to evaluate the therapeutic effect as well as the adverse effects. For example, when oral hypoglycemic drugs are used by patients with diabetes mellitus, the therapeutic goal is usually to maintain the blood glucose level within the normal range. Inadequate reduction of the blood glucose level to the normal range may necessitate increasing the dose of the oral hypoglycemic drugs; the appearance of adverse effects may call for holding or reduction of the oral hypoglycemic doses. Also, the goal for using antihypertensive drugs in patients with high blood pressure is to maintain the patient's blood pressure within the normal range with minimal adverse effects.

For many drugs, it is possible to assess the success or the failure of therapy by monitoring the patient clinically. However, this is not readily accomplished for drugs such as antiepileptic drugs when the incidence of seizures is infrequent or in psychiatric conditions that are not easy to evaluate. Also, when the drug adverse effect is serious or irreversible, it is not possible to use these adverse effects as monitoring parameters, as in the case of digoxin, which has serious cardiac toxicities, and aminoglycosides, which have irreversible ototoxicity. Furthermore, sometimes it is difficult to find reliable monitoring parameters for drugs used for prophylaxis of serious conditions. In these cases, monitoring the patients for the desired therapeutic effects or the undesired toxic effects may be inadequate to achieve optimal patient care. Another approach for monitoring drug therapy is to monitor the drug blood concentration. This approach may be useful if the drug blood concentration is correlated with the incidence and intensity of the desired therapeutic effects and with the undesired toxic effects of the drug. In this way, the drug blood concentration serves as an intermediate therapeutic endpoint and for prophylaxis of toxicity. The drug blood concentration can also serve as an additional piece of information to guide and to assess drug therapy.

17.3 DRUG BLOOD CONCENTRATION VERSUS DRUG DOSE

After systemic administration of a drug, it reaches the systemic circulation, and the rate of change of the drug blood concentration will be governed by the pharmacokinetic principles. This means that administration of the same dosing regimen of the same drug to different individuals should produce different blood concentrations because of the variability in the pharmacokinetic behavior of the drug in these individuals. The drug in the systemic circulation will be distributed to all parts of the body and can reach its site of action to exert its therapeutic effect. Also, the drug distributes to all parts of the body and can cause adverse effects. The intensity of the therapeutic and the toxic effects of most drugs depend on their concentrations at the site of action, which is usually at equilibrium with the drug in the blood as presented in Figure 17.1. Based on this discussion, the correlation between the drug blood concentration and the drug effects is much stronger than the correlation between the drug dose and the drug effects.

There are many examples that show the close correlation between the drug blood concentration and the incidence and the intensity of its therapeutic and toxic

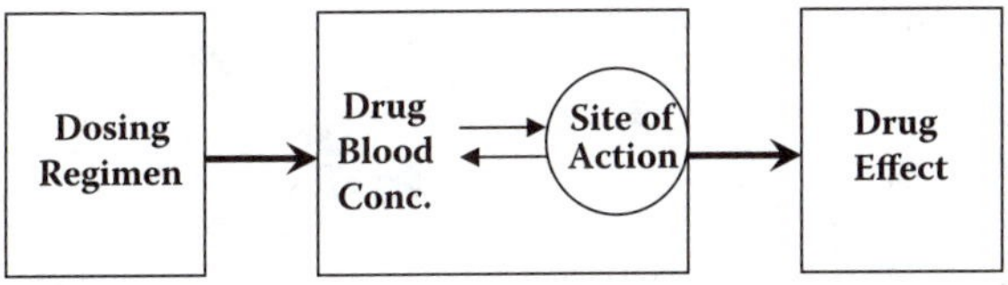

FIGURE 17.1 A schematic presentation of the relationship among the dosing regimen, the drug blood concentration, the drug concentration at the site of action, and the drug effect.

effects. Good correlation exists between the pharmacological effect of theophylline as measured by the pulmonary function test (PEFR, peak expiratory flow rate) and theophylline blood concentrations. As the theophylline blood concentration increases, the pulmonary function improves, and when the theophylline concentration decreases, the pulmonary function decreases. Also, a good correlation exists between the plasma warfarin concentration at steady state and the pharmacological effect of warfarin as measured by the prothrombin time. The prothrombin time follows the warfarin steady-state plasma concentrations, with the increase in warfarin plasma concentration resulting in prolongation of the prothrombin time.

This may indicate that, as the drug blood concentration increases, the intensity of the therapeutic effect increases, and higher drug blood concentration may be more beneficial to obtain better therapeutic effects. However, this is not usually true because as the drug blood concentration increases, the drug becomes more effective, and at the same time more side effects and toxicity start to occur. For example, as the phenytoin concentration increases above 20 mg/L, patients develop nystagmus. When the phenytoin plasma concentration reaches 30–40 mg/L, the incidence of ataxia increases; mental changes usually occur as the phenytoin concentration exceeds 40 mg/L. The appearance of toxic effects usually requires holding or decreasing the drug dosage to decrease its blood concentration. So, the drug blood concentration should be kept within the range of concentrations that produce the maximum therapeutic effect and the minimum adverse effects. This range of drug blood concentrations is known as the *therapeutic range*.

17.4 THERAPEUTIC RANGE

The *therapeutic range* is defined as the range of drug concentration in the blood within which the probability of the desired clinical response is relatively high and the probability of the unacceptable toxicity is relatively low. Figure 17.2 represents a hypothetical example that shows that the probability of the desired therapeutic effect is low when the drug concentration is low and the probability of toxicity is low. As drug blood concentration increases, the probability of the therapeutic effect increases, then stays relatively constant. Over the same concentration range, the probability of toxicity increases more slowly, and then the probability of toxicity increases more rapidly as the drug blood concentration increases. In Figure 17.2,

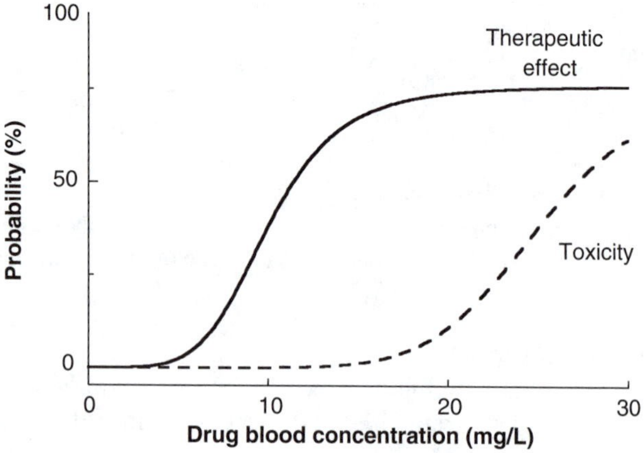

FIGURE 17.2 The therapeutic range is chosen to achieve the highest probability of the therapeutic effect and the lowest probability of toxicity.

if one selected 10 mg/L as the lower end of the range, then the minimum probability of the desired therapeutic effect would be about 40%. If 20 mg/L was chosen as the upper end of the therapeutic range, then the maximum probability of response would be about 80%. Over this same concentration range, the probability of unacceptable toxicity would remain less than about 10%. So, the therapeutic range should not be considered in absolute terms because it represents the range of drug blood concentration within which the majority of patients show pharmacological response with minimum incidence of adverse effects. It is important to note that some patients may start showing the desired therapeutic effect when the drug blood concentration is below the therapeutic range, and some patients may not show any therapeutic effects even if the drug blood concentration is within the therapeutic range. Also, a few patients may develop toxicity when their drug blood concentration is within the therapeutic range, and some patients may not develop toxicity even if their drug blood concentration is slightly above the therapeutic range.

The drug therapeutic and adverse effects are usually correlated with the drug concentration at the site of action. This means that the therapeutic range should be expressed in terms of the drug concentration at the site of action rather than the drug blood concentration. Most drugs are monitored at steady state, and at steady state equilibrium exists between the drug concentration in all parts of the body. This does not mean that the drug concentration is similar in all parts of the body at steady state, but it means that the ratio of the drug blood concentration to the drug concentration in any particular organ is relatively constant at steady state. The decrease in blood drug concentration should be accompanied by a proportional decrease in the drug concentration in all tissues, including the site of action at steady state. So, when the drug concentration in blood is in the therapeutic range, the drug concentration at the site of action will not be known, but this concentration should produce the optimal therapeutic effect with minimal toxicity.

17.5 VARIABILITY IN DRUG PHARMACOKINETICS AND RESPONSE

The correlations between the blood drug concentrations and the therapeutic and toxic effects are much better than the correlations between the drug dosing regimen and the therapeutic and toxic effects. This is because of the interpatient variability in drug pharmacokinetics and response. There are many examples that support this observation. For example, some patients require less than 2 mg/day of warfarin, and others require more than 10 mg/day of warfarin to produce the same therapeutic effect (the same prothrombin time). Also, after administration of the same dose of tolbutamide to a group of diabetes patients, the reduction in the blood glucose concentration ranges from 10 to 50% of the baseline blood glucose level, indicating variable response. These two examples illustrate the fact that doses are not usually correlated with the therapeutic effects because of the variability in the drug disposition in different patients. Because of the large interindividual variability, drugs should not be administered to patients at fixed doses. Doses should be tailored according to the specific patient's condition. The large difference in response between patients results from many factors, such as body weight, age, drug interactions, genetic factors, pregnancy, diseases, and factors related to the drug formulations and many other factors.

17.5.1 Body Weight

Administration of the same dose of the drug to patients with different body weights may produce different drug plasma concentrations. Dosage adjustment based on body weight can decrease the variability in drug concentrations between individuals. In extremely thin or obese patients, adjusting the dose based on lean body weight may be necessary to decrease variability in drug concentrations.

17.5.2 Age

17.5.2.1 Pediatrics

The physiological differences between children and adults can result in differences in drug pharmacokinetics. Neonates and infants have higher gastric pH, higher gastric motility, and a lower level of bile acids, which can affect drug absorption. Also, neonates and infants have higher total body water and lower albumin concentration, which can affect the drug distribution and the plasma protein binding of drugs. The kidney function is not fully developed, and the enzymatic capacity is generally lower (sometimes higher) in neonates and infants, which can affect the elimination of drugs.

17.5.2.2 Geriatrics

The physiological changes associated with aging can significantly affect the pharmacokinetics of drugs. The increase in gastric pH and the decrease in gastrointestinal blood flow associated with aging can affect drug absorption. The change in body composition in older individuals (decreased muscles and increased fat) can affect drug distribution. The decrease in kidney function and in the enzymatic capacity in older individuals can affect the elimination of drugs. Also, older patients use more drugs, which increases the probability of drug–drug interactions.

17.5.3 Drug–Drug Interactions

Administration of multiple drugs can result in drug–drug interactions that can alter the absorption, distribution, or elimination of one or more of the administered drugs. These drug interactions result in alteration in the drug concentration in plasma and at the site of action. This alteration can lead to modification of the therapeutic effect of the interacting drugs.

17.5.4 Genetic Factors

Inherited variability in pharmacokinetics because of a lower level or absence of an enzyme can affect the metabolic rate and the metabolic profile of some drugs. For example, the rate of isoniazid metabolism is dependent on the acetylator phenotype. Rapid acetylators eliminate isoniazid faster than slow acetylators. Also, the amount of morphine formed after administration of codeine is lower in poor metabolizers (patients with abnormally lower CYP2D6).

17.5.5 Pregnancy

Pregnancy is a condition associated with physiological changes that can affect the absorption, distribution, and elimination of drugs. The increase in gastric pH, the decrease in gastric emptying rate, and the slower gastric motility associated with pregnancy can affect the rate and extent of drug absorption. The significant increase in plasma volume during pregnancy can increase drug volume of distribution, and the decrease in albumin serum concentration can decrease the protein binding of drugs. The increase in cardiac output in general and the renal blood flow in particular during pregnancy increases the renal elimination rate of drugs such as ampicillin, digoxin, and lithium.

17.5.6 Diseases

The physiological and pathological changes caused by diseases can alter drug pharmacokinetics. Diseases that affect the eliminating organs can significantly affect the rate of drug elimination. For example, kidney dysfunction can alter the renal excretion of drugs that are eliminated by the kidney, and liver failure can alter the rate of drug metabolism. Also, the physiological changes associated with some diseases can affect the distribution and elimination of drugs. For example, patients with congestive heart failure have reduced cardiac output and reduced liver blood flow, which decreases the hepatic elimination of drugs such as lidocaine.

It is clear that drug pharmacokinetic behavior is different in different patient populations. Within each population there is also interindividual variability in drug pharmacokinetics. This difference in drug pharmacokinetics in different patients is one of the main causes of variability in patient response to drug therapy. This difference necessitates individualization of the dosing regimen for each patient to ensure optimal drug response.

17.5.7 Other Factors

Many other factors can affect the drug disposition and response, including nonlinear disposition, factors related to the drug formulation, environmental factors, dietary factors, occupational exposure, stress, smoking, and seasonal variations.

17.6 ADVANTAGES OF THERAPEUTIC DRUG MONITORING

The advantages of TDM are summarized in this section.

17.6.1 Facilitate Rapid Achievement of an Appropriate Dosing Regimen

The use of drug blood concentration measurement can help in choosing the proper dosage for patients in a short time. This is extremely useful in emergency situations.

17.6.2 Evaluate Existing Dosing Regimen

Drug blood concentration measurement can serve as a guide to determine if the patient is receiving an adequate dose of the drug and if the dose should be increased or decreased.

17.6.3 Prophylaxis against Toxicity

Drug blood concentration measurement can serve as a means to adjust the drug dosing regimen to achieve plasma drug concentrations within the therapeutic range. This is important to avoid the empirical change in drug dose that may expose the patient to drug toxicities.

17.6.4 Distinguish between Pharmacokinetic and Pharmacodynamic Causes of Therapeutic Failure

Drug blood concentration measurement can help to determine the cause of therapeutic failure. One can determine whether the drug is not effective because it does not reach the systemic circulation in adequate concentrations to exert its therapeutic effect (pharmacokinetic failure) or because the drug is not effective in this particular patient's condition (pharmacodynamic failure).

17.6.5 Cost-Effectiveness

Although application of the TDM service may seem costly, it is very cost-effective. Pharmacoeconomic studies have shown that the use of drug blood concentration measurement results in decreases in the incidence of toxicity, the incidence of complications, the length of hospital stay, and the length of the sick period, which decreases the overall health care cost.

17.7 CANDIDATE DRUGS FOR THERAPEUTIC DRUG MONITORING

TDM is necessary for drugs with some common characteristics, which are discussed next.

17.7.1 Drugs with Low Therapeutic Index

Drugs in which the ratio of the minimum toxic concentration to the minimum effective concentration is low require accurate determination of the drug dosage to avoid drug toxicity or subtherapeutic effects. TDM can serve as a means to choose the appropriate dosing regimen in this case.

17.7.2 Drugs with Great Variability in Their Pharmacokinetic Properties

The correlation between the drug blood concentration and drug dose in drugs with great variability in pharmacokinetic properties is usually poor. This makes it difficult to choose the drug dosing regimen that can maintain the drug blood concentration within the therapeutic range. TDM can serve as a guide to choose the appropriate dosing regimen required to achieve drug blood concentrations within the therapeutic range.

17.7.3 Drugs Used in Patients Who Are at High Risk of Toxicity

Patients at high risk of toxicity because of concurrent disease, multiple drug therapy, or any other factors may benefit greatly from TDM. Some drugs may have active metabolites (i.e., their metabolites have a similar pharmacological effect, such as procainamide), and other drugs may have toxic metabolites (e.g., carbamazepine). In these cases, both the parent drug and the metabolite drug concentrations should be monitored. For drugs that are highly bound to plasma protein or their protein binding is variable (e.g., phenytoin), the free unbound plasma drug concentrations are correlated much better with the pharmacological effects and the toxic effects when compared with the total drug concentrations. In these cases, measuring the unbound drug blood concentration may be necessary.

17.8 METHODS FOR MEASURING DRUG BLOOD CONCENTRATIONS

There are several analytical techniques that can be used to determine drug concentrations in biological fluids. High-performance liquid chromatography, gas chromatography, and radioimmunoassay are techniques that can be used to determine the drug concentrations in biological fluids. These techniques are accurate, sensitive, specific, and precise. However, they require complex sample-handling procedures. Other techniques, such as enzyme immunoassays and fluorescence polarization immunoassay, are also used for determination of the drug concentration in biological fluids. These techniques are fast and require simple sample-handling procedures and have reasonable accuracy, sensitivity, and specificity, which make them suitable for routine determination of drug blood measurement in clinical settings.

17.9 ESTABLISHING A THERAPEUTIC DRUG MONITORING SERVICE

17.9.1 Major Requirements

The most important requirement for the establishment of a TDM service in any health care institution is the availability of trained personnel to run the service. These personnel should have basic knowledge of the pharmacokinetic principles and the clinical pharmacokinetics of the drugs that will be monitored. Another important requirement for this service is the availability of a sensitive, accurate, specific, and rapid method of drug analysis in blood and other biological fluids.

17.9.2 Procedures

Application of TDM as a mean of individualization of drug therapy usually proceeds through several steps, discussed next.

17.9.2.1 Determination of Initial Dosing Regimen

Determination of the initial dosing regimen is achieved by using the patient's specific information, including age, sex, weight, organ function, nutritional status, and use of other medications, to estimate the patient's pharmacokinetic parameters for the drug under consideration. The estimated drug pharmacokinetic parameters for the patient are used to calculate the initial dosage requirements for the patient that should achieve steady-state concentration within the therapeutic range. So, the pharmacokinetic parameters used in the calculation of the initial dosing regimen are the pharmacokinetic parameters of the drug in a population similar to that of the patient monitored.

17.9.2.2 Determination of the Patient's Specific Pharmacokinetic Parameters

After the start of drug therapy, the next step should be the determination of the patient's specific pharmacokinetic parameters of the drug. This is usually achieved by planning a sampling strategy for blood or other body fluids that will allow calculation of the patient's specific drug pharmacokinetic parameters. The number of samples and the timing of these samples can be different depending on the drug monitored. For some drugs, such as aminoglycosides, multiple blood samples can be obtained at specific time points after administration of the first dose. Other drugs, such as digoxin and phenytoin, should be monitored by obtaining a single blood sample at steady state. Knowledge about the clinical pharmacokinetics of the drug will be helpful in determining the number and timing of the samples. The obtained blood samples should be analyzed for the drug concentration in the blood. The measured concentrations can be used to determine the patient's specific pharmacokinetic parameters of the drug.

17.9.2.3 Calculation of the Dosage Requirements Based on the Patient's Specific Pharmacokinetic Parameters of the Drug

The calculated patient's specific pharmacokinetic parameters are used to determine the dose and dosing interval for the drug required to achieve a steady-state drug concentration within the therapeutic range in the monitored patient. This calculated dosing regimen is specific for this particular patient because it is calculated based on the patient's specific pharmacokinetic parameters. Recommendations should be made to adjust the dosing regimen to achieve the desired therapeutic concentration. If the patient continues to receive the drug for a long time, such as in the treatment of chronic diseases (e.g., epilepsy and cardiovascular diseases), then it is important to obtain follow-up blood samples periodically to make sure that the recommended dosing regimen achieves the desired drug blood concentrations. Further dosage adjustment can be made based on the results of these follow-up samples.

In summary, optimization of drug therapy can be achieved empirically, sometimes at considerable expense, time, and occasional toxicity. However, drug blood concentration measurement can serve as a therapeutic endpoint to guide and assess drug therapy and as prophylaxis for toxicity.

QUESTIONS

17.1. Define TDM and the therapeutic range.
17.2. Enumerate the sources of variability in drug pharmacokinetics and response.
17.3. What are the advantages of TDM?
17.4. What are the characters that make a drug a candidate for TDM?
17.5. What are the general requirements for establishing a TDM service?
17.6. Please describe the procedures for individualization of drug therapy.

Solutions to Practice Problems

CHAPTER 2

2.1. a. Drug A because the half-life is dose independent.
b. $k = 0.1155\ hr^{-1}$
c. Drug A: Increasing the dose increases the initial rate of drug elimination, while elimination rate constant and half-life remain constant (dose independent); Drug B: Increasing the dose does not affect the elimination rate and the elimination rate constant, while the half-life increases.

2.2. a. A plot of the amount versus time is straight line on the Cartesian scale, so the elimination follows zero-order kinetics.
b. The elimination rate constant = 11 mg/hr.
c. The half-life immediately after drug administration = 18.2 hr.
d. If the dose is 600 mg the elimination rate constant will be 11 mg/hr.
e. The amount of drug remaining 20 hours after administration of 400 mg = 180 mg.
f. No drug will be remaining 40 hours after administration of 400 mg.

2.3. a. A plot of the amount versus time is straight line on the semilog scale, so the elimination follows first-order kinetics.
b. The elimination rate constant, $k = 0.4617\ hr^{-1}$.
c. The dose is equal to the y-intercept = 500 mg.
d. The equation: $A = 500\ mg\ e^{-0.4617\ t}$.
e. The amount of the drug after 10 hours = 4.94 mg.
f. The half-life = 1.5 hr.

2.4. a. Half-life = 3 hr, $k = 0.231\ hr^{-1}$, Vd = 30 L, and $CL_T = 6.93$ L/hr.
b. The AUC = 144.1 mg-hr/L.
c. If the dose is only 500 mg, Cp_0 will be 16.65 mg/L, and the AUC will be 72.05 mg-hr/L. Half-life, k, Vd, and CL_T will not change.
d. The dose = 1500 mg

2.5. a. Half-life = 0.9 hr, $k = 0.77\ hr^{-1}$, Vd = 50 L, $CL_T = 38.5$ L/hr, AUC = 5.195 mg-hr/L
b. The concentration will be 0.5 mg/L after 2.7 hours.
c. If the dose is only 400 mg, Cp_0 will be 8 mg/L, and the AUC will be 10.39 mg-hr/L. Half-life, k, Vd, and CL_T will not change.
d. The plasma concentration after 10 hours = 0.0018 mg/L.

2.6. Calculate the plasma concentrations at different time points by substitution in the equation for different values for time. Plot the concentrations on semilog graph paper.

2.7. a. Half-life = 3 hr, k = 0.2303 hr^{-1}, Vd = 400 L, CL_T = 92.12 L/hr, AUC = 4.342 mg-hr/L

b. The slope will be the same and the y-intercept will be 2.5 mg/L.

c. The concentration will be 0.25 mg/L after 6 hours.

d. The dose = 1600 mg.

2.8. a. Half-life = 5 hr, k = 0.1382 hr^{-1}, Vd = 0.5 L/kg, CL_T = 0.0691 L/hr/kg, AUC = 72.46 mg-hr/L.

b. The slope will be the same and the y-intercept will be 40 mg/L.

c. The concentration will be 1 mg/L after 16.69 hours.

d. The initial concentration should be 5.238 mg/L, so the dose = 2.62 mg/kg.

2.9. a. Ampicillin, largest k

b. Ampicillin, smallest Vd

c. Propranolol, highest clearance (k x Vd)

d. Propranolol, largest Vd

e. Ampicillin, fastest rate of elimination

2.10. a. Before renal disease: Half-life = 2 hr, k = 0.3465 hr^{-1}, Vd = 20 L, CL_T = 6.93 L/hr, AUC = 86.6 mg-hr/L; After renal disease: Half-life = 4 hr, k = 0.1733 hr^{-1}, Vd = 20 L, CL_T = 3.47 L/hr, AUC = 173 mg-hr/L

b. The renal disease decreased the efficiency of the kidney for eliminating the drug. This is reflected in the lower total body clearance, smaller elimination rate constant and longer half-life.

2.11. a. Half-life = 7 hr, k = 0.099 hr^{-1}, Vd = 40 L, CL_T = 3.96 L/hr, AUC = 202 mg-hr/L

b. The plasma concentration after 14 hr = 5 mg/L.

c. The slope should be the same –0.043 hr^{-1}.

d. The initial plasma concentration = 10 mg/L.

2.12. a. Half-life = 3 hr

b. The MEC is dose independent = 2 mg/L

c. Duration = 9 hr

d. Dose = 60 mg

e. The concentration will always be lower than the MEC, so no effect is observed.

CHAPTER 4

4.1. a. k = 0.13 hr^{-1}, half-life = 5.33 hr

b. t_{max} = 6 hr

c. C_{max} = 207 mg/L

4.2. a. t_{max}: Drug A = 2.0 hr, Drug B = 2.0 hr
b. C_{max}: Drug A = 33.44 mg/L, Drug B = 16.72 mg/L

4.3. a. t_{max} = 2.746 hr
b. C_{max} = 50.66 mg/L
c. t_{max} will be the same, C_{max} = 10.1 mg/L

4.4. a. Cp after 6 hr = 10 mg/L
b. Half-life = 6 hr
c. $k_a = 0.624\ hr^{-1}$
d. Vd = 29.2 L
e. t_{max} = 3.32 hr
f. C_{max} = 11.69 mg/L
g. Slope = $-0.05\ hr^{-1}$

4.5. a. Half-life = 4.5 hr
b. Vd = 59.6 L
c. CL_T = 9.18 L/hr
d. t_{max} = 2.28 hr, C_{max} = 5.9 mg/L
e. AUC = 54.5 mg-hr/L

4.6. a. ka = $0.693\ hr^{-1}$
b. Equation: Cp = 154 ng/ml $(e^{-0.332\,t} - e^{-0.693\,t})$
c. t_{max} = 2.04 hr, C_{max} = 40.7 ng/ml

4.7. a. A plot of the fraction remaining to be absorbed versus time is linear on semilog graph paper indicating first-order absorption.
b. $k_a = 0.347\ hr^{-1}$

4.8. a. $k_a = 1.0\ hr^{-1}$
b. Half-life = 3 hr, Vd = 50 L

CHAPTER 5

5.1. Bioequivalent drug products should have the same active therapeutic moiety.

5.2. Bioequivalent drug products should have the same rate and extent of drug absorption. Sustained release tablets and immediate release tablets have different rates of drug absorption.

5.3. F = 0.638

5.4 a. $F_{capsule}$ = 0.4
b. F_{IM} = 0.9
c. $F_{suspension}/F_{capsule}$ = 1.25
d. IV > IM > suspension > capsule
e. No, bioequivalent drug products have the same dosage form.

5.5. a. Formulation A, because it has shorter t_{max}.
b. F_A/F_B = 0.75. This means that the absolute bioavailability of formulation A is only 75% of the absolute bioavailability of formulation B.

5.6. a. Half-life = 2.31 hr, Vd = 20 L
b. The syrup has the fastest absorption rate
c. Absolute bioavailability: Syrup = 0.921, Capsules = 0.691, Tablets = 0.577
d. $F_{capsule}/F_{syrup} = 0.75$
e. $F_{tablet}/F_{capsule} = 0.835$

5.7. a. Half-life = 4 hr
b. AUC = 64.6 mg-hr/L
c. $F_{tablet} = 0.54$
d. $CL_T = 4.17$ L/hr, Vd = 24 L

5.8. a. Half-life = 9 hr, Vd = 20 L
b. Bioavailability = 0.36

5.9. a. Bioavailability = 0.809
b. AUC = 43.3 mg-hr/L

CHAPTER 6

6.1. Loading dose = 450 mg, Infusion rate = 52 mg/hr

6.2. a. At steady state rate of elimination = rate of administration = 70 mg/hr
b. $Cp_{ss} = 10.1$ mg/L
c. k = 0.231 hr^{-1}
d. Cp_{ss} is not affected by loading dose = 10.1 mg/L
e. Approximately 15 hr
f. $Cp_{ss} = 20.2$ mg/L

6.3. a. Half-life = 7 hr, Vd = 40.4 L
b. Loading dose = 485 mg, Infusion rate = 48 mg/hr

6.4. a. Half-life = 5 hr
b. Vd = 45.2 L
c. $Cp_{ss} = 16$ mg/L
d. $Cp_{ss} = 32$ mg/L

6.5. a. $Cp_{ss} = 16$ mg/L
b. Elimination rate = 100 mg/hr
c. Half-life = 5 hr
d. $Cp_{ss} = 16$ mg/L
e. $Cp_{ss} = 32$ mg/L

6.6. a. Elimination rate = 60 mg/hr
b. Half-life = 7 hr
c. Vd = 30.3 L
d. Loading dose = 455 mg, Infusion rate = 45 mg/hr

6.7. a. Elimination rate = 20 mg/hr
b. $Cp_{ss} = 4.95$ mg/L
c. k = 0.1155 hr^{-1}

d. Cp_{ss} = 4.95 mg/L
e. Approximately 30 hr
f. Cp_{ss} = 9.9 mg/L

CHAPTER 7

7.1. a. $Cp_{ss\ max}$ = 18.16 mg/L, $Cp_{ss\ min}$ = 8.16 mg/L
b. $Cp_{average}$ = 12.5 mg/L
c. Dose = 400 mg every 8 hr

7.2. a. Half-life = 13.3 hr
b. Vd = 20 L
c. $Cp_{average}$ = 20 mg/L

7.3. a. $Cp_{average}$ = 16.67 mg/L
b. $Cp_{average}$ = 16.67 mg/L
c. Dose = 240 mg every 12 hr

7.4. a. $Cp_{average}$ = 9 mg/L
b. Dose = 444.4 mg
c. Dose = 333.3 mg
d. $Cp_{ss\ max}$ = 27.8 mg/L, $Cp_{ss\ min}$ = 13.9 mg/L

7.5. a. $Cp_{average}$ = 20 mg/L
b. $Cp_{average}$ = 40 mg/L
c. CL_T = 2.5 L/hr
d. Dose = 750 mg every 8 hr
e. $Cp_{average}$ = 25 mg/L

7.6. a. $Cp_{ss\ max}$ = 16.58 mg/L, $Cp_{ss\ min}$ = 6.58 mg/L
b. $Cp_{average}$ = 10.8 mg/L
c. $Cp_{ss\ max}$ = 33.16 mg/L, $Cp_{ss\ min}$ = 13.16 mg/L

7.7. a. Half-life = 6 hr
b. Vd = 15 L
c. $Cp_{average}$ = 21.6 mg/L
d. Approximately 30 hr
e. At steady state rate of elimination = rate of administration = 450 mg

7.8. a. Half-life = 9.43 hr, Vd = 40 L
b. Dose = 1268 mg

7.9. a. Loading dose = 600 mg
b. Dosing interval = 11.5 hr ≅ 12 hr
c. Dose = 308 mg ≅ 300 mg
d. $Cp_{average}$ = 13.9 mg/L
e. Dosing regimen = 400 mg every 12 hr

7.10. a. Dosing interval = 11.5 hr ≅ 12 hr
b. Dose = 613.4 mg ≅ 600 mg
c. $Cp_{average}$ = 14.3 mg/L

CHAPTER 8

8.1. a. Amount = 720 mg
b. Renal excretion rate = 30 mg/hr = 0.5 mg/min
c. Cr CL = 50 ml/min
d. CL_R = Cr CL = 50 ml/min

8.2. a. Renal excretion rate = 140.7 μg/hr
b. Renal excretion rate = 25 μg/hr
c. CL_R = 50 ml/hr
d. Slope = -k/2.303 = –0.3 hr^{-1}

8.3. a. Bioavailability = 0.875

8.4. a. Half-life = 1.61 days
b. CL_R = 140 L/day, CL_T = 215 L/day
c. Fraction = 0.65
d. Amount = 1.165 mg
e. k_m = 0.15 day^{-1}

8.5. a. Half-life = 3 hr
b. CL_R = 7 L/hr
c. Fraction = 0.6
d. k_m = 0.091 hr^{-1}

CHAPTER 9

9.1. Metabolite 1: Formation rate limited; Metabolite 2 and Metabolite 3: Elimination rate limited

9.2. a. CL_T = 4.33 L/hr, AUC = 23 μmol hr/L
b. CL_R = 0.866 L/hr
c. Fraction = 0.3
d. CL_T = 3.0 L/hr
e. CL_R = 3.0 L/hr
f. Formation clearance metabolite 1 = 1.3 L/hr; Formation clearance metabolite 2 = 2.165 L/hr
g. AUC of drug = 69 μmol-hr/L; AUC of metabolite 1 = 30 μmol-hr/L
h. Amount of metabolite 1 = 100 μmol, amount of metabolite 2 = 0 μmol
i. Ratio = 0.433
j. No, because we do not have information about the elimination rate constants of the parent drug and the metabolite.

9.3. a. Fraction metabolized = 0.924, $CL_{T(m)}$ = 10.87 L/hr, $Vd_{(m)}$ = 35.7 L, Metabolite formation clearance = 7.65 L/hr, formation rate constant = 0.1159 hr^{-1}
b. $Cp_{ss(m)}$ = 21 μmol/L
c. Ratio = 0.82

9.4. a. $CL_{T(m)}$ = 8 L/hr, $Vd_{(m)}$ = 20 L
b. Fraction = 0.546

c. Metabolite formation clearance = 2.87 L/hr, formation rate constant = 0.109 hr^{-1}
d. Amount = 800 mg
e. Cp_{ss} = 12.7 mg/L, $Cp_{ss(m)}$ = 4.55 mg/L

9.5. a. CL_R = 4.16 L/hr
b. CL_m = 9.70 L/hr
c. Formation clearance = 9.702 L/hr
d. $CL_{T(m)}$ = 7 L/hr, $CL_{m(m)}$ = 0 L/hr, and $CL_{R(m)}$ = 7 L/hr
e. $k_{(m)}$ = 0.233 hr^{-1}, $k_{(m)} < k$ (i.e., elimination rate limited)
f. AUC = 8.66 μmol-hr/L, $AUC_{(m)}$ = 12 μmol-hr/L
g. Ratio = 1.39

CHAPTER 10

10.1. a. Half-life = 7.9 hr, Vd = 24.6 L
b. Dose = 285 mg every 12 hr
c. Half-life in failure = 16.6 hr, $Cp_{ss\ max}$ = 23.5 mg/L, $Cp_{ss\ min}$ = 14.2 mg/L. The maximum and the minimum concentrations change due to the reduction in dose, but the average concentrations resulting from the full dose and the reduced dose before and after developing the renal failure are similar.

10.2. a. Vd = 24 L
b. CL_T = 0.91 L/hr
c. Dose = 219 mg every 12 hr
d. $Cp_{ss\ max}$ = 25.0 mg/L, $Cp_{ss\ min}$ = 15.86 mg/L

10.3. a. Half-life = 7.5 hr, Vd = 11.76 L
b. CL_R = 0.65 L/hr
c. Half-life in failure = 12.5 hr
d. $Cp_{ss\ max}$ = 52.5 mg/L, $Cp_{ss\ min}$ = 27.0 mg/L

10.4. a. CL_R = 19.39 L/hr
b. Half-life = 5.45 hr
c. Dose = 1.65 gm every day
d. $Cp_{ss\ max}$ = 10.0 mg/L, $Cp_{ss\ min}$ = 4.67 mg/L

10.5. a. $Cp_{average}$ = 20.9 mg/L
b. $Cp_{ss\ max}$ = 33.6 mg/L, $Cp_{ss\ min}$ = 11.89 mg/L
c. The IV dose = 260 mg every 12 hr
d. $Cp_{ss\ max}$ = 39.4 mg/L, $Cp_{ss\ min}$ = 28.1 mg/L

CHAPTER 11

11.1. a. V_{max} = 590 mg/day, K_m = 9.8 mg/L
b. Concentration = 30 mg/L, half-life = 2.34 days
c. Cp_{ss} = 10.1 mg/L
d. Dose = 396 mg/day

11.2. a. V_{max} = 630 mg/day, K_m = 7.2 mg/L
b. Dose = 425mg/day

c. Half-life = 0.986 day

d. Elimination rate when Cp = K_m is equal to $^1/_2$ V_{max} = 315 mg/day

11.3. a. V_{max} = 640 mg/day, K_m = 5.6 mg/L

b. Dose = 466 mg/day

c. Half-life = 1.01 day, CL_T = 31.1 L/day

d. Cp_{ss} = 13.3 mg/L

11.4. a. V_{max} = 790 mg/day, K_m = 5.6 mg/L

b. Enzyme induction will increase V_{max} without affecting K_m. New V_{max} = 830 mg/day, K_m = 5.6 mg/L

c. Dose = 648 mg/day

11.5. a. V_{max} = 340 mg/day, K_m = 8.8 mg/L

b. Cp_{ss} = 17.2 mg/L

c. Half-life = 1.1 day, CL_T = 13.0 L/day

CHAPTER 12

12.1. The drug concentration will be different in different tissues depending on the affinity of the drug to each tissue.

12.2. During the alpha-phase the decline in drug concentration is due to the distribution and elimination processes, while during the beta-phase the decline in drug concentration is due to the elimination process only.

12.3. a. After 0.5 hr: Cp = 10.1 mg/L; after 3 hr: Cp = 4.32 mg/L; after 12 hr: Cp = 1.60 mg/L

b. Cp (mg/L) = 36 $e^{-12.8t}$ + 12 $e^{-0.11t}$

12.4. a. α $t_{1/2}$ = 0.0775 hr; β $t_{1/2}$ = 3.65 hr; V_c – 14.26 L; AUC = 3.885 mg-hr/L; CL_T = 19.3 L/hr; k_3 = 1.353 hr^{-1}; k_2 = 1.255 hr^{-1}; k_1 = 6.52 hr^{-1}; Vd_{ss} = 88.3 L; Vd_β = 101.6 L

b. Cp (8 hr) = 0.14 mg/L; Amount remaining = 14.2 mg

12.5 a. A = 53.0 mg/L; B = 17 mg/L; α = 1.34 hr^{-1}; β = 0.13 hr^{-1}; α $t_{1/2}$ = 0.52 hr; β $t_{1/2}$ = 5.3 hr; V_c = 7.14 L; AUC = 170.0 mg-hr/L; CL_T = 2.94 L/hr; k_3 = 0.412 hr^{-1}; k_2 = 0.423 hr^{-1}; k_1 = 0.635 hr^{-1}; Vd_{ss} = 17.8 L; Vd_β = 22.6 L

b. Cp (12 hr) = 3.57 mg/L

c. Cp_o = 210 mg/L

d. A, B, and AUC

e. A = 159 mg/L, B = 51 mg/L, AUC = 510 mg-hr/L

f. Infusion rate = 29.4 mg/hr

12.6 a. A = 1.356 mg/L; B = 0.431 mg/L; α = 0.124 min^{-1}; β = 0.0072 min^{-1}; α $t_{1/2}$ = 5.59 min; β $t_{1/2}$ = 96.0 min; V_c = 28.0 L; AUC = 70.8 mg-min/L; CL_T = 0.706 L/min; k_3 = 0.0252 min^{-1}; k_2 = 0.0354 min^{-1}; k_1 = 0.0706 min^{-1}; Vd_{ss} = 83.8 L; Vd_β = 98.0 L

b. The equation describes the best curve that describe the best profile

c. Amount = 7.5 mg

d. The concentration when 5 mg is remaining = 0.051 mg/L

CHAPTER 13

13.1. a. Regimen: 75 mg every 8 hr administered as IV infusion of 1 hr duration
b. $Cp_{ss\ max}$ = 6.02 mg/L; $Cp_{ss\ min}$ = 0.998 mg/L

13.2. a. Half-life = 2.22 hr
b. Vd = 15 L
c. Regimen: 130 mg every 8 hr administered as IV infusion of 1 hr duration
d. $Cp_{ss\ max}$ = 8.1 mg/L, $Cp_{ss\ min}$ = 0.9 mg/L

13.3. a. Half-life = 3.0 hr
b. Vd = 15 L
c. Regimen: 140 mg every 8 hr administered as IV infusion of 1 hr duration
d. $Cp_{ss\ max}$ = 9.89 mg/L, $Cp_{ss\ min}$ = 1.96 mg/L

13.4. a. CrCL = 26.7 ml/min
b. 22%
c. Estimated half-life = 11.36 hr
d. Half-life = 8.5 hr, Vd = 14 L
e. Cp_{max} = 5.15 mg/L
f. $Cp_{ss\ max}$ = 8.25 mg/L, $Cp_{ss\ min}$ = 3.37 mg/L
g. Concentration increases due to drug accumulation
h. Regimen: 90 mg every 24 hr administered as IV infusion of 1 hr duration

13.5. a. Half-life = 3 hr, Vd = 10.18 L
b. Regimen: 95 mg every 12 hr administered as IV infusion of 1 hr duration
c. $Cp_{ss\ max}$ = 8.9 mg/L, $Cp_{ss\ min}$ = 0.70 mg/L
d. The half-life will be approximately 6 hr

13.6. a. Estimated half-life = 9.2 hr
b. Four samples should be obtained: before drug administration, then 1, 4, and 10 hr after drug administration.
c. Half-life = 9 hr, Vd = 8.57 L
d. Regimen: 65 mg every 24 hr administered as IV infusion of 0.5 hr duration
e. $Cp_{ss\ max}$ = 8.67 mg/L, $Cp_{ss\ min}$ = 1.48 mg/L

CHAPTER 14

14.1. a. MRT = 5.97 hr
b. CL_T = 4.14 L/hr
c. Vd_{ss} = 24.7 L

14.2. a. The extent of absorption: C > A > B
b. The rate of absorption: B > A > C

14.3. a. $MRT_{IV} = 6.59$ hr
b. $MRT_{capsule} = 9.9$ hr, $MRT_{tablet} = 9.1$ hr
c. $MAT_{capsule} = 3.31$ hr, $MAT_{tablet} = 2.51$ hr
d. $CL_T = 7.41$ L/hr, $Vd_{ss} = 48.9$ L

CHAPTER 15

15.1. Small variability in the extraction ratio for high extraction ratio drugs results in significant variability in the drug bioavailability.

15.2. Enzyme induction significantly affects the hepatic clearance of low extraction ratio drugs and has little effect on the hepatic clearance for high extraction ratio drugs.

15.3. a. $CL_H = 38.96$ ml/min
b. $CL_H = 38.5$ ml/min
c. $CL_H = 85.0$ ml/min

15.4. a. $CL_H = 1.33$ L/min
b. $CL_H = 0.923$ L/min
c. Extraction ratio: Before CHF = 0.89, After CHF = 0.92
d. Bioavailability: Before CHF = 0.11, After CHF = 0.08

15.5. Note: The arrows represent the significant change in the CL_T, half-life, or bioavailability, while small or minor changes are considered no change.

a. Effect of Enzyme Induction

Drug	CL_T	Half-life	Bioavailability
A	↑	↓	↔
B	↔	↔	↔
C	↔	↔	↓
D	↑	↓	↔
E	↔	↔	↔
F	↑	↓	↔
G	↑	↓	↔
H	↔	↔	↓

b. Effect of Enzyme Inhibition

Drug	CL_T	Half-life	Bioavailability
A	↓	↑	↔
B	↔	↔	↔
C	↔	↔	↑
D	↓	↑	↔
E	↔	↔	↔
F	↓	↑	↔
G	↓	↑	↔
H	↔	↔	↑

c. Effect of Displacement from the Plasma Protein Binding Sites

Drug	CL_T	Half-life	Bioavailability
A	↑	↓	↔
B	↔	↔	↔
C	↔	↔	↔
D	↑	↓	↔
E	↔	↔	↔
F	↔	↔	↔
G	↔	↔	↔
H	↔	↔	↔

d. Effect of the Decrease in Hepatic Blood Flow

Drug	CL_T	Half-life	Bioavailability
A	↔	↔	↔
B	↔	↔	↔
C	↓	↑	↓
D	↔	↔	↔
E	↔	↔	↔
F	↔	↔	↔
G	↔	↔	↔
H	↓	↑	↓

CHAPTER 16

16.1. a. Duration = 5 hr
b. Duration = 11 hr

16.2. a. Duration = 4.5 hr
b. The minimum effective dose = 14.1 mg

16.3. a. The minimum effective dose = 9.9 mg/kg
b. Half-life = 3.4 hr

Index

A

B

C

D

G

H

I

K

L

M

N

O

P

R

T

U

V

W

Z